Diagnostic Methods for Cirrhosis and Portal Hypertension

Annalisa Berzigotti · Jaime Bosch
Editors

Diagnostic Methods for Cirrhosis and Portal Hypertension

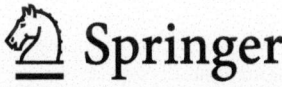 Springer

Editors
Annalisa Berzigotti
Inselspital, University of Bern
UVCM, DMLL, Hepatology Inselspital,
University of Bern
Berne
Switzerland

Jaime Bosch
Hospital Clinic
Hepatic Hemodynamic Laboratory Hospital
Clinic
Barcelona
Spain

ISBN 978-3-030-10239-5   ISBN 978-3-319-72628-1   (eBook)
https://doi.org/10.1007/978-3-319-72628-1

Printed on acid-free paper

This Springer imprint is published by Springer Nature
The registered company is Springer International Publishing AG
The registered company address is: Gewerbestrasse 11, 6330 Cham, Switzerland

Preface

The past years have witnessed an enormous advancement in all areas of hepatology, from molecular pathophysiology to diagnostic techniques and therapy, to the point that we have now effective therapies for most liver diseases and noninvasive diagnostic tests are creating new gold standards for diagnosis that before required difficult and demanding invasive techniques.

These changes are paramount most especially in the diagnosis of cirrhosis and portal hypertension. We come from an era when cirrhosis was diagnosed based on liver biopsy to one when pathologists prefer to use the term "advanced chronic liver disease" instead of "cirrhosis," thus underlining the dynamic nature of disease process. In this scenario, different disease stages are better defined on the basis of clinical, imaging, and hemodynamic characteristics than by the biopsy findings that correlate poorly with patient outcome. This is well illustrated by the fact that with similar liver biopsy findings, patient prognosis can be very good (as exemplified by the compensated patient without portal hypertension) or extremely poor (as in the case of the decompensated patient with multiple complications).

The above considerations emphasize one of the major requirements in modern medicine, that is, diagnostic tests should be able to inform on prognosis, therefore providing the basis for both risk stratification at the time of diagnosis and personalizing treatment.

This approach has been used to devise this book that reviews the more recent advances in the diagnostic methods for cirrhosis, the main complication of portal hypertension, and non-cirrhotic causes of portal hypertension. We are making special emphasis on new noninvasive methods and on the use of these tests in the different stages of cirrhosis and different complications of portal hypertension. After being part of the standard of care for the adult population, noninvasive diagnostic methods are increasingly used in the pediatric population with cirrhosis and/or portal hypertension, and this aspect as well as the specificities of diagnostics in Western and Eastern countries is taken into account.

Our aim is to offer to the general hepatologists and hepatologists in training the current state of the art regarding the many different techniques available and under development for clinical decision making. We hope the reader will find in the different chapters of this book—all written by well-known opinion leaders in their fields—a concise but comprehensive and updated, clinically focused guide to answer difficult questions, such as when to think about rare causes of non-cirrhotic portal hypertension (e.g., long-lasting porto-sinusoidal disease), when to start endo-scopic surveillance in a given patient, or when to shift from a completely noninva-sive assessment to an invasive measurement of HVPG in different clinical scenarios (e.g., sustained virological response after treatment with direct-acting antivirals).

We would like to acknowledge the commitment and efforts of all the authors from different disciplines (hepatology, endoscopy, radiology, pathology) and from the different areas of the world that have contributed to this book. They provide an outstanding example of what interdisciplinary collaboration can bring into the com-plex field of hepatology.

We hope that this book will be helpful for hepatologists and physicians interested in liver diseases in order to select the most appropriate diagnostic methods for their patients with cirrhosis and/or portal hypertension.

Berne, Switzerland   Annalisa Berzigotti
Barcelona, Spain   Jaime Bosch

Contents

Cirrhosis and Portal Hypertension: Staging and Prognosis

1

Guadalupe Garcia-Tsao

Cirrhosis is considered the end-stage of chronic liver disease of any etiology with a broad spectrum of clinical manifestations, from an entirely asymptomatic stage to a stage characterized by multiorgan failure. The clinical manifestations of cirrhosis are due mostly to portal hypertension and its hemodynamic consequences and/or to liver insufficiency.

Numerous prognostic studies over the years have indicated that the natural history of cirrhosis does not represent, as in most disease states, a continuum of a single entity but that cirrhosis is an entity that progresses across different stages, each with different prognosis, predictors of death and pathophysiological mechanisms.

A systematic review of 116 prognostic studies in cirrhosis had already demonstrated that cirrhosis is a heterogeneous disease with median survival times that ranged widely between 1–186 months [1]. This review also showed that, when patients are classified into two stages depending on the presence or absence of clinically evident liver-related events (specifically ascites, variceal hemorrhage, hepatic encephalopathy [HE] and/or jaundice), 1-year survival in patients without these events (compensated patients) is 95% (interquartile range 91–98%) while in those with any of these events (decompensated patients), it is 61% (interquartile range 56–70%) [1]. This systematic review also revealed that predictors of death are different in patients with compensated compared with those with decompensated cirrhosis [1].

From another perspective, analysis of individual patient data from two prospective Italian cohort studies including over 1600 patients demonstrated a median survival of greater than 12 years in patients with compensated cirrhosis, while patients with decompensated cirrhosis have a median survival of 1.8 years [1].

G. Garcia-Tsao, M.D.
Section of Digestive Diseases, Yale University School of Medicine, New Haven, CT, USA

Digestive Diseases Section, VA-CT Healthcare System, West Haven, CT, USA
e-mail: guadalupe.garcia-tsao@yale.edu

© Springer International Publishing AG, part of Springer Nature 2018
A. Berzigotti, J. Bosch (eds.), *Diagnostic Methods for Cirrhosis and Portal Hypertension*, https://doi.org/10.1007/978-3-319-72628-1_1

These results have been confirmed in a recent prospective study that analyzed a concurrent cohort of patients with cirrhosis (both compensated and decompensated) and showed that decompensation was, by far, the strongest predictor of death in cirrhosis. Furthermore, both stages have different predictors of death (age for compensated; Model for End-Stage Liver Disease [MELD] score for decompensated), and predictors that were common to both stages (albumin, platelet count) have different strengths of association [2].

Therefore, compensated cirrhosis and decompensated cirrhosis should be considered as two different disease entities, with different probabilities of death and different predictors of death and should be described, studied and managed separately.

Within these two main stages of cirrhosis, recent advances have provided further granularity that has allowed sub-staging of compensated and decompensated cirrhosis not only regarding prognosis but also regarding the predominant pathogenic mechanisms (Fig. 1.1). Before detailing this sub-staging, it is important to briefly summarize the pathophysiology of the complications of cirrhosis.

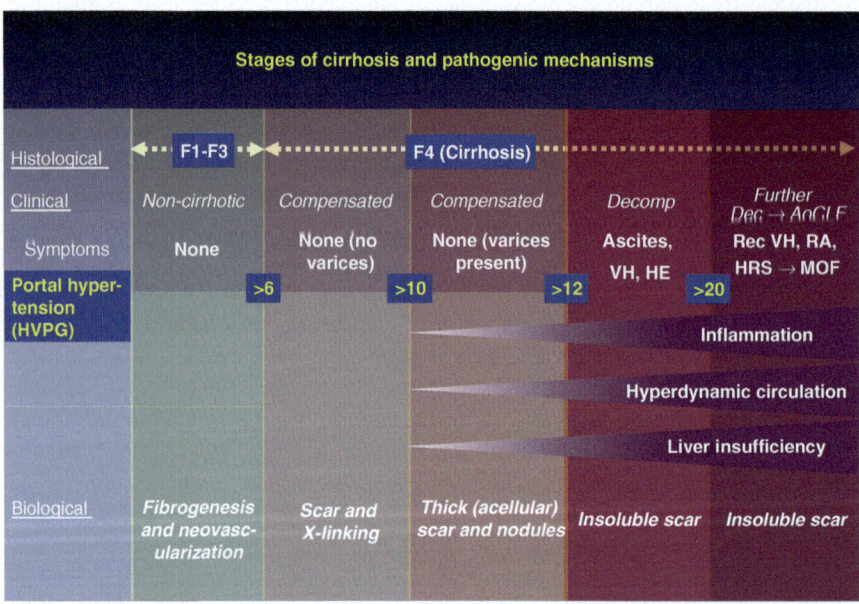

Fig. 1.1 Stages of cirrhosis and pathogenic mechanisms. The figure shows the different stages of chronic liver disease from a non-cirrhotic stage to a stage of further (late) decompensation with the severity of portal hypertension and the different pathogenic mechanisms at each stage, as well as the biology of fibrogenesis at each stage. *VH* variceal hemorrhage, *HE* hepatic encephalopathy, *Rec* recurrent, *RA* refractory ascites, *HRS* hepatorenal syndrome, *MOF* multiorgan failure, *HVPG* hepatic venous pressure gradient, an indirect measure of portal hypertension

1.1   Pathophysiology of the Complications of Cirrhosis

It is important to summarize the pathophysiology of cirrhosis and its complications because the main pathogenic mechanism(s), and therefore the targets of therapy, are different depending on the prognostic stage.

The pathophysiological process that leads to cirrhosis in patients with chronic liver disease consists of progressive fibrogenesis. However, at least initially, different types of chronic liver disease lead to different patterns of fibrosis and may therefore lead to different clinical manifestations [3]. For example, in primary biliary cirrhosis, where the process is predominantly portal and therefore fibrosis is mainly portal-to-portal, the initial clinical complications may be secondary to pre-sinusoidal portal hypertension (varices and variceal hemorrhage without liver insufficiency or ascites) while in alcoholic cirrhosis and non-alcoholic steatohepatitis, where fibrosis is sinusoidal, initial complications will be secondary to sinusoidal portal hypertension and liver insufficiency (ascites, in addition to varices and variceal hemorrhage). Eventually however, cirrhosis of all etiologies will end up by involving the sinusoids and will affect liver function.

Cirrhosis is characterized by a disrupted liver architecture mainly secondary to fibrous tissue that surrounds regenerative nodules (structural abnormalities) which leads to increased intravascular resistance. This increased intrahepatic resistance is compounded by active intrahepatic vasoconstriction due to contraction of activated stellate cells and endothelial dysfunction (functional abnormalities) and leads to an increase in portal pressure [4]. In turn, portal hypertension leads to the formation of portosystemic collaterals and to splanchnic vasodilatation which increases blood flow into the portal system that maintains the portal hypertensive state. Increased flow through gastroesophageal collaterals results in their growth and potential rupture (variceal hemorrhage) as well as shunting of neurotoxic substances such as ammonia into the systemic circulation and brain (encephalopathy). Vasodilatation leads to a decrease in effective arterial blood volume which stimulates baroreceptors and leads to secretion of neurohumoral systems and activation of the sympathetic nervous system that in turn lead to sodium and water retention, increased blood volume and a hyperdynamic circulatory state. Additionally, these vasoactive substances cause further intrahepatic vasoconstriction and worsen portal hypertension. While increased hepatic sinusoidal pressure forces fluid into the peritoneum, sodium and water retention, by replenishing the intravascular volume, perpetuate ascites formation. Later on, relative cardiac dysfunction leads to worsening vasodilatation (clinically manifested as arterial hypotension) and further activation of neurohumoral systems that can lead to hyponatremia and renal dysfunction. In more advanced stages, liver insufficiency leads to jaundice and coagulopathy and worsening hepatic encephalopathy, a state of multi-organ failure. Inflammation (secondary to covert or overt infection) plays an important role in the circulatory/cardiac dysfunction of cirrhosis [5].

1.2   Compensated Stage of Cirrhosis

Compensated cirrhosis is defined as cirrhosis in the absence of ascites, variceal hemorrhage, HE or jaundice. The patient is asymptomatic. In fact, one of the challenges in this stage is to establish the diagnosis of cirrhosis as is discussed in other chapters in this book. Importantly, the patient in whom ascites is controlled by diuretics or the patient in whom HE is controlled by ammonia-lowering therapies is not a compensated patient. Even though these symptomatic therapies may initially resolve some of the clinical complications, the pathogenic mechanisms that led to their development are still in place and prognosis is not improved by therapy. Because compensated patients have a very low probability of death (10% in 20 years) before becoming decompensated [6] the overarching goal of therapy in patients with compensated cirrhosis is to prevent decompensation rather than to prevent death [7].

In patients with compensated cirrhosis, liver insufficiency is minimal or absent and **portal hypertension (PH)** is the predominant pathogenic mechanism leading to decompensation (Fig. 1.1). All relevant studies looking at the prognostic significance of the severity of portal hypertension in cirrhosis have measured portal pressure by hepatic vein catheterization with calculation of the hepatic venous pressure gradient (HVPG).

An HVPG ≥6 mmHg defines portal hypertension, and therefore the presence of cirrhosis. This is true in diseases in which the resistance to portal flow is located at the sinusoids, such as alcoholic and/or viral-related cirrhosis [8] and cirrhosis secondary to nonalcoholic steatohepatitis. In portal-based diseases (cholestatic liver diseases) there will be an important pre-sinusoidal component of portal hypertension that is not reflected by the HVPG which, at least initially, will underestimate the actual portal pressure. Therefore, patients with cholestatic liver disease have been routinely excluded from therapeutic or prognostic studies using HVPG.

An HVPG ≥10 mmHg defines clinically significant portal hypertension (CSPH) because patients are at a significantly higher risk of developing gastroesophageal varices [9] and at a significantly higher risk of developing clinical decompensation [10] and HCC [11]. The probability of developing decompensation at 2 and 5 years in patients with an HVPG ≥10 mmHg is 13% and 29%, respectively, while in patients with an HVPG <10 mmHg it is only 6% and 15%, respectively [10]. An HVPG ≥10 mmHg has been therefore termed "clinically significant portal hypertension" (CSPH) and it is now recommended that patients with compensated cirrhosis be classified in two broad categories: those with mild PH and those with CSPH [12].

Although it has been considered that, histologically, cirrhosis is an "all or nothing" phenomenon, recent studies have shown that thickness of fibrous septa and the proportion of a liver biopsy composed by fibrous tissue correlate with the severity of portal hypertension. Specifically, studies performed in patients with mostly viral cirrhosis that analyze the correlation between histological characteristics and HVPG measurements performed at the time or near the time of the liver biopsy, show that patients with mild PH are more likely to have thin fibrous septa, while patients with CSPH are more likely to have thick fibrous septa [13, 14]. A quantitative assessment of liver biopsy also shows that 90% of patients with a fibrosis area <15% have mild PH [14, 15].

The two sub-stages of compensated cirrhosis not only differ in their probability of developing varices/decompensation and in the amount of fibrous tissue on a biopsy but, as described below, pathophysiological mechanisms are also different and the targets and goals of therapy will therefore be different (Table 1.1).

1. Compensated cirrhosis with mild portal hypertension

Patients with mild PH are defined by an HVPG >5 but <10 mmHg. The predominant mechanism at this stage is the increase in intrahepatic resistance, the initial mechanism leading to PH in cirrhosis. Evidence of this is the recent demonstration that the portal pressure-lowering response to non-selective beta-blockers (NSBB), which act by causing splanchnic vasoconstriction and decreasing flow, is significantly lower in patients with mild PH than in those with CSPH [16]. NSBB will only reduce portal pressure when a hyperdynamic circulatory state is present and, as also demonstrated in that study, a hyperdynamic state, while present in patients with CSPH, was not present in those with mild PH [16]. Therapies at this stage should target intrahepatic mechanisms, that is, should lead to removal of fibrous tissue and/or to amelioration of intrahepatic vasoconstriction, including amelioration of endothelial dysfunction (Table 1.1).

In patients with mild PH, the goals of therapy are to prevent the development of CSPH and, because these patients have less fibrous tissue, regression to a non-cirrhotic stage is a conceivable goal. Treatment of etiology is currently the main therapy at this stage and has been shown, in a small number of patients, to decrease HVPG to normal levels (i.e. below 6 mmHg) in a significant proportion of patients [17]. However, whether this indicates regression to a non-cirrhotic stage and/or whether progression to CSPH is prevented in this setting remains to be determined.

2. Compensated cirrhosis with clinically significant portal hypertension

Patients with compensated cirrhosis and CSPH are defined by an HVPG ≥10 mmHg. In patients with CSPH, in addition to increased intrahepatic resistance an important mechanism is an increase in portal venous inflow. At this stage, the hyperdynamic circulation has already developed [16] and therefore NSBB will be useful in reducing portal pressure. Acting on intrahepatic resistance will probably result in an added/synergistic portal pressure lowering effect.

In patients with CSPH, the goals of therapy are to prevent clinical decompensation. About a third to half of patients with compensated cirrhosis have varices when first diagnosed [6, 9]. Patients with varices (without ascites, HE or jaundice) that have not bled are still in the low-mortality compensated stage, however both evolution to decompensation and mortality are higher in patients with varices compared to those without varices [6, 18, 19]. Notably, because these studies had not stratified patients into those with mild and CSPH (a recent concept), subgroups of patients without varices in these studies likely included patients with mild PH. Patients with varices by definition have CSPH because it has been shown that all patients with

Table 1.1 Stages and substages of cirrhosis

Main stage	Sub-stages	Definition	Mechanism(s)/Targets of therapy	Goals of therapy
Compensated	Mild PH	HVPG >5 <10 mmHg	– Intrahepatic resistance (thin fibrous septa)	– Prevent progression to CSPH/varices – Regression of cirrhosis?
	CSPH, no varices	HVPG ≥10 mmHg	– Intrahepatic resistance (thick fibrous septa) – Increased flow (splanchnic vasodilatation)	Prevent decompensation
	CSPH, varices	Gastroesophageal varices	– Increased flow (splanchnic vasodilatation) – Increased resistance (thick fibrous septa)	Prevent variceal hemorrhage and/or decompensation
Decompensated	Early	VH, ascites, encephalopathy	– Vasodilatation – Inflammation and bacteria – Liver dysfunction – Intrahepatic resistance	Ameliorate decompensating event Prevent further decompensation Prevent death (if more than one complication)
	Late	Recurrent VH, HypoNa, HRS, SB?, recurrent HE, jaundice	– Vasodilatation – Decreased cardiac output – Inflammation and bacteria – Liver dysfunction	Ameliorate decompensating event Prevent death
	AOCLF	Multiorgan failure	– Inflammation and bacteria – Liver dysfunction	Prevent death

gastroesophageal varices have an HVPG of at least 11–12 mmHg [20, 21]. This likely applies to patients with portosystemic collaterals on imaging and these should also be considered as having CSPH [7].

CSPH can therefore be sub-staged into those with and without varices. In both, the main goal of therapy is still to prevent clinical decompensation but in patients with medium/large varices, a main objective is to also to prevent the first episode of variceal hemorrhage (Table 1.1).

A recent placebo-controlled study was the first to use this stratification strategy by including patients with CSPH with no or small varices and randomizing them NSBB or placebo and showed that NSBB were associated with a significantly lower rate of clinical decompensation (mostly ascites) [22]. In patients with CSPH and medium/large varices a number of randomized trials demonstrate that NSBB (compared to no therapy) prevent first variceal hemorrhage [23, 24] with a lower decompensation rate and a lower mortality in those that demonstrate a reduction in portal pressure [25–27].

1.3 Decompensated Stage of Cirrhosis

This is the symptomatic stage of cirrhosis and is defined by the presence of ascites, variceal hemorrhage, HE or jaundice. The development of jaundice is clear evidence of liver insufficiency and of a decompensated stage but it is extremely rare to have jaundice as the initial decompensating and it is more common in the setting of further decompensation and acute-on-chronic liver failure as described below.

The diagnosis of cirrhosis at the decompensated stage is not challenging and is usually established by physical examination and/or routine tests. The main pathogenic mechanisms are the **hyperdynamic circulatory state** and **portal hypertension** [28].

Of the decompensating events, overt ascites is clearly the most common, accounting for 60–80% of initial clinical events, followed by gastrointestinal hemorrhage, while HE and jaundice occur as the first clinical event in only a minority of patients [6, 29]. Ascites is the only complication that could be considered continuous (diuretics may control ascites but, in general, it will recur when diuretics are discontinued), while both variceal hemorrhage and encephalopathy are episodic (at least initially) and, if they occur in an otherwise compensated patient and if the acute episode resolves, the patient can return to a "compensated" stage (although in both cases, particularly with variceal hemorrhage, specific therapy to prevent recurrence may affect the "natural" history).

Even though each of the individual complications of cirrhosis has an impact on survival, the magnitude of the impact is different. Decompensated patients with ascites have a significantly poorer outcome than those presenting with variceal hemorrhage as the only decompensating event [19]. This was confirmed in an Italian prospective inception cohort study of 464 patients in which patient flow across stages was assessed by competing risk analysis [6]. In this study, decompensated patients were placed in three strata: (1) bleeding without other complications; (2) first non-bleeding decompensation (mainly ascites); and (3) two decompensating events [6]. Five-year mortality rates for each of these three stages was 20%, 30% and 88% respectively. The mortality rate difference between patients who present with variceal hemorrhage (no other complication) and those that present with one non-bleeding complication was not large, similar to findings in another cohort followed for a median of 33 months in which a poor outcome (death or LT) was 20% in patients with variceal hemorrhage and 36% in those with ascites [29].

1. Decompensated cirrhosis with one vs. two or more decompensating events

Based on the above, one way of substaging decompensated cirrhosis is to classify patients into those presenting with only one decompensating event vs. those presenting with two or more decompensating events.

However, unlike compensated cirrhosis, where pathogenic mechanisms are common to each substage, pathogenic mechanisms and therefore the targets of therapy in decompensated cirrhosis differ depending on the specific decompensating event.

In patients presenting with variceal hemorrhage, the main mechanism is portal hypertension, with an HVPG >20 mmHg being the most important predictor of rebleeding and death [30, 31] . Therefore, the main target of therapy is the increased splanchnic flow (splanchnic vasoconstrictors) and the bleeding varix (endoscopic band ligation) but acting on increased intrahepatic resistance would also be important. While acting on fibrogenesis at this stage would likely be futile because scar tissue is insoluble (Fig. 1.1), ameliorating intrahepatic vasoconstriction would be a target of therapy that would have an additive effect to splanchnic vasoconstrictors [32]. The goals of therapy in patients with variceal hemorrhage are to stop the hemorrhage and prevent rebleeding while also preventing the other complications (ascites, HE) (Table 1.1). Therapies such as the combination of NSBB (acting on flow), local therapy (endoscopic variceal ligation) and simvastatin (amelioration of endothelial dysfunction) and therapies such as the transjugular intrahepatic portosystemic shunt (TIPS) that resolve portal hypertension by bypassing the site of increased resistance (i.e. the liver) have been shown to improve survival in selected patients [33, 34].

In patients presenting with ascites, the main mechanisms are sinusoidal hypertension and sodium retention which is due to vasodilatation and the hyperdynamic circulatory state. The target should therefore be vasodilatation (or mechanisms leading to vasodilatation such as bacterial translocation) and the goal of therapy would be not only to eliminate the fluid (as it will improve quality of life) but mostly to prevent the development of complications that reflect a worsening vasodilation such as refractory ascites, hyponatremia and hepatorenal syndrome while also preventing the other complications (variceal hemorrhage, HE) and improving survival. Unfortunately, because treatments for ascites have so far targeted mechanisms that are further down in the pathophysiological cascade (removing fluid, increasing sodium excretion), current therapies have not resulted in improvements in survival or prevention of other complications.

In patients presenting with HE, the main mechanisms are portosystemic shunting (as a result of portal hypertension) and liver insufficiency. In a patient who is otherwise compensated, the main mechanism is shunting and finding a shunt that could be occluded becomes a target of therapy that has been shown to improve HE [35] but without an effect on other complications or on survival. Because liver insufficiency plays an important role in the pathogenesis of hepatic encephalopathy, improving liver perfusion (by acting on intrahepatic resistance) may have some role in not only preventing HE but other complications and could potentially improve survival. No examples of this strategy are available.

In patients presenting with two or more decompensating events, prevention of death is the main target of therapy. In this setting, the use of NSBB together with local therapy (ligation) in patients with Child B/C cirrhosis has shown to have a better survival than local therapy alone [36]. Also, patients with more than one complication (variceal hemorrhage and ascites) in whom portal pressure is reduced with NSBB, have a lower rate of decompensation and death [27].

2. Decompensated cirrhosis with early vs. late decompensation

Another way to stratify patients with decompensated cirrhosis would be to classify them into those who are decompensated by virtue of having ascites (controlled with diuretics), first variceal hemorrhage or first precipitant-induced HE and those that have other complications that denote a more advanced liver disease, i.e. a later stage of "further decompensation" with ascites that is no longer responsive to diuretics (refractory ascites), hyponatremia, hepatorenal syndrome (HRS), recurrent variceal hemorrhage, recurrent/persistent HE, and jaundice.

There is evidence demonstrating that refractory ascites has a higher mortality than diuretic-responsive ascites [37], that the presence of hyponatremia is associated with a significantly poorer survival in patients on the liver transplant waiting list, independent of MELD score [38] and that HRS type 1 (acute kidney injury in cirrhosis) has a higher mortality than HRS type 2 (kidney failure associated mostly with refractory ascites) which in turn has a higher mortality than refractory ascites [39]. In fact, while the median survival in patients with decompensated cirrhosis is 2 years, in those with refractory ascites it is 7 months and in those with untreated HRS it is 1 month.

Therefore, patients who die of decompensated cirrhosis often do so after development of "further decompensation", that is, when worsening of the pathophysiological mechanisms (portal hypertension, hyperdynamic circulatory state and/or liver insufficiency) lead to a subsequent complication after the initial event (Fig. 1.1). Specifically, patients with ascites will develop refractory ascites, hyponatremia or hepatorenal syndrome (HRS) as a result of worsening vasodilatation (and decreasing mean arterial pressure), activation of neurohumoral systems and a relative decrease in cardiac output [40]; patients with variceal hemorrhage will develop recurrent variceal hemorrhage as a result of worsening portal pressure and/or worsening of the hyperdynamic circulatory state [30, 41]; and patients will develop recurrent/persistent HE, coagulopathy and jaundice as a result of further impairment in liver function. Inflammation resulting from an overt infection such as spontaneous bacterial peritonitis or covert infection such as that occurring with bacterial translocation may be the most important driving forces in the development of late decompensation and therefore it would represent a main target in patients with decompensated cirrhosis [42, 43].

Goals of therapy in the stage of early decompensation are to prevent further decompensation and thereby prevent death (primarily). Randomized trials using norfloxacin [44] or enoxaparin [45] that have an effect in preventing bacterial translocation/inflammation have been shown to prevent/delay the development of HRS [44] and other complications [45] with a resultant improvement in survival.

The goal of therapy in the stage of late decompensation would be to prevent death. In this stage, therapies that improve vasodilatation (i.e. terlipressin) in HRS [46], bypass the site of increase resistance and increase the effective arterial blood volume (i.e. TIPS) in refractory ascites [47] or replace the sick liver (i.e. liver transplantation) have accomplished the goal of improving survival.

1.4   Acute-on-Chronic Liver Failure

The presence of acute deterioration of pre-existing cirrhosis with multiorgan failure has recently been termed "acute-on-chronic liver failure" (AoCLF). Most of the complications of the "further" decompensated stage represent an "organ failure" with HRS representing the kidney, hypotension (resulting from extreme vasodilatation) representing the circulatory system, encephalopathy representing the nervous system, coagulopathy and jaundice representing liver failure. Together with hypoxemia (which could be related to hepatopulmonary syndrome), these are the six organ failures that have been used in a European consortium to define AoCLF 30% [48]. However, because AoCLF can occur in patients at any stage of cirrhosis, whether they are previously compensated or decompensated, it is now considered a distinct stage of cirrhosis.

The entity occurs in hospitalized patients and usually follows a precipitating event, most commonly an infection or alcoholic hepatitis although a precipitant cannot be identified in up to 40% of the cases. In a North American consortium organ failures have been defined as grade III/IV encephalopathy (West Haven criteria), shock (MAP <60 mm Hg or a decrease of 40 mmHg in SBP despite fluid resuscitation and adequate cardiac output), need for mechanical ventilation and need for dialysis or other forms of renal replacement therapy [49]. When using either definition (European or NorthAmerican), the presence of two or more organ failures is associated with a very high 28-day mortality (>30%) [48, 49].

From the pathophysiologic perspective, marked systemic inflammatory response is the main driving force of AoCLF. Markers of inflammation such as white cell count are significantly higher in patients with ACLF and is an independent predictor of mortality. Innate immune dysfunction affecting neutrophils and circulating monocytes is present and it is hypothesized that the severity of the inflammatory response predisposes to immune failure and increased risk of infection [50].

The main target of therapy is therefore this inflammatory state and the goal of therapy is to prevent death. Because this is a newly described entity there are no clear examples of therapies that would address inflammation and led to a decrease in survival, although data from a prospectively collected database of patients with AoCLF demonstrated that NSBB users had a lower white blood cell count and had a lower mortality compared to non-users [51].

References

1. D'Amico G, Garcia-Tsao G, Pagliaro L. Natural history and prognostic indicators of survival in cirrhosis. A systematic review of 118 studies. J Hepatol. 2006;44:217–31.
2. Ripoll C, Bari K, Garcia-Tsao G. Serum albumin can identify patients with compensated cirrhosis with a good prognosis. J Clin Gastroenterol. 2015;49:613–9.
3. Rosselli M, MacNaughtan J, Jalan R, Pinzani M. Beyond scoring: a modern interpretation of disease progression in chronic liver disease. Gut. 2013;62(9):1234–41.
4. Bosch J, Groszmann RJ, Shah VH. Evolution in the understanding of the pathophysiological basis of portal hypertension: how changes in paradigm are leading to successful new treatments. J Hepatol. 2015;62(1S):S121–30.
5. Bernardi M, Moreau R, Angeli P, Schnabl B, Arroyo V. Mechanisms of decompensation and organ failure in cirrhosis: from peripheral arterial vasodilation to systemic inflammation hypothesis. J Hepatol. 2015;63(5):1272–84.
6. D'Amico G, Pasta L, Morabito A, D'Amico M, Caltagirone M, Malizia G, et al. Competing risks and prognostic stages of cirrhosis: a 25-year inception cohort study of 494 patients. Aliment Pharmacol Ther. 2014;39(10):1180–93.
7. de Franchis R, Baveno VI Faculty. Expanding consensus in portal hypertension. Report of the Baveno VI Consensus Workshop: stratifying risk and individualizing care for portal hypertension. J Hepatol. 2015;63(3):743–52.
8. Perello A, Escorsell A, Bru C, Gilabert R, Moitinho E, Garcia-Pagan JC, et al. Wedged hepatic venous pressure adequately reflects portal pressure in hepatitis C virus-related cirrhosis. Hepatology. 1999;30:1393–7.
9. Groszmann RJ, Garcia-Tsao G, Bosch J, Grace ND, Burroughs AK, Planas R, et al. Beta-blockers to prevent gastroesophageal varices in patients with cirrhosis. N Engl J Med. 2005;353:2254–61.
10. Ripoll C, Groszmann R, Garcia-Tsao G, Grace N, Burroughs A, Planas R, et al. Hepatic venous pressure gradient predicts clinical decompensation in patients with compensated cirrhosis. Gastroenterology. 2007;133(2):481–8.
11. Ripoll C, Groszmann RJ, Garcia-Tsao G, Bosch J, Grace N, Burroughs A, et al. Hepatic venous pressure gradient predicts development of hepatocellular carcinoma independently of severity of cirrhosis. J Hepatol. 2009;50(5):923–8.
12. Garcia-Tsao G, Abraldes J, Berzigotti A, Bosch J. Portal hypertensive bleeding in cirrhosis: risk stratification, diagnosis and management – 2016 practice guidance by the American Association for the Study of Liver Diseases. Hepatology. 2017;65(1):310–35.
13. Nagula S, Jain D, Groszmann RJ, Garcia-Tsao G. Histological-hemodynamic correlation in cirrhosis—a histological classification of the severity of cirrhosis. J Hepatol. 2006;44(1):111–7.
14. Kumar M, Sakhuja P, Kumar A, Manglik N, Choudhury A, Hissar S, et al. Histological subclassification of cirrhosis based on histological-haemodynamic correlation. Aliment Pharmacol Ther. 2008;27(9):771–9.
15. Sethasine S, Jain D, Groszmann RJ, Garcia-Tsao G. Quantitative histological-hemodynamic correlations in cirrhosis. Hepatology. 2012;55(4):1146–53.
16. Villanueva C, Albillos A, Genesca J, Abraldes JG, Calleja JL, Aracil C, et al. Development of hyperdynamic circulation and response to beta-blockers in compensated cirrhosis with portal hypertension. Hepatology. 2016;63(1):197–206.

17. Mandorfer M, Kozbial K, Schwabl P, Freissmuth C, Schwarzer R, Stern R, et al. Sustained virologic response to interferon-free therapies ameliorates HCV-induced portal hypertension. J Hepatol. 2016;65(4):692–9.
18. Bruno S, Zuin M, Crosignani A, Rossi S, Zadra F, Roffi L, et al. Predicting mortality risk in patients with compensated HCV-induced cirrhosis: a long-term prospective study. Am J Gastroenterol. 2009;104(5):1147–58.
19. Zipprich A, Garcia-Tsao G, Rogowski S, Fleig WE, Seufferlein T, Dollinger MM. Prognostic indicators of survival in patients with compensated and decompensated cirrhosis. Liver Int. 2012;32(9):1407–14.
20. Lebrec D, De Fleury P, Rueff B, Nahum H, Benhamou JP. Portal hypertension, size of esophageal varices, and risk of gastrointestinal bleeding in alcoholic cirrhosis. Gastroenterology. 1980;79:1139–44.
21. Garcia-Tsao G, Groszmann RJ, Fisher RL, Conn HO, Atterbury CE, Glickman M. Portal pressure, presence of gastroesophageal varices and variceal bleeding. Hepatology. 1985;5(3):419–24.
22. Villanueva C, et al. . β-Blockers to prevent the decompensation of cirrhosis in patients with clinically significant portal hypertension. AASLD 2016 abstract.
23. Poynard T, Cales P, Pasta L, Ideo G, Pascal JP, Pagliaro L, et al. Beta-adrenergic antagonists in the prevention of first gastrointestinal bleeding in patients with cirrhosis and oesophageal varices. An analysis of data and prognostic factors in 598 patients from four randomized clinical trials. N Engl J Med. 1991;324:1532–8.
24. D'Amico G, Pagliaro L, Bosch J. Pharmacological treatment of portal hypertension: an evidence-based approach. Semin Liver Dis. 1999;19:475–505.
25. Villanueva C, Aracil C, Colomo A, Hernandez-Gea V, Lopez-Balaguer JM, Alvarez-Urturi C, et al. Acute hemodynamic response to beta-blockers and prediction of long-term outcome in primary prophylaxis of variceal bleeding. Gastroenterology. 2009;137(1):119–28.
26. Hernandez-Gea V, Aracil C, Colomo A, Garupera I, Poca M, Torras X, et al. Development of ascites in compensated cirrhosis with severe portal hypertension treated with beta-blockers. Am J Gastroenterol. 2012;107(3):418–27.
27. Turco L, et al. A reduction in the hepatic venous pressure gradient (HVPG) prevents clinical outcomes in compensated and decompensated cirrhosis: A meta-analysis. EASL 2017 abstract.
28. Iwakiri Y, Groszmann RJ. The hyperdynamic circulation of chronic liver diseases: from the patient to the molecule. Hepatology. 2006;43(2 Suppl 1):S121–31.
29. Bruno S, Saibeni S, Bagnardi V, Vandelli C, De LM, Felder M, et al. Mortality risk according to different clinical characteristics of first episode of liver decompensation in cirrhotic patients: a nationwide, prospective, 3-year follow-up study in Italy. Am J Gastroenterol. 2013;108(7):1112–22.
30. Moitinho E, Escorsell A, Bandi JC, Salmeron JM, Garcia-Pagan JC, Rodes J, et al. Prognostic value of early measurements of portal pressure in acute variceal bleeding. Gastroenterology. 1999;117:626–31.
31. Abraldes JG, Villanueva C, Banares R, Aracil C, Catalina MV, Garci A-P, et al. Hepatic venous pressure gradient and prognosis in patients with acute variceal bleeding treated with pharmacologic and endoscopic therapy. J Hepatol. 2008;48(2):229–36.
32. Abraldes JG, Albillos A, Banares R, Turnes J, Gonzalez R, Garcia-Pagan JC, et al. Simvastatin lowers portal pressure in patients with cirrhosis and portal hypertension: a randomized controlled trial. Gastroenterology. 2009;136(5):1651–8.
33. Abraldes JG, Villanueva C, Aracil C, Turnes J, Hernandez-Guerra M, Genesca J, et al. Addition of simvastatin to standard therapy for the prevention of variceal rebleeding does not reduce rebleeding but increases survival in patients with cirrhosis. Gastroenterology. 2016;150(5):1160–70.
34. Garcia-Pagan JC, Di PM, Caca K, Laleman W, Bureau C, Appenrodt B, et al. Use of early-TIPS for high-risk variceal bleeding: results of a post-RCT surveillance study. J Hepatol. 2013;58(1):45–50.

35. Laleman W, Simon-Talero M, Maleux G, Perez M, Ameloot K, Soriano G, et al. Embolization of large spontaneous portosystemic shunts for refractory hepatic encephalopathy: a multi-center survey on safety and efficacy. Hepatology. 2013;57(6):2448–57.
36. Albillos A, Zamora J, Martinez J, Arroyo D, Ahmad I, de la Pena J, et al. Stratifying risk in the prevention of recurrent variceal hemorrhage: results of an individual patient meta-analysis. Hepatology. 2017;66(4):1219–31.
37. Salerno F, Borroni G, Moser P, Badalamenti S, Cassara L, Maggi M, et al. Survival and prognostic factors of cirrhotic patients with ascites: a study of 134 outpatients. Am J Gastroenterol. 1993;88:514–9.
38. Kim WR, Biggins SW, Kremers WK, Wiesner RH, Kamath PS, Benson JT, et al. Hyponatremia and mortality among patients on the liver-transplant waiting list. N Engl J Med. 2008;359(10):1018–26.
39. Alessandria C, Ozdogan O, Guevara M, Restuccia T, Jimenez W, Arroyo V, et al. MELD score and clinical type predict prognosis in hepatorenal syndrome: relevance to liver transplantation. Hepatology. 2005;41(6):1282–9.
40. Garcia-Tsao G, Parikh CR, Viola A. Acute kidney injury in cirrhosis. Hepatology. 2008;48(6):2064–77.
41. Abraldes JG, Aracil C, Catalina MV, Monescillo A, Banares R, Villanueva C, et al. Value of HVPG predicting 5-day treatment failure in acute variceal bleeding. Comparison with clinical variables. J Hepatol. 2006;44(Suppl 2):S12. (abstract)
42. Wiest R, Das S, Cadelina G, Garcia-Tsao G, Milstien S, Groszmann RJ. Bacterial translocation to lymph nodes of cirrhotic rats stimulates eNOS-derived NO production and impairs mesenteric vascular contractility. J Clin Invest. 1999;104:1223–33.
43. Schrier RW, Arroyo V, Bernardi M, Epstein M, Henriksen JH, Rodes J. Peripheral arterial vasodilation hypothesis – a proposal for the initiation of renal sodium and water retention in cirrhosis. Hepatology. 1988;8:1151–7.
44. Fernandez J, Navasa M, Planas R, Montoliu S, Monfort D, Soriano G, et al. Primary prophylaxis of spontaneous bacterial peritonitis delays hepatorenal syndrome and improves survival in cirrhosis. Gastroenterology. 2007;133(3):818–24.
45. Villa E, Camma C, Marietta M, Luongo M, Critelli R, Colopi S, et al. Enoxaparin prevents portal vein thrombosis and liver decompensation in patients with advanced cirrhosis. Gastroenterology. 2012;143(5):1253–60.
46. Gluud LL, Christensen K, Christensen E, Krag A. Systematic review of randomized trials on vasoconstrictor drugs for hepatorenal syndrome. Hepatology. 2010;51:576–84.
47. Bureau C, Thabut D, Oberti F, Dharancy S, Carbonell N, Bouvier A, et al. Transjugular intrahepatic portosystemic shunts with covered stents increase transplant-free survival of patients with cirrhosis and recurrent ascites. Gastroenterology. 2017;152(1):157–63.
48. Moreau R, Jalan R, Gines P, Pavesi M, Angeli P, Cordoba J, et al. Acute-on-chronic liver failure is a distinct syndrome that develops in patients with acute decompensation of cirrhosis. Gastroenterology. 2013;144(7):1426–37.
49. Bajaj JS, O'Leary JG, Reddy KR, Wong F, Biggins SW, Patton H, et al. Survival in infection-related acute-on-chronic liver failure is defined by extrahepatic organ failures. Hepatology. 2014;60(1):250–6. https://doi.org/10.1002/hep.27077.
50. Albillos A, Lario M, Alvarez-Mon M. Cirrhosis-associated immune dysfunction: distinctive features and clinical relevance. J Hepatol. 2014;61(6):1385–96.
51. Mookerjee RP, Pavesi M, Thomsen KL, Mehta G, MacNaughton J, Bendtsen F, et al. Treatment with non-selective beta-blockers is associated with reduced severity of systemic inflammation and improved survival of patients with acute-on-chronic liver failure. J Hepatol. 2016;64(3):574–82. Epub 2015 Oct 28

Part I

Gold-Standard Invasive Diagnostic Methods

Liver Biopsy Diagnosis of Cirrhosis

2

Zachary D. Goodman

2.1 Introduction

The ability of the liver to regenerate is well known, and many acute injuries heal without the formation of scars. Many chronic liver diseases, however, result in collagen production, usually termed fibrosis, as a reaction to the disease, and this scarring, in conjunction with hepatocellular regeneration and vascular alterations produces cirrhosis with its complications. Consequently the evaluation of fibrosis has always been a major function of liver biopsy interpretation.

Descriptions of cirrhotic livers observed in postmortem examinations can be found in the works of Vesalius, Morgangi and others from the seventeenth to nineteenth centuries, but the term "cirrhosis" is attributed to Rene Laennec [1], who is better known for the invention of the stethoscope and his contributions to thoracic medicine.

Although at first cirrhosis was an autopsy diagnosis, the advent of percutaneous liver biopsy enabled diagnosis in living patients. Needle biopsies of the liver for various indications were reported in the nineteenth and early twentieth century, and by the mid-twentieth century this had become a standard method of investigation of liver disease. A 1954 report from the Armed Forces Institute of Pathology stated that cirrhosis was diagnosed in 12% of liver biopsies submitted for consultation [2].

Although indications have varied and undergone refinement over the years, liver biopsy remains an essential component in the evaluation of liver disease [3], and it is a standard by which other modalities are judged. It is best used in conjunction with clinical evaluation, blood tests and imaging to provide a complete assessment of the patient. Depending on the underlying disase, liver biopsy can provide useful

Z.D. Goodman
Liver Pathology Research and Consultation, Center for Liver Diseases, Inova Fairfax Hospital, Falls Church, VA, USA
e-mail: Zachary.Goodman@inova.org

© Springer International Publishing AG, part of Springer Nature 2018
A. Berzigotti, J. Bosch (eds.), *Diagnostic Methods for Cirrhosis and Portal Hypertension*, https://doi.org/10.1007/978-3-319-72628-1_2

and often critical information on diagnosis, staging, prognosis and management of the patient. In a patient with hepatic decompensation, liver biopsy may reveal the underlying etiology and determine whether the decompensation was caused by progression of the disease to cirrhosis. This is especially true in a patient presenting with the new onset of compications of portal hypertension. On the other hand, in a patient with compensated liver disease, biopsy may reveal clinically unsuspected cirrhosis.

2.2   Fibrosis and Cirrhosis—Definitions

Fibrosis in liver disease is usually defined as an abnormal increase in collagen fibers and other components of the extracellular matrix in response to chronic injury. Scars are the result of collagen deposition in excess of collagen resorption as part of the wound healing response to injury. Scars have a natural tendency to contract and to remodel in response to mechanical stresses and other local factors. Hepatocytes have a natural tendency to regenerate to maintain liver cell mass and function. The combined effect of ongoing injury, liver cell death, scarring and regeneration produce the tissue changes that are termed cirrhosis.

Cirrhosis is a morphologic term with a relatively official definition [4]. It was defined by a committee convened by the World Health Organization in 1977 as "a diffuse process characterized by fibrosis and the conversion of normal liver architecture into structurally abnormal nodules." Key features are that it must be *diffuse* and involve the entire liver; there must be *fibrosis*; there must be *loss of normal architecture*; and *nodules* must be present. Absence of any of these cardinal features means that cirrhosis cannot be diagnosed. The well-known clinical complications of cirrhosis, such as variceal hemorrhage, ascites, coagulopathy and encephalopathy result from the portal hypertension and hepatocellular insufficiency caused by the cirrhosis and the underlying disease that produced it. However, a strict morphologic definition distinguishes cirrhosis from precirrhotic fibrosis and the various other diseases that can cause noncirrhotic portal hypertension and hepatic insufficiency. These include congenital hepatic fibrosis (fibrosis and ductal plate malformation without loss of architecture); nodular regenerative hyperplasia (hepatocellular nodules without fibrosis); and hepatoportal sclerosis, also called idiopathic portal hypertension or noncirrhotic portal fibrosis (portal hypertension with only minimal histologic changes). A correct diagnosis requires a specimen that is both adequate and correctly interpreted.

2.3   Biopsy Examination of Liver Tissue

There are several important issues to consider in successful liver biopsy evaluation of a patient with clinical evidence of portal hypertension and suspected cirrhosis. These include (a) the liver biopsy method and instrument used; (b) the size and condition of the specimen; (c) techniques for the detection of fibrosis; and (d) methods of tissue analysis.

Biopsy Methods, Size and Condition of the Specimen. The AASLD Guideline for liver biopsy recommends that the specimen have enough tissue for accurate diagnosis, grading and staging [3]. Based on evidence from studies of chronic hepatitis C, a biopsy should have at least the equivalent of an undamaged and unfragmented 2 cm core of tissue obtained with 16 gauge needle. The principal ways to obtain liver tissue for evaluation are listed in Table 2.1. As invasive procedures, all have some potential drawbacks as well as merits. Wedge liver biopsies obtained during surgical procedures may have abundant tissue, but care must be taken to avoid excessive use of electrocautery, which can markedly distort the specimen. Laparoscopy can be used to visualize the liver surface and direct biopsies to areas of abnormalities, but this raises the possibility that the biopsy may not be representative of the entire liver. All needle biopsies are potentially subject to sampling variability, but this can be minimized by adhering to the AASLD guideline, obtaining larger biopsies and performing two or more passes. Very narrow gauge needles (19 g or smaller) are frequently used for transjugular and sometimes other biopsies, resulting in further increase in sampling variability. Multiple passes may overcome sampling error in most cases, but some will remain uncertain. Instruments such as Meghini and Klatskin needles that rely on suction to extract the specimen may cause it to break into small fragments, especially when there is advanced fibrosis or cirrhosis [5]. Tissue obtained with cutting needles is less likely to fragment but may yield less tissue per pass.

Tissue obtained by one of these biopsy methods is immersed in a fixative, most often 10% neutral buffered formalin (formaldehyde) for routine processing. This

Table 2.1 Methods of obtaining liver tissue for pathologic examination

Source of tissue	Advantages	Disadvantages
Surgical biopsy	Direct examination of viscera by surgeon Large amount of tissue obtainable	Risks of surgery and anesthesia
Laparoscopically-directed (cutting needle)	Direct visualization of liver Adequate sampling	Time and cost Complications (usually minor) in 2.5%
CT or ultrasound-directed (fine needle)	Good for focal lesions Adequate tissue from many tumors	Small amount of tissue Inadequate for most inflammatory diseases
Transjugular (transvenous)	Safest when there is high risk of hemorrhage or percutaneous route is hampered by ascites or obesity	Technically more difficult Expense
Percutaneous (Blind) or ultrasound-directed	Relatively simple procedure Adequate tissue for most diffuse inflammatory diseases	Random sampling, may not be representative
Suction needle (Menghini, Jamshidi, etc.)	Larger biopsies than cutting needles from noncirrhotic livers	Specimen fragmentation, especially in cirrhosis
Cutting needle (Trucut, and spring-loaded cutting needle biopsy "guns")	Less fragmentation than with suction needles Ease of use	

causes time-dependent chemical reactions that produce cross-linking of proteins with hardening and preservation of the tissue. The tissue is then dehydrated by immersion in graded ethanol followed by lipid extraction in xylene, and immersion in hot melted paraffin to infiltrate the tissue so that it can be sectioned. The paraffin containing tissue is then cooled and hardened to form the blocks that can be attached to a microtome which is used to cut sections that are typically 4 µm thick. The sections mounted on glass microscope slides can then be stained by a variety of methods to allow evaluation of the tissue and pathologic changes. Other fixatives and processing protocols can be used for special requirements, or the tissue can be snap frozen without fixation or processing and sections cut with a cryostat to stain for lipids or for substances too labile to survive processing.

Techniques for Detection of Fibrosis. In the gross liver specimen, as examined at autopsy or in a surgical resection or endstage liver explanted prior to transplantation, fibrosis is visible as firm, grayish-white or tan scars. On a cut surface, the scars tend to be depressed, while parenchymal nodules in cirrhotic livers often bulge above the cut surface. In histologic sections large scars are readily seen in the routine hematoxylin and eosin stain, but they may be difficult to distinguish from areas of necrosis and stromal collapse, while areas of early fibrosis are often undetectable. Special stains that demonstrate connective tissue are therefore essential for the evaluation of fibrosis. **Masson's trichrome** is the most widely used stain in the United States and many other countries. Type I collagen, which forms the supporting connective tissue of portal areas, hepatic vein tributaries and Glisson's capsule, and which is the major type of collagen in scar tissue, appears blue (Fig. 2.1). **Reticulin**

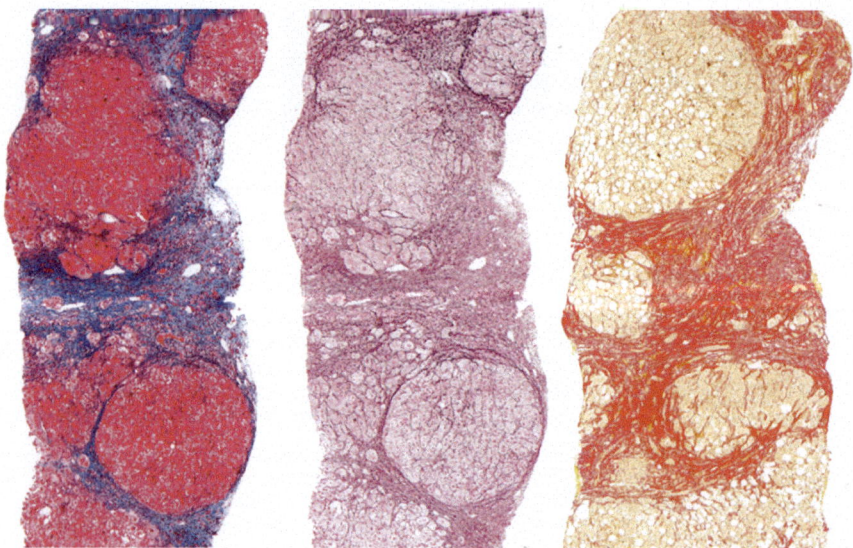

Fig. 2.1 Stains for detection of fibrosis. This cirrhotic liver is stained with Masson trichrome (*left*), in which fibrous tissue is *blue*; with Gordon-Sweet's reticulin stain (*center*), in which the fibrous tissue is *black*; and with *Sirius red* (*right*), which stains the connective tissue *red*

stain includes several variants of silver impregnation techniques that can be used to produce black staining of type III collagen fibers, which form the reticulin framework of sinusoids and which are present where Type I collagen is found (Fig. 2.1). **Sirius red** produces bright red staining of collagen (Fig. 2.1). Futhermore, stain binding is stoichiometric which allows quantification of the collagen by morphometric techniques. Others include the van Gieson, stain, popular in some laboratories, produces red staining of type I collagen. In Gomori's trichrome, collagen is green. Elastic fibers, present normally in Glisson's capsule and in portal tracts but also found in mature scars, can be demonstrated by several stains, including the orcein and Victoria blue stains that are used to detect hepatitis B surface antigen. The Movat pentachrome can be used to distinguish collagen (yellow staining) and elastic fibers (black) from other extracellular matrix components (blue-green). Finally, immunostains, using specific antibodies, can be used to demonstrate the numerous specific components of the extracellular matrix.

2.4 Progression of Liver Disease to Cirrhosis

Normal human liver has very little connective tissue visible by light microscopy. Collagen is present in Glisson's capsule, in major anatomical septa and in portal areas. Portal areas occupy only about 4–6% of the two-dimensional area of histologic sections, and most of the portal space is occupied by blood vessels and bile ducts, so that stainable collagen accounts for less than 1%. With aging, there appears to be increased density of the portal connective tissue of no clinical significance, and some increase in collagen surrounding bile ducts.

Our understanding of the progression of liver diseases is largely based on cross-sectional data from liver biopsies in many patients used to construct logical sequences of progression. There is relatively little data from repeated biopsies of uniform cohorts of patients, and therapeutic interventions that follow initial diagnoses may change the natural history. Nevertheless, progression of most chronic liver diseases is believed to be caused by increasing fibrosis leading eventually to cirrhosis. Activation of stellate cells with subsequent production of collagen is generally thought to be the major cause of progression, but other mechanisms may play a role.

Different types of diseases produce different patterns of fibrosis as the disease progresses. These can be divided into those diseases that are portal-based and those that begin in acinar zone 3 and thus are central-based. The major portal-based diseases that lead to cirrhosis include chronic hepatitis (viral and autoimmune), chronic cholestatic diseases (primary biliary cholangitis, primary sclerosing cholangitis, and chronic mechanical obstruction of any cause) and hemochromatosis. Central-based diseases include steatohepatitis (alcoholic or nonalcoholic) and chronic venous outflow obstruction of any cause.

Portal-based diseases. In chronic viral and autoimmune hepatitis, the primary disease process is immune-mediated hepatocellular injury leading to cell death through apoptosis, both within the parenchyma and at the interface between the portal areas and the parenchyma. Fibrosis mainly occurs as a consequence of the

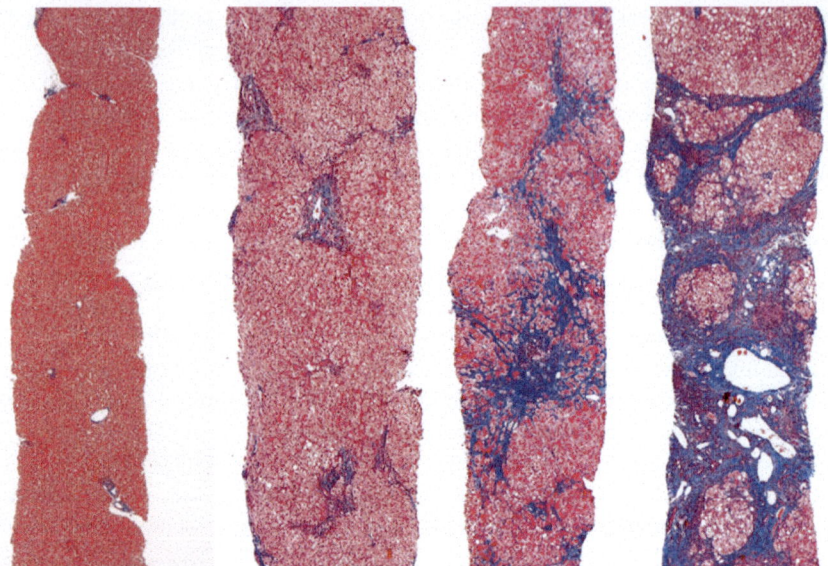

Fig. 2.2 Progression of fibrosis in chronic hepatitis C, a disease with portal-based fibrosis demonstrated with Masson trichrome stains. The four biopsies are from diffent patients with progressively more severe disease. From left to right, the first has no fibrosis (Ishak stage 0), second has fibrosis of most portal tracts (Ishak stage 2), third has extensive bridging fibrosis (Ishak stage 4), and the fourth on the right has established cirrhosis (Ishak stage 6)

injury at the interface ("interface hepatitis"). The portal area enlarges, sometimes maintaining a round contour, but often extending through zone 1 of the acinus as a broad-based area of fibrosis, or "active septum" that may eventually join a similar septum extending from the adjacent portal area (Fig. 2.2) to create a portal-portal bridge.

Bridging fibrosis is a term that is often misused. The portal tracts form a tree-like structure within the liver, and portal triads in a histologic section represent cross-sections of the branches of the tree. Fibrous expansion of portal areas makes them more likely to be cut tangentially so that they traverse the section and may be misinterpreted as bridging fibrosis. These tangentially cut portal tracts are often called portal-portal septa, but they contain pre-existing bile ducts and hepatic artery branches which run the length of the structure, allowing them to be distinguished from true bridges, which are scars that traverse parenchyma in planes of section that should have no fibrous tissue. Similarly, a tangential section at a branch point of the biliary tree in a patient with fibrous portal expansion may show liver parenchyma surrounded by fibrous tissue in the plane of section, even though in three dimensions it would not form a true nodule. Care must be taken to avoid an erroneous diagnosis of cirrhosis in such cases.

Severe exacerbations of the hepatitis can produce confluent necrosis of acinar zone 3, producing *portal-central bridging necrosis*, which may lead to stromal collapse and post-necrotic scarring, creating a so-called "passive septum." It has also been postulated that vascular occlusion may be superimposed, producing larger areas of parenchymal extinction and accelerating the disease process [6]. The scars that are produced by these processes tend to contract, like scars anywhere in the body, and consequently the hepatic architecture becomes distorted. The scars extend in three dimensions to envelope pre-existing acini and acinar agglomerates, creating cirrhotic nodules of varying size (Fig. 2.2).

Chronic biliary tract diseases also produce periportal injury that leads to fibrosis of acinar zone 1. This may be due to the cholestasis itself and the toxic effects of bile acids and other bile components, but there may also be an element of interface hepatitis, especially in primary biliary cholangitis. Fibrosis typically extends along acinar zone 1, usually associated with activation of portal myofibroblasts and ductular proliferation. The septa thus formed link adjacent portal tracts, producing fairly regular nodules of parenchyma, often with a terminal hepatic venule in the center.

In hemochromatosis the fibrosis is thought to follow hepatocyte death due to massive iron overload. Since the iron accumulation is most severe in the periportal hepatocytes, these are the first to die, stimulating a fibrogenic response, producing thick portal-portal bridges. Untreated patients have continuing hepatocyte loss with scarring, eventually producing very small cirrhotic nodules with central veins incorporated into the scars and obliteration of acinar landmarks.

Central-based diseases. In steatohepatitis, whether due to alcohol or NASH, fibrosis begins in the sinusoids surrounding the terminal hepatic venule, reflecting collagen synthesis by activated stellate cells. The venule wall becomes thickened, and collagen along with other components of the extracellular matrix is deposited in the space of Disse, predominantly in zone 3 of the acinus, producing a typical pattern of pericellular fibrosis. Disease progression results in ever-increasing sinusoidal fibrosis in zone 3, extending from central veins to portal areas (Fig. 2.3). The portal connective tissue also appears to increase, although the mechanism for this is not clear. Hepatocyte death, probably through apoptosis, causes the sinusoidal fibrosis to condense into fibrous bridges, which appear central-portal in some planes of section and portal-portal in others. Alcohol inhibits hepatocellular regeneration,

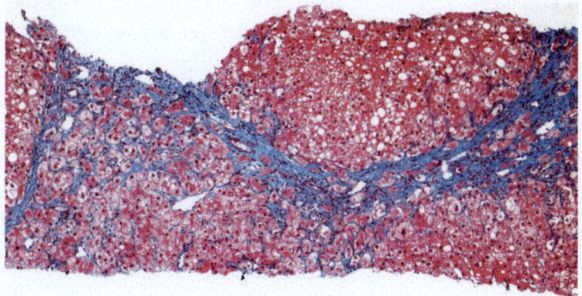

Fig. 2.3 Bridging fibrosis in nonalcoholic steatohepatitis. Masson trichrome stain shows sinusoidal fibrosis surrounding individual liver cells in acinar zone 3 with condensation into a bridge of fibrous tissue extending from a portal tract (right of field) to a central vein (left of field)

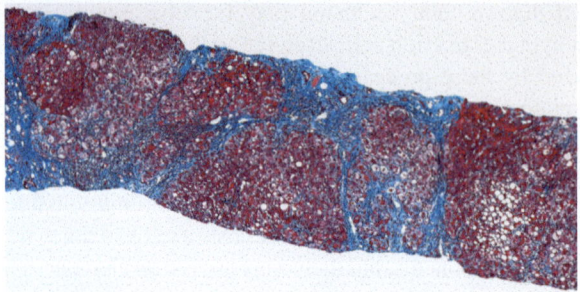

Fig. 2.4 Cirrhosis in nonalcoholic steatohepatitis (cutting needle biopsy). Masson trichrome stain shows regenerative nodules of hepatocytes with a mild degree of residual steatosis surrounded by fibrous septa. The biopsy was performed with a Tru-cut cutting needle, which shows the true architecture of the liver tissue, including both regenerative nodules and fibrosis

so that in alcoholic hepatitis there may be tremendous fibrosis with preservation of acinar structures but without true cirrhosis. However, the fibrous bridges, like scars in other body sites, tend to contract, and there is often ductular proliferation within the areas of scarring, so that the hepatic architecture becomes distorted. Occlusion of outflow veins may occur at any stage of the disease and probably is a factor in progression to cirrhosis. Hepatocellular regeneration, producing nodules of liver cells surrounded by fibrosis, results in the full picture of cirrhosis (Fig. 2.4).

Chronic venous outflow obstruction also produces fibrosis with a central-based pattern. The congestion and hepatocyte atrophy produces central vein thickening and sinusoidal fibrosis very similar to that seen in steatohepatitis. The fibrosis is predominantly in zone 3, and the resulting central-central and central-portal bridging fibrosis produces a cirrhosis with a pattern of so-called reverse lobulation.

2.5   Histologic Diagnosis of Cirrhosis

Cirrhosis, as has been noted, is defined by WHO as a diffuse process characterized by fibrosis and conversion of the normal liver architecture into structurally abnormal nodules [4]. Three basic morphologic categories are recognized on the basis of the size of the cirrhotic nodules. The micronodular type includes those cases in which almost all nodules are less than 3 mm in diameter. In the macronodular type, most nodules are greater than 3 mm in diameter and usually show striking variation in size. The mixed pattern is characterized by approximately equal numbers of micro- and macronodules. Regenerative nodules are not essential for the diagnosis of cirrhosis; in both biliary cirrhosis and hemochromatosis, for example, regeneration may be minimal or absent.

The diagnosis of cirrhosis may be difficult to establish by percutaneous needle biopsy, particularly if the pattern is macronodular. Cutting needles (e.g., Tru-cut) are preferred because these obtain specimens that include the fibrous septa and the parenchymal nodules (Fig. 2.4). Suction techniques (e.g., Menghini needles) are limited by preferential sampling of parenchyma as the biopsy needle rebounds from the fibrous septa. There are, however, a number of microscopic clues to the diagnosis, even in this type of specimen. Suction biopsies from cirrhotic livers are commonly fragmented, and the fragments have rounded edges. Fibrous septa can course through the fragments, but these are sometimes represented by thin strips hugging margins of the fragments. Stains for collagen (Fig. 2.5) are frequently necessary to detect them. Such stains are also valuable for distinguishing fibrosis from collapsed reticulin that follows extensive necrosis and for demonstrating thick liver plates in regenerative nodules of the cirrhotic liver. Reticulin stains usually demonstrate a very irregular pattern because of alterations in the growth of hepatocytes. Many cell plates are greater than one cell in thickness, and the compressed sinusoidal spaces may be nearly invisible. Hepatocytes are pleomorphic, unless the process is entirely inactive. An alteration of the spatial relationship between the portal vessels and central veins is typical. Micronodular cirrhosis is less difficult to establish by needle biopsy than is macronodular cirrhosis because the diameter of the biopsy needle usually exceeds that of the small cirrhotic nodules. The capsule of the liver in many

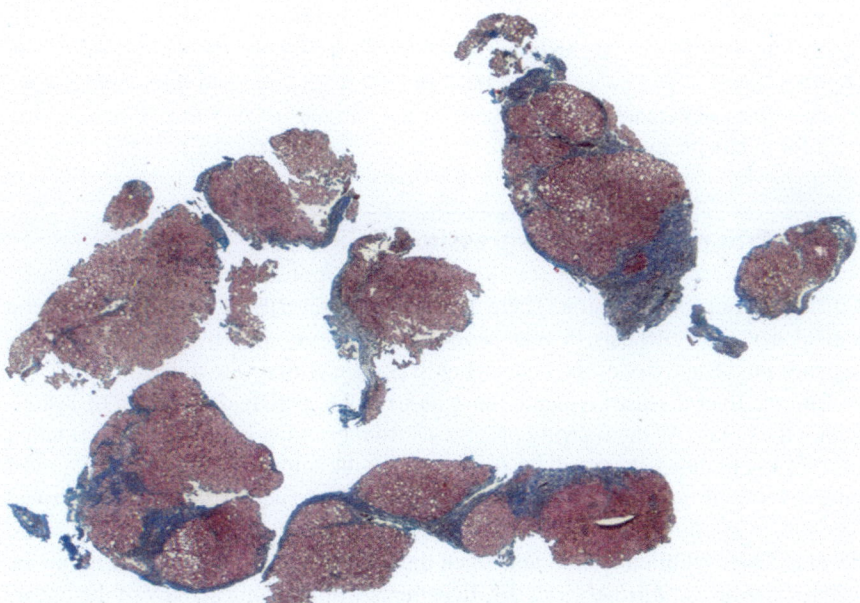

Fig. 2.5 Cirrhosis in chronic hepatitis C (suction needle biopsy). Masson trichrome stain shows a fragmented specimen shows a fragmented specimen with delicate bands of blue-staining fibrous tissue on the dges of several fragments and occasionally traversing and enveloping a fragment. Only a few complete nodules can be seen and the architecture is not accurately represented because much of the fibrous tissue remained in the liver while the parenchymal nodules were prefertially aspirated by this Menghini needle biopsy. The trichrome stain shows sufficient nodularity for a diagnosis of probable cirrhosis, but the fragmentation makes it impossible to be certain whether the cirrhosis is incomplete, established or advanced, and such a specimen is not suitable for morphometry to quantify the fibrosis

noncirrhotic patients is thickened by an increase in fibrous tissue, vessels, and duct-ules. A small biopsy specimen from such an area (particularly a superficial wedge biopsy) should be interpreted with caution and not diagnosed as cirrhosis.

An advantage of liver biopsy over noninvasive fibrosis assessments is that the biopsy can determine whether the cirrhosis is fully developed or incomplete, the basic morphologic type (i.e., micronodular, macronodular, or mixed), the degree of activity, and often the presumptive cause. Biopsy specimens showing occasional nodules or extensive fibrosis may be judged to represent early or incomplete cir-rhosis, but the designation cirrhosis should be reserved for those with complete loss of acinar architecture. An assessment of the activity should take into account the degree of hepatocellular degeneration and necrosis and the amount of inflammation in the parenchyma of the nodules.

Although it is not always possible, an etiologic diagnosis can often be estab-lished or suggested by changes observed in hematoxylin and eosin-stained sections alone (e.g., interface hepatitis and plasma cells in autoimmune hepatitis; fat, bal-looning degeneration and Mallory-Denk bodies in alcoholic or nonalcoholic steato-hepatitis; absence of bile ducts and chronic cholestasis indicating biliary cirrhosis secondary to primary biliary cholangitis (PBC) or primary sclerosing cholangitis). Special stains, however, are an important auxiliary technique. Particularly useful are copper stains for Wilson's disease and PBC, the PAS stain and immunostains for α_1-antitrypsin deficiency, immunostains of the antigens of hepatitis B, and an iron stain for hemochromatosis.

2.6 Progression and Regression of Cirrhosis

Cirrhosis is not a static lesion. There are degrees of severity of cirrhosis, and after a patient develops cirrhosis, it may worsen, stabilize, or improve. In general, this depends on the activity of the underlying liver disease that caused the cirrhosis.

Chronic liver diseases typically have an irregular, patchy distribution of lesions within the organ. As the scarring progresses from bridging fibrosis to the formation of complete nodules, there will be areas in which the acinar architecture is preserved intermixed with areas of complete nodularity. Livers such as this may be termed *incomplete cirrhosis*. As the disease progresses, areas of preserved architecture become fewer within the liver, and when the liver is completely nodular, it may be said to have an e*stablished cirrhosis*. In patients with ongoing activity of the under-lying disease, the cirrhotic nodules remain small, and the cirrhosis is typically *micronodular*. With further progression, hepatic parenchyma continues to be lost while the scars of the cirrhosis widen and broad areas of extinction appear, produc-ing what may be termed an *advanced cirrhosis*. Although it is rare to have serial biopsies to document the sequence, it is likely that this type of disease progression is the cause of increasing portal hypertension and hepatocellular insufficiency that results in clinical decompensation in patients with cirrhosis.

Resolution of the underlying disease can result in considerable improvement in fibrosis, even in patients with cirrhosis. This has been observed in alcoholics who stop drinking, in hemochromatosis after phlebotomy to remove excess iron, in hepatitis C after a sustained virological response to interferon-ribavirin therapy, and in hepatitis B following prolonged antiviral therapy or spontaneous seroconversion. It is a principle of pathology that scars remodel as necessary to serve their function of wound healing, and after an injury is healed, the scars tend to contract and resolve. In cirrhosis, this results in the conversion of a micronodular cirrhosis, in which the nodules tend to be small and uniform into a macronodular cirrhosis, a change that often occurs even in patients whose underlying disease remains active [7]. *Incomplete septal cirrhosis* is a term that has been used for livers in which are generally nodular but which have relatively delicate and incomplete fibrous septa, although it is unclear whether this is really a stage in the development of cirrhosis, a regressing cirrhosis [8], or perhaps a form of nodular regenerative hyperplasia in a liver with a some underlying fibrosis. It has even been suggested, based on repeated biopsies in some patients, that cirrhosis can resolve completely. It seems likely, however, that this may be due to the difficulty of diagnosing macronodular cirrhosis or incomplete septal cirrhosis in a needle biopsy.

2.7   Staging of Fibrosis

Stage of a disease process indicates how far the disease has progressed in the course of its natural history. At the end stage, the disease has run its course, and the patient dies or the affected organ fails. In most liver diseases, the end stage is decompensated cirrhosis with its complications. The various staging systems that have been devised for use in chronic liver disease all provide stages that progress from normal liver architecture through stages of increasing fibrosis to cirrhosis. The presumption is that progressive stages are associated with worsened prognosis and decreased survival. This has been demonstrated for cirrhosis of many etiologies, but it is less well established for the precirrhotic stages of liver disease. Nevertheless, establishment of the stage of disease is a primary function of the liver biopsy.

Staging by liver biopsy. There are two principal purposes for staging fibrosis. The first, and by far the most common, is for management and prognosis of an individual patient. The second is to gather data as part of a clinical trial and in studies that have attempted to define the natural history of fibrosis progression in some liver diseases. The criteria for diagnosis and classification of cirrhosis and precirrhotic fibrosis were established in autopsy specimens, where the entire liver can be carefully sectioned, inspected grossly, and samples taken from multiple areas. However, in living patients, needle biopsies are the mainstay of histologic evaluation for diagnosis, grading and staging of liver diseases. Although the same terminology is used, needle biopsies are inherently subject to sampling variability, and this is compounded by small biopsies and narrow gauge needles. For management of an individual patient it is usually sufficient to know whether the patient has cirrhosis or significant precirrhotic fibrosis, characterized by bridging fibrosis. A number of semiquantitative scores have been used in clinical trials and in retrospective analyses (Table 2.2). These have a range from four categories with the Knodell score [9]

Table 2.2 Semiquantitative fibrosis staging systems for use in clinical trials of chronic hepatitis

Fibrosis	Knodell	Scheuer	Metavir	Batts-Ludwig	Ishak	Laennec
None	0	0	0	0	0	0
Portal (few)	1	1	1	1	1	1
Portal (most)	1	1	1	2	2	1
Periportal ± short septa	1	2	1	2	2	1
Few bridges or septa	3	3	2	3	3	2
Numerous bridges or septa	3	3	3	3	4	3
Incomplete cirrhosis	4	4	4	4	5	4a
Cirrhosis, definite or probable	4	4	4	4	6	4b
Cirrhosis, advanced	4	4	4	4	6	4c

to five with the Scheuer [10], Metavir [11] and Batts-Ludwig [12] scores; to seven with the Ishak score [13] and eight with the Laennec score [14]. Although a seven and eight category scales are less reproducible than one with fewer categories, they have the potential to convey more information. Consequently, the range of the Ishak and Laennec scores give better chance of detecting a change that may be inapparent using simpler scores, as long as there is a sufficient number of patients for statistical significance, so this approach is recommended for clinical trials of chronic viral hepatitis. In chronic hepatitis C, increasing Ishak stage from stages 2 through 6 was shown to predict a stepwise increasing likelihood of adverse clinical outcomes [15], while in patients with late stage disease of mixed etiology, the Laennec score had similar predictive value [14]. In biliary diseases, the four-stage system proposed by Ludwig et al. [16, 17] for use in primary biliary cholangitis and primary sclerosing cholangitis has correlated with patient survival in long term follow up studies and been used successfully in clinical trials. It is noteworthy that stages 1 and 2 correspond to early-stage, stage 3 to mid-stage, and stage 4 to late-stage disease. Similarly, in steatohepatitis, the NASH CRN staging has four categories of increasing fibrosis that correlate with survival [18, 19]. Expansion of these scales to similar seven or eight categories would undoubtedly increase their predictive value.

Morphometry is a way to quantify morphologic features in a specimen on a continuous scale, rather than as discrete stages. Current methods use computer-assisted digital image analysis programs to calculate the proportion of the tissue section composed of the structure of interest, in this case fibrous tissue [20–22]. The methods for this are time consuming compared to simple histologic scoring, and the necessary equipment and expertise are not widely available, but in studies to evaluate progression or regression of fibrosis, it seems appropriate to measure the amount of fibrosis as precisely as possible. Unfragmented and preferably large specimens are necessary for this, since specimen fragmentation tends to under-represent the fibrous septa in fibrotic and cirrhotic liver. Furthermore, sampling variability makes precise quantification of the amount of fibrous tissue by morphometry of little value in a needle biopsy from an individual patient. However, in a clinical trial, measurement of the amount of fibrosis in needle biopsy samples from many patients can be used to estimate the amount and distribution of fibrosis in the cohort as a whole with a high degree of accuracy. In one study of patients with advanced fibrosis and cirrhosis (Ishak stages 4–6) due to chronic hepatitis C, fibrosis quantifed by morphometry was shown to increase on average by 58% per year [20], indicating that changes in the average amount of fibrosis measured by morphometry can be a much more sensitive technique for demonstrating progression or regression of fibrosis than histologic staging.

Importance of biopsy size and condition. Since the size of the liver biopsy sample is proportional to the size of needle used, 18 gauge or wider needles are essential for evaluating hepatic architecture. Furthermore, several studies have shown a significant loss of diagnostic accuracy in biopsies less than 2.5 or 2.0 cm in length [23–25]. Although it is widely held that a 1.5 cm needle core is adequate for assessing most liver diseases, it has been found in various series that a single 1.5 cm specimen can fail to recognize cirrhosis in 15–40% of cases [23, 24, 26, 27]. Of course, this means that 60–85% of the time, a 1.5 cm biopsy is sufficient to recognize cirrhosis, and if it is recognizable, the biopsy has virtually 100% positive predictive value. If there is a 15% prevalence of cirrhosis in the population of patients subjected to liver biopsy, then failure to recognize 40% means that the negative predictive value is 93%, so while not perfect, a 1.5 cm long needle biopsy is still as good or better than most of the noninvasive tests, even with the worst reported results. Nevertheless it has been shown that reduced size biopsies tend to lower grade and stage in chronic HCV specimens Table 2.3), and it has been suggested that a minimum of 11 complete portal tracts is necessary for accurate grading and staging [24]. Since most 2 cm long needle biopsies will contain at least 11 portal tracts, this is the basis of the AASLD recommendation. To assess for the presence of cirrhosis, it has also been shown that cutting needles are superior to suction-type needles, which often produce fragmented specimens that may be nondiagnostic [5]. Fragmented specimens always raise the possibility of cirrhosis, and in a patient with a strong clinical suspicion of cirrhosis, a fragmented biopsy with delicate rims of

Table 2.3 Relationship of biopsy size to diagnostic accuracy for evaluation of fibrosis as reported by Colloredo et al. [24] in 161 liver biopsies, assuming that a biopsy >3 cm long is accurate

Biopsy length	Cirrhosis[a]	No cirrhosis	Positive predictive value	Negative predictive value	Diagnostic accuracy
>3 cm	18 (11.2%)	143 (88.8%)	1.00	1.00	100%
1.5 cm	12 (7.4%)	149 (92.6%)	1.00	0.96	96%
1.0 cm	8 (4.9%)	153 (95.1%)	1.00	0.93	94%
Biopsy length	**Significant fibrosis[b]**	**No significant fibrosis**	**Positive predictive value**	**Negative predictive value**	**Diagnostic accuracy**
>3 cm	66 (41.0%)	95 (59.0%)	1.00	1.00	100%
1.5 cm	51 (31.6%)	110 (68.4%)	1.00	0.86	91%
1.0 cm	32 (19.8%)	129 (80.2%)	1.00	0.74	78%

[a]Cirrhosis = Stage 5 or 6 of Ishak fibrosis score
[b]Significant fibrosis = Bridging fibrosis (Ishak stage 3–4) or cirrhosis

fibrosis around the tissue fragments can be considered diagnostic of cirrhosis (Fig. 2.5). However, noncirrhotic liver tissue may also fragment, especially when drawn through a suction needle, so fragmentation is not synonymous with cirrhosis (Fig. 2.5). Thus, long and wide, (>2 cm long with a 16 gauge needle) biopsies are desirable for optimal results, and if cirrhosis is suspected, a cutting needle rather than a suction needle should be used.

References

1. Laennec RTH. Traite de l'Auscultation Mediate, et des Maladies des Poumon et du Coeur. Paris: Chaude; 1819.
2. Smetana HF. The histologic diagnosis of viral hepatitis by needle biopsy. Gastroenterology. 1954;26:612–25.
3. Rockey DC, Caldwell SH, Goodman ZD, Nelson RC, Smith AD. Liver biopsy. Hepatology. 2009;49:1017–44.
4. Anthony PP, Ishak KG, Nyak NC, Poulsen HE, Scheuer PJ, Sobin LS. The morphology of cirrhosis: definition, nomenclature, and classification. Bull World Health Organ. 1977;55:521–40. (reprinted in J Clin Pathol. 1978;31:395–414)
5. Sherman KE, Goodman ZD, Sullivan ST, Faris-Young S. Liver biopsy in cirrhotic patients. Am J Gastroenterol. 2007;102:789–93.
6. Wanless IR. Vascular disorders. In: MacSween RNM, Burt AD, Portmann BC, Ishak KG, Scheuer PJ, Anthony PP, editors. Pathology of the liver. 4th ed. London: Churchill Livingstone; 2002. p. 539–73.
7. Fauerholdt L, Schlichting P, Christensen E, Poulsen H, Tygstrup N, Juhl E. Conversion of micronodular cirrhosis into macronodular cirrhosis. Hepatology. 1983;3:928–31.
8. Wanless IR, Nakasimia E, Sherman M. Regression of human cirrhosis. Morphologic features and the genesis of incomplete septal cirrhosis. Arch Pathol Lab Med. 2000;124:1599–607.
9. Knodell RG, Ishak KG, Black WC, Chen TS, Craig R, Kaplowitz N, Kiernan TW, Wollman J. Formulation and application of a numerical scoring system for assessing histological activity in asymptomatic chronic active hepatitis. Hepatology. 1981;1:431–5.
10. Scheuer PJ. Classification of chronic viral hepatitis: a need for reassessment. J Hepatol. 1991;13:372–4.
11. Bedossa P, Bioulac-Sage P, Callard P, Chevallier M, Degott C, Deugnier Y, Fabre M, Reynes M, Voight JJ, Zafrani ES. Interobserver and intraobserver variations in liver biopsy interpretation in patients with chronic hepatitis C. Hepatology. 1994;20:15–20.
12. Batts KP, Ludwig J. Chronic hepatitis: an update on terminology and reporting. Am J Surg Pathol. 1995;19:1409–17.
13. Ishak KG, Baptista A, Bianchi L, Callea F, De Groote J, Gudat F, Denk H, Desmet V, Korb G, MacSween RNM, Phillips MJ, Portmann BG, Poulsen H, Scheuer PJ, Sachmidt M, Thaler H. Histological grading and staging of chronic hepatitis. J Hepatol. 1995;22:696–9.
14. Kim SU, Oh HJ, Wanless IR, Lee S, Han KH, Park YN. The Laennec staging system for histological sub-classification of cirrhosis is useful for stratification of prognosis in patients with liver cirrhosis. J Hepatol. 2012;57:556–63.
15. Everhart JE, Wright EC, Goodman ZD, Dienstag JL, Hoefs JC, Kleiner DE, Ghany MG, Mills AS, Nash SR, Govindarajan S, Rogers TE, Greenson JK, Brunt EM, Bonkovsky HL, Morishima C, Litman HJ. Prognostic value of Ishak fibrosis stage: findings from the hepatitis C antiviral long-term treatment against cirrhosis trial. Hepatology. 2009;51:585–94.
16. Ludwig J, Dickson ER, McDonald GS. Staging of chronic non-suppurative destructive cholangitis (syndrome of primary biliary cirrhosis). Virchows Arch A. 1978;379:103–12.
17. Ludwig J, Barham SS, LaRusso NF, Elveback LR, Wiesner RH, McCall JT. Morphologic features of chronic hepatitis associated with primary sclerosing cholangitis and chronic ulcerative colitis. Hepatology. 1981;1:632–40.

18. Kleiner DE, Brunt EM, Van Natta M, Behling C, Contos MJ, Cummings OW, Ferrell LD, Liu YC, Torbenson MS, Unalp-Arida A, Yeh M, McCullough AJ, Sanyal AJ. Design and validation of a histological scoring system for nonalcoholic fatty liver disease. Hepatology. 2005;41:1313–21.
19. Younossi Z, Stepanova M, Rafiq N, Makhlouf H, Younoszai Z, Agrawal R, Goodman Z. Pathologic criteria for non-alcoholic steatohepatitis (NASH): inter-protocol agreement and ability to predict liver-related mortality. Hepatology. 2011;53:1874–82.
20. Goodman ZD, Becker RL, Pockros PJ, Afdhal NH. Progression of fibrosis in chronic hepatitis C: evaluation by morphometric image analysis. Hepatology. 2007;45:886–94.
21. Goodman ZD, Stoddard AM, Bonkovsky HL, Fontana RJ, Ghany MG, Morgan TR, Wright EC, Brunt EM, Kleiner DE, Shiffman ML, Everson GT, Lindsay KL, Dienstag JL, Morishima C. HALT-C Trial Group: fibrosis progression in chronic hepatitis C: morphometric image analysis in the HALT-C trial. Hepatology. 2009;50:1738–49.
22. McHutchison J, Goodman Z, Patel K, Makhlouf H, Rodriguez-Torres M, Shiffman M, Rockey D, Husa P, Chuang WL, Levine R, Jonas M, Theodore D, Brigandi R, Webster A, Schultz M, Watson H, Stancil B, Gardner S. Farglitazar lacks antifibrotic activity in patients with chronic hepatitis C infection. Gastroenterology. 2010;138:1365–73.
23. Holund B, Poulsen H, Schlichting P. Reproducibility of the liver biopsy diagnosis in relation to the size of the specimen. Scand J Gastroenterol. 1980;15:329–35.
24. Colloredo G, Guido M, Sonzogni A, Leandro G. Impact of liver biopsy size on histological evaluation of chronic viral hepatitis: the smaller the sample, the milder the disease. J Hepatol. 2003;39:239–44.
25. Schiano TD, Azeem S, Bodian CA, Bodenheimer HC Jr, Merati S, Thung SN, Hytiroglou P. Importance of specimen size in accurate needle liver biopsy evaluation of patients with chronic hepatitis C. Clin Gastroenterol Hepatol. 2005;3:930–5.
26. Abdi W, Millan JC, Mezey E. Sampling variability on percutaneous liver biopsy. Arch Intern Med. 1979;139:667–9.
27. Regev A, Berho M, Jeffers LJ, Milikowski C, Molina EG, Pyrsopoulos NT, Feng ZZ, Reddy KR, Schiff ER. Sampling error and intraobserver variation in liver biopsy in patients with chronic HCV infection. Am J Gastroenterol. 2002;97:2614–8.

Hepatic Venous Pressure Measurement and Other Diagnostic Hepatic Hemodynamic Techniques

3

Annalisa Berzigotti and Jaime Bosch

3.1 Introduction

Portal hypertension is a very common complication of advanced chronic liver disease (ACLD), and almost invariably occurs during its natural history [1]. Its relevance is due to the fact that it is responsible for the main complications of cirrhosis, including the formation of oesophageal and gastric varices; variceal bleeding; bleeding from portal hypertensive gastropathy, enteropathy and colopathy; ascites; spontaneous bacterial peritonitis; hepatorenal syndrome; hepatic encephalopathy; hepato-pulmonary syndrome; porto-pulmonary hypertension; splenomegaly and hypersplenism [1]. It is important to remark that these are the complications that most often lead to death or require liver transplantation in patients with cirrhosis.

It is important to note that all complications of cirrhosis can be prevented by preventing the portal pressure to increase above certain thresholds. Similarly, once present, the complications of portal hypertension can be solved by effectively decreasing the portal pressure. These concepts are of paramount importance since they represent the rational for the use of treatments aimed at decreasing or at preventing the increase of portal pressure [2], and for the use of changes in portal pressure as surrogates of clinical outcomes in the initial assessment of new treatments for both ACLD and of the complications of portal hypertension. This is why the measurement of portal pressure is a key parameter for understanding the progression of ACLD, for prognostic stratification and for assessing the effects of therapy.

A. Berzigotti • J. Bosch (✉)
Swiss Liver Center, Hepatology, University Clinic for Visceral Surgery and Medicine, Inselspital, University of Bern, Bern, Switzerland
e-mail: Annalisa.berzigotti@insel.ch; Jbosch@clinic.cat

© Springer International Publishing AG, part of Springer Nature 2018
A. Berzigotti, J. Bosch (eds.), *Diagnostic Methods for Cirrhosis and Portal Hypertension*, https://doi.org/10.1007/978-3-319-72628-1_3

3.1.1   Direct vs. Indirect Measurement of Portal Pressure

The portal venous system carries the outflow blood from splanchnic organs to the liver; therefore, its access is not anatomically simple.

Direct measurements of portal pressure are based on introducing a catheter or a needle into the portal vein. This requires its catheterisation under direct vision (at laparotomy), through its percutaneous puncture under ultrasound or radiologic guidance (either direct, trans-hepatic, or trans-venous), or by trans-esophageal or trans-gastric puncture under endoscopic ultrasound guidance.

All these methods are invasive and involve some risk for the patients, so its use is reserved to specific or special situations. The best example is in the evaluation of non-cirrhotic or pre-hepatic portal hypertension, or during an invasive procedure required for another reason (i.e., an abdominal operation). Another limitation of these techniques is that they require a separate procedure for measuring the pressure at the inferior vena cava or hepatic vein in order to be able to express the results in terms of a pressure gradient (see below).

Indirect Measurements of portal pressure are measurements done out of the portal vein system but reflecting the portal vein pressure. Historically, the first used was the measurement of the splenic pulp pressure by percutaneous spleen puncture. This is very rarely (if ever) used currently in clinical practice, but is very frequently used in studies in rats or mice. The second is the measurement of the hepatic venous pressure gradient (HVPG) at hepatic vein catheterization, which is by far, the most widely used technique to determine portal pressure in clinical practice, and that is what the rest of this chapter is dealing with.

Non-invasive estimation of portal pressure. Since both direct and indirect techniques for the measurement of portal pressure are all invasive methods it has been long desired to have a reliable, non-invasive way of determining portal pressure. Such a "portal sphygmomanometer" is not yet available, but several candidate non-invasive diagnostic methods are under intensive investigation. Most attempts are based on the use of imaging techniques, micro-bubble based ultrasound techniques, elastographic methods, and determination of metabolic, biochemical or heamotologic parameters quantitatively related to the degree of liver dysfunction. These methods are covered in specific chapters of this book.

3.1.2   HVPG: What Is It and How It Works?

HVPG stands for Hepatic Venous Pressure Gradient, and represents the difference between the "wedged" (or "occluded") and the "free" hepatic vein pressure at retrograde hepatic vein catheterization (WHVP and FHVP respectively). This was first used by Myers and Taylor in 1951, and since then has been proved as the simpler, safer and more reliable indirect technique for the determination of portal venous pressure in patients with chronic liver disease.

The scientific basis of this measurement is the same as the measurement of the wedged pulmonary "capillary" pressure, an index of left atrial pressure. The hepatic vein "wedged" pressure is obtained by advancing a catheter into the hepatic vein as far as it could go, until it totally occludes the lumen of the vein. When blood flow in a hepatic vein is stopped by the 'wedged' catheter, the static column of blood transmits the pressure from the preceding communicated vascular territory, in this case, the hepatic sinusoids. Thus, WHVP is a measure of hepatic sinusoidal pressure and not of portal pressure itself. However, WHVP adequately reflects portal pressure in alcoholic liver disease, non-alcoholic steatohepatitis (NASH), hepatitis C- and hepatitis B-related cirrhosis [1]. These entities are, by far, the most frequent etiologies of chronic liver disease in developed countries. Other liver diseases may cause portal hypertension without increasing WHVP; these are mainly diseases involving the portal tracts and occluding or constricting portal venules, as it happens in hepatic schistosomiasis, primary biliary cholangitis, and so called "idiopathic intrahepatic portal hypertension" and its related lesions [3].

The technique of measurement of WHVP was improved by the introduction of occlusion balloon catheters [4]. In this case, "wedging" of the catheter is achieved by inflating a small balloon at the tip of the catheter (Fig. 3.1a). This allows occlusion of a much larger hepatic vein, and therefore the measurement of sinusoidal pressure averages a much larger portion of the liver, which translates into increased accuracy and decreased variability of the measurements, which become easier and more reliable. Indeed, a high variability of HVPG values between different hepatic veins has been reported using end-hole, non-balloon catheters. The "free" hepatic vein pressure (FHVP) is recorded after releasing the balloon. The HVPG is recorded as WHVP minus FHVP. Hepatic vein catheterization represents a safe and relatively simple technique to perform accurate measurements of portal pressure in patients with liver disease [3].

Physiologically, intravascular pressure in any vascular territory should not be expressed as an absolute pressure, but as a pressure gradient, which is the difference in pressure between the inflow and outflow of the system, and represents the perfusion pressure of this particular vascular territory. Portal pressure should therefore be expressed as the portal pressure gradient (PPG), the pressure difference between the portal vein and the inferior vena cava, which represents the perfusion pressure within the portal-hepatic circulation. Since WHVP is equal to the portal pressure, then the HVPG is equal to the PPG. The normal HVPG/PPG value is up to 5 mmHg. Expressing portal pressure as the PPG is not modified by changes in intra-abdominal pressure that will increase both the portal pressure and the inferior vena cava (IVC) pressure, but will not significantly modify the HVPG. Of even greater practical importance, expressing portal pressure measurements as the PPG or HVPG provides an internal zero level, which is not affected by the position of the external pressure transducer to which the catheter is connected to measure intravascular pressure (see below).

Fig. 3.1 Measurement of wedged hepatic venous pressure (WHVP). (Panel **a**) Balloon occluded venography showing adequate occlusion of the hepatic vein for the measurement of the WHVP; the *arrow* indicates the balloon. Note that there is no reflux of the contrast dye and that the measurement is obtained in a large area of the liver. This makes balloon occlusion more reliable than «wedging» a straight end-hole catheter into a small hepatic vein. (Panel **b**) Hepatic vein venography showing communicant vessels between two hepatic veins (*arrows*). This finding precludes adequate occlusion of the venous outflow, and therefore does not allow an accurate measurement of the WHVP. Veno-venous communication are very characteristic of non-cirrhotic portal hypertension

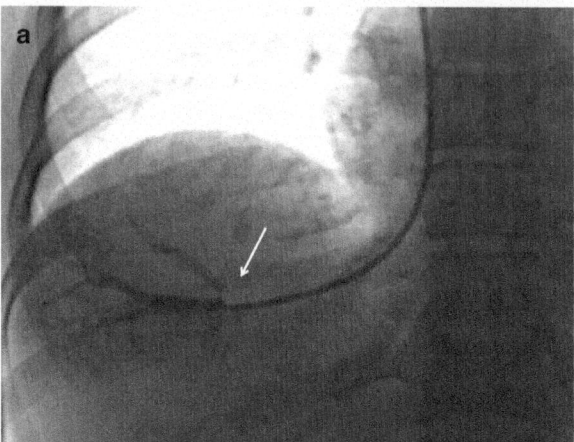
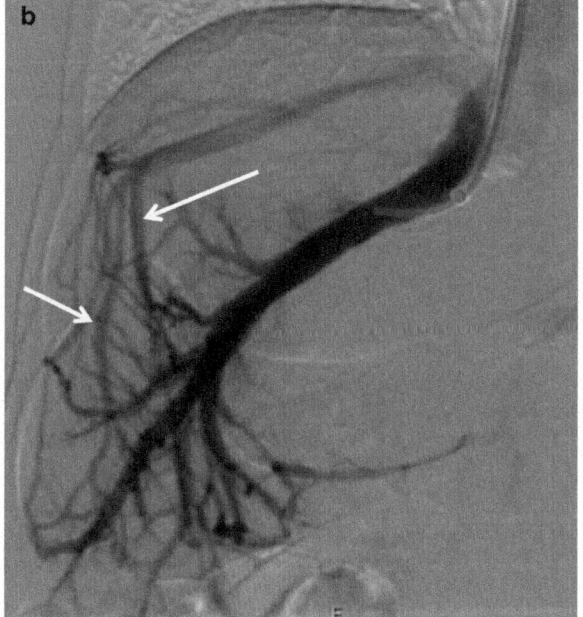

3.2   The Technique

Accuracy. *Anything worth doing should be done right* [5]. This quotation is especially true regarding measurements of HVPG due to the fact that this procedure is invasive and relatively costly, and therefore making it wrong is both an expensive error and kind of professional misconduct. Moreover, accuracy in the measurement is a must for many of its applications, since even a small deviation can lead to different conclusions: it is not the same to measure a HVPG of 9.5 mmHg than one of 10.5, and the significance of a decline of HVPG from 14 to 12 mmHg is not the same as a decline from 14 to 13 mmHg.

Generally speaking, the aim is to be able to measure HVPG with a precision of up to 0.5 mmHg. Greater is not possible: even if an instrument may give measurements of greater precision in ideal *in vitro* conditions, the physiologic fluctuation of pressures according to heart cycle and respiration makes that the best estimate of hepatic venous pressures cannot be of <0.5 mmHg. Thus, measurements should be rounded to the next half mmHg (12.3 would be 12.5, and 13.7 would be 13.5). In order to increase accuracy, measurements are done by triplicate, which allows averaging the measurements or discarding a given measurement if it has artifacts interfering with a correct interpretation.

3.2.1 Technical Requirements

Hepatic vein catheterization is most frequently done in a vascular radiology suit, although the laboratories with more experience worldwide are not in radiology departments, but in the hands of hepatologists. The X-ray equipment required does not need to be sophisticated high-performance angiographic machine, but any plain digital C-arm equipment will make it. These typically cost between around 150,000 € or $.

The lab shall be equipped with a vital signs monitor, for continuous monitoring of electrocardiogram, heart rate, non-invasive measurement of arterial pressure and oxygen saturation by pulse oxymetry. This should be complemented with a hemodynamic recorder system that can print on line and/or store electronically the tracings of intravascular pressure measurements. There are many of these equipments on the market, ranging from very sophisticated ones designed for cardiac catheterization labs to very simple but excellent ones. The only requirements are that these could print and/or store the pressure tracings, and that these can be set at the adequate magnification and speed (see below).

3.2.2 Catheters

As already explained, balloon-tipped catheters are preferable to straight end-hole catheters since allow more accurate and consistent measurements [6]. There are many of such catheters in the market; the only requirement is that the balloon is not totally terminal, to avoid it obstructing the lumen of the catheter if inflated in a small hepatic vein.

3.2.3 Vascular Access

Hepatic vein catheterization requires a access to the systemic venous circulation; the most commonly approaches are through the right jugular vein or right femoral vein, but large enough peripheral veins can also be used (e.g. basilic vein in the right arm). Usually, the transjugular approach is the preferred one, as it is simple and allows performing a transjugular liver biopsy as part of the procedure.

The procedure shall be done in aseptic conditions and under local anesthesia. The patient should have a peripheral i.v. drip for drug administration in case this is needed during the procedure. The venous puncture shall be done under ultrasound guidance. This minimizes the risk of hurting other structures and diminishes local complications [7], which are the most commonly observed (see below).

Sedation. Deep sedation is not required and can interfere with correct measures, so it should not be used. A slight conscious sedation (midazolam 0.02 mg/kg i.v.) can be used to improve the patient's comfort and does not modify hemodynamic measurements [8]. Larger doses should not be used since they affect the HVPG measurements. If a transjugular biopsy is part of the procedure, pressure measurements shall be done first, with the patient awake and able to cooperate. After completing the hemodynamic measurements, the patient can be given 25 mcg Fentanyl i.v. to improve comfort and analgesia before proceeding to the liver biopsy [9].

Hepatic vein catheterization. The main right hepatic vein is the preferred vein for the hemodynamic measurements, as it is easy to enter and large. It is accessed under fluoroscopy, which is usually quite simple. Care should be taken not to make loops in the right atrium to enter the right ventricle, as this make cause arrhythmias. Usually these are limited to a few ectopic beats, but a severe and potentially lethal arrhythmia can be precipitated. If necessary, a guide wire is advanced first to the IVC, and then a multipurpose catheter advanced in the hepatic vein; the multipurpose catheter is substituted afterwards by the balloon catheter over the wire. Once in the hepatic vein, correct occlusion of the hepatic vein when inflating the balloon should be first checked by the manual injection of 5–10 cc of diluted contrast media (Fig. 3.1a). At this moment, it should be noted the hepatic vein is correctly occluded by the balloon, revealing a typical 'wedged' pattern and that there is no reflux of contrast around the balloon or washout through communications with other hepatic veins (Fig. 3.1b). If either is observed, the balloon catheter should be repositioned deeper in the hepatic vein and the contrast injection repeated after inflating the balloon to check if the problem has been overcome. If washout trough other hepatic veins trough small hepatic vein communications are detected this should be carefully noted, as its presence may point to the existence of portal-sinusoidal disease (previously known as "idiopathic" or "non-cirrhotic intrahepatic" portal hypertension) rather than cirrhosis as the underlying disease causing portal hypertension.

3.2.4   Pressure Measurements: Specifications for a Correct Measurement and Frequent Mistakes

The technique to obtain HVPG values is relatively straightforward; however, achieving accurate measurements requires specialist training, as the procedure differs from those used in heart catheterization laboratories, interventional radiology rooms and intensive care units. Hemodynamic measurements shall be obtained in specific conditions. These include paying attention to all the following:

(a) Time of the day: better during morning hours, as portal pressure follows a circadian rhythm, decreasing during afternoon and evening and rising over the night. In case measurements are done pm, take a note on the history as to plan next measurement at approximately the same time.

(b) <u>Fasting</u>: patients shall be fasting for at least 6 h. Even a small meal causes a postprandial hyperemia that does not modify portal pressure in normal subjects, but that cause a marked increase in portal pressure (HVPG) when there is portal hypertension due to increased resistance and endothelial dysfunction that makes the hepatic circulation unable to dilate in response to an increased blood flow.

(c) <u>Setting the recorder</u>: Hepatic venous pressures range between 0 and 50 mmHg; most commonly between zero and 30 mmHg. So the *full scale* in the recorder should be set for that range of pressures (Fig. 3.2a). 1 mmHg should ideally be mirrored by a 1 mm scale. The recorder and pressure transducer should be checked using *calibration steps* against known pressures before its use to detect any malfunctioning. The *zero level* should be checked paying attention to both the position of the transducer (that should be fixed at the mid-axillary line with

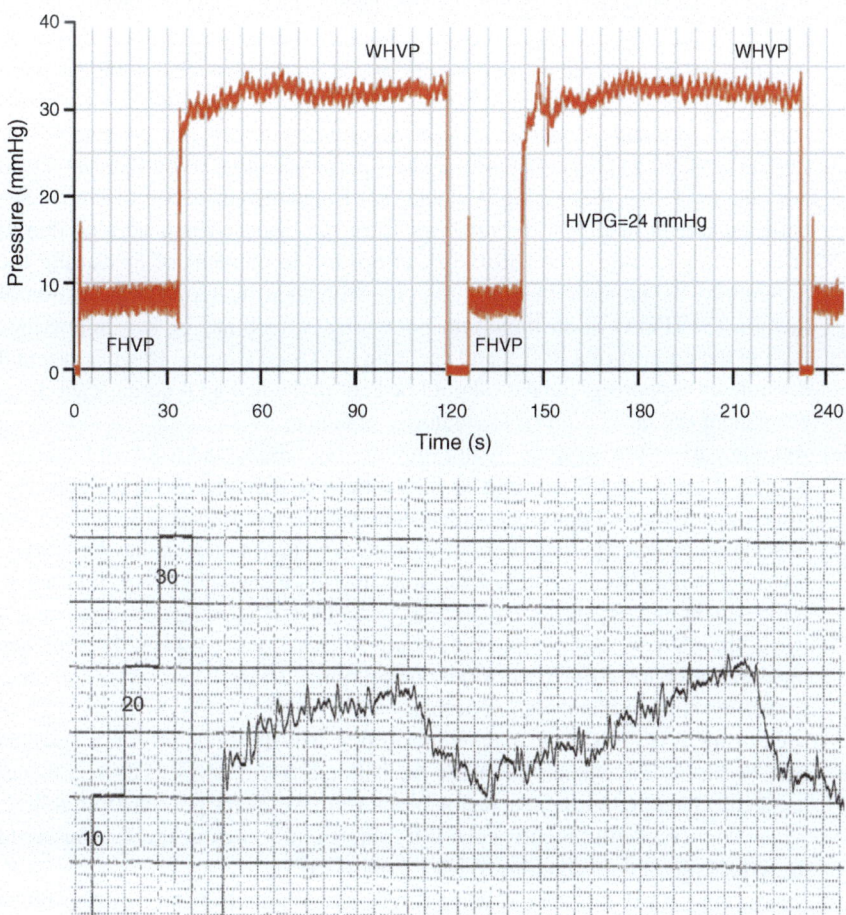

Fig. 3.2 HVPG Tracings. (Panel **a**) Correct HVPG Tracing. Note that the scale is set at 40 mmHg, and that the 0 value is correctly recorded. (Panel **b**) Incorrect measurement of the WHVP: notice the marked fluctuation due to deep breathing. This is most commonly due to excessive sedation

the patient lying supine) and at the recording, that should read 0 when transducer is open to air (atmospheric pressure). *Recorder speed* should be set to "low" speeds, of about 1–7 mm/s (not at the 25/50 mm/s used for EKG or cardiac hemodynamic measurements, the reason for it being the long time required for stabilization of the WHVP after inflating the balloon, frequently of over 1 min. At high speed this takes 3 m of recording for a single measurement!). *Oscillating and filtered ("mean") pressures*: some equipment allow printing both the oscillating pressure (that shows fine fluctuations of the tracing due to the heart cycle and respiration) and an electronically averaged or filtered pressure (mean pressure). If this is the case print both. The oscillating will show you very easily if there are artifacts, while the filtered or "mean" pressure—if stable—facilitates the reading of the exact pressure. Some electronic equipment allows post-processing an automatically derive the mean pressure from the oscillating tracing.

(d) Screen measurements vs. measurements from printed tracings. Most pressure measurement systems show pressure tracings on the screen, together with instant point measurements. This is very useful for the physician doing the measurement to observe if the morphology of the tracing is adequate and if stabilizes appropriately. However, screen measurements are not acceptable for several reasons: (1) they represent a short period of time, so by themselves do not guarantee that the tracing is stable; (2) frequently there are discrepancies between screen readings and readings from print-outs, which may be due to errors in appreciating the zero level, errors in the moment of measuring the pressure by the monitor, that may coincide with an artifact, or a combination of factors; (3) HVPG is an important parameter, sometimes of key importance (i.e., in the context of a RCT), and according to Good Clinical Practice original documents supporting the data should be kept in the patient records. Therefore, permanent tracing should be mandatorily obtained.

(e) Ask the patient to cooperate by not moving, not talking and ask him breathing quietly. If the patient is sleeping he should be waked up and asked to cooperate. This is due to the fact that sleeping (especially if the patient is in a deep sleep due to sedation or if the patient is snoring) makes the pressure cycle having marked pressure oscillations that preclude accurate measurements (Fig. 3.2b). Take a note if the patient moves, speaks, coughs, etc. as to discard a tracing with artefacts.

(f) Rinse the catheter with saline before any measurement, especially after any injection of contrast dye (that should be minimized before hemodynamic measurements since it increases pressures).

(g) Measuring WHVP: Check under fluoroscopy that the catheter is not "pushed out" by blood flow when you inflate the balloon. If this happens correct placement and check for correct occlusion of the vein. Allow the pressure to stabilize, which very frequently requires one full minute and sometimes more. Failure to do so leads to underestimating WHVP (and HVPG).

(h) Measuring FHVP: this should be paid special attention as most mistakes relate to incorrect measurements of FHVP due to having the catheter to much introduced in the hepatic vein. The FHVP should be measured close to the junction of the hepatic vein and inferior vena cava (IVC). It is paramount to have the

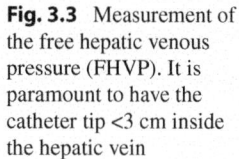

Fig. 3.3 Measurement of
the free hepatic venous
pressure (FHVP). It is
paramount to have the
catheter tip <3 cm inside
the hepatic vein

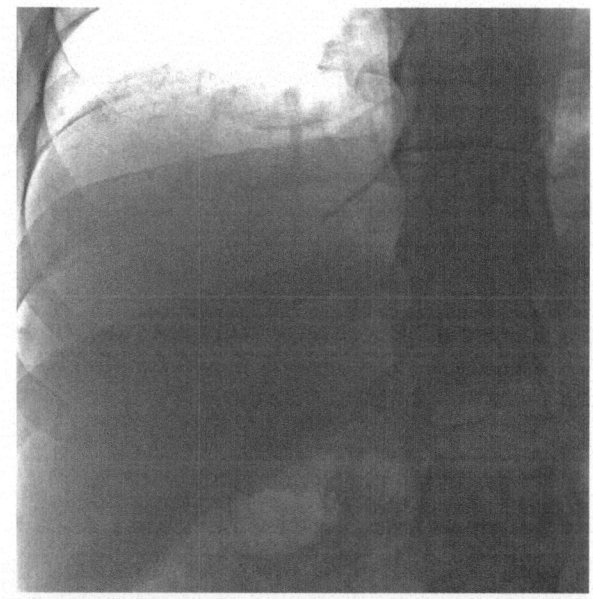

catheter tip <3 cm inside the hepatic vein when measuring FHVP (Fig. 3.3). This is due to the fact that in cirrhosis the hepatic veins are frequently irregular due to liver nodularity and this causes the FHVP to be falsely higher when measured well inside the hepatic veins, leading to underestimate the HVPG. Very commonly the site appropriate for measuring the WHVP is too far into the hepatic vein for an adequate measurement of the FHVP. Care should be paid in these cases at repeating the free pressure measurement at a "withdrawn" position, close to the IVC. This is especially important in patients with ascites or obese.

(i) <u>Measure IVC pressure and right atrial pressure (RAP)</u>: These should be measured to get more information on the hemodynamic condition of the patient (i.e., high pressures point towards fluid overload or heart failure) and as internal checks: the IVC pressure at the level of hepatic veins should not differ over 2 mmHg from the FHVP, and should be 0.5–2 mmHg greater than RAP. If this is not so, probably something is wrong: check that the position of the transducer relative to patient has not changed, repeat measurements to discard poor positioning of the catheter tip during IVC measurements, since the hepatic veins drain frequently in the thoracic IVC, which is very short, making that the catheter can slip into the right atrium—leading to a falsely low IVC pressure- or to the abdominal IVC—leading to a falsely high IVC pressure.

It should be kept in mind that all studies in portal hypertension from which the HVPG has been shown to bear a close correlation with clinical events and prognosis have calculated the HVPG as the difference between WHVP and FHVP. Several studies have shown that using the RAP to calculate the HVPG leads to an overestimation and results in loss of prognostic information [10], so this should not be done.

3.2.5 Limitations

HVPG does not reflect the PPG in diseases where the increased resistance is located at presinusoidal sites, such as portal vein thrombosis or liver diseases affecting predominantly the portal tracts, such as schistosomiasis, initial stages of primary biliary cirrhosis, or porto-sinusoidal disease (previously termed "idiopathic portal hypertension"). In these cases, a direct measurement of portal pressure could be indicated if clinical consequences are expected.

3.2.6 Associated Procedures

In addition to pressure measurements, hepatic vein catheterization allows for the performance of a wedged hepatic retrograde portography using CO_2 as a contrast agent (Fig. 3.4). This will demonstrate the portal vein in most instances. In fact, inability to demonstrate the portal vein on CO_2 retrograde portography strongly suggests the presence of presinusoidal portal hypertension. Hepatic vein catheterization also allows for the performance of a transjugular liver biopsy, which adds very little time, discomfort, and risk to the procedure and can be done on a day-hospital basis. TJLB obtained with Tru-Cut needles allow obtaining large samples fully adequate for histological examination. Furthermore, at hepatic vein catheterization it is also possible to measure the hepatic blood flow using indocyanine green (ICG) as the indicator, as well as the intrinsic clearance of ICG, a quantitative liver function test that assesses the overall hepatic metabolic activity.

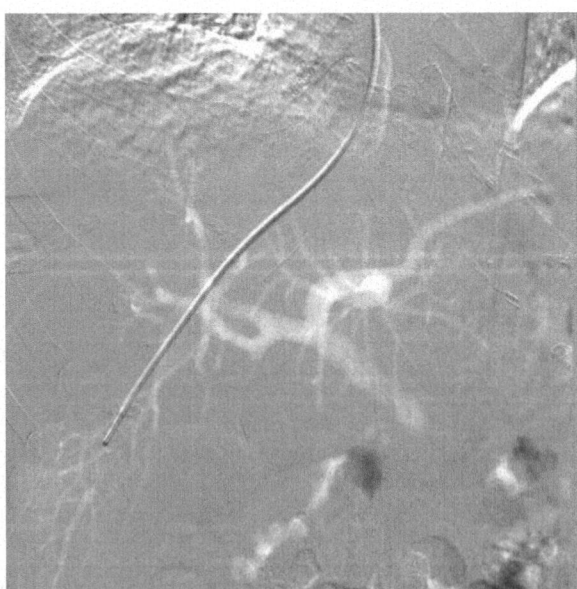

Fig. 3.4 Wedged retrograde portography using CO_2 as contrast agent. The intrahepatic portal vein and the portal vein trunk are clearly visualized

3.2.7   Contraindications

There is no absolute contraindication to hepatic vein catheterisation and HVPG measurement. In case of known allergy to iodinated contrast dye CO_2 can be used as an alternative contrast, or an appropriate pre-medication can be implemented. It should be stressed that jugular vein puncture can be safely conducted in patients with moderate coagulation disorders, which are very common in patients with portal hypertension, and the procedure does not usually require replacement therapy. Platelet or fresh frozen plasma replacement can be considered in patients with proven severe coagulation disorders (e.g. thrombocytopenia $<20 \times 10^9$/L, INR >2.5 or clear spontaneous bleeding tendency).

3.2.8   Tolerability, Radiation Exposure and Complications

HVPG measurement is usually very well tolerated [9]; similar to any other invasive procedure experienced operators achieve maximal patients' comfort. Radiation exposure is low on average, and is comparable to that of a standard thorax radiograph [11]. Care should be paid to limit fluoroscopy time to the minimum in obese patients, since they are more prone to accumulate high radiation doses [11].

Complications occur in less than 1% of patients and major complications are very rare [11]. They include: (a) local injury at the venous access site (hematoma, arteriovenous fistulae, Horner's syndrome, transient brachial paralysis and pneumothorax), and (b) cardiac arrhythmias caused by the contact of the catheters with the right atrium walls. A recent meta-analysis confirmed that first group of complications are notably reduced by using ultrasound-guided puncture instead of anatomical landmark access technique [7]. Arrhythmias are usually transient or easily corrected. In the authors' experience, placing a long guidewire into the inferior vena cava immediately after the venous access has been obtained is usually easy and allows avoiding potentially pro-arrhythmic manoeuvres in the heart, since the catheter is later safely moved onto the guidewire.

No death has been reported due to complications related to HVPG alone. On the other hand, casualties are described after TJLB in 0.09% of cases due to intraperitoneal bleeding, subcapsular hematoma or hemobilia [12].

3.3   Applications

3.3.1   Classification of Portal Hypertension

In patients with newly diagnosed portal hypertension of unclear origin, HVPG provide data useful for locating the site of increased resistance where PH takes onset. According to the HVPG measurement findings, portal hypertension is classified as pre-sinusoidal (normal or minimally increased WHVP and FHVP, with a normal or slightly increased HVPG), sinusoidal (increased WHVP and normal FHVP, leading to increased HVPG) and post-sinusoidal (increased WHVP and FHVP with normal or slightly increased HVPG). The finding of intrahepatic veno-venous collaterals vessels is frequently observed in vascular liver diseases (e.g. idiopathic portal hypertension) and is an important cause of WHVP underestimation, and as such it should be always reported. In patients with long-lasting known chronic liver disease a HVPG over 6 mmHg strongly suggests cirrhosis. HVPG between 6 and 9 mmHg indicate subclinical sinusoidal portal hypertension, while values equal or above 10 mmHg indicate clinically significant portal hypertension (CSPH, see below).

3.3.2   Correlation with Degree of Fibrosis and Other Histological Parameters

Given that it is a quantitative parameter reflecting portal pressure in a large part of the liver, and that portal pressure is largely dependent from fibrosis-induced increases in hepatic resistance, it has been suggested that HVPG could be a better method for staging chronic hepatitis. HVPG correlates with the severity of liver fibrosis in patients with HCV-related CLD [13, 14] and in patients with cirrhosis of any etiology [15–17], and in the setting of recurrent HCV hepatitis after liver transplantation, HVPG ($\geq$6 mmHg) had a higher accuracy than liver biopsy is identifying patients at risk of developing decompensated cirrhosis [14].

Furthermore, it has been shown that HVPG decreases in patients with hepatitis C who attain a sustained virologic response [18, 19]. Given these observation, it can be postulated that HVPG is a valid indicator of patients remaining at risk of complications after antiviral therapy for hepatitis C [20]. In patients with alcoholic hepatitis very high values of HVPG are usually observed, suggesting that inflammation and hepatocyte ballooning contribute to further increase portal pressure in this setting.

3.3.3   Risk Stratification in Advanced Chronic Liver Disease

Compensated ACLD. HVPG is the single most accurate prognostic marker in patients with advanced chronic liver disease and has been extensively validated [21]. Patients with HVPG <10 mmHg have a negligible risk of developing the complications typical of cirrhosis, while above this threshold (CSPH) all the complications of the disease can appear, including development of varices [22] and of clinical decompensation [23]. Patients also show an increased risk of developing hepatocellular carcinoma [24]. In compensated patients with normal bilirubin levels and single hepatocellular carcinoma undergoing surgical resection, the presence of CSPH prior to surgery is an independent and strong risk factor for postoperative liver failure/clinical decompensation [25], and is associated with a higher risk of 3- and 5-year mortality [26]. Therefore, in patients with compensated ACLD without overt clinical signs of portal hypertension and potentially resectable hepatocellular carcinoma, HVPG measurement is required to select the best treatment option [27].

A HVPG $\geq$12 mmHg is needed for variceal bleeding to develop [28, 29]. Markedly higher values, i.e. HVPG $\geq$16 mmHg were associated with an increased risk of death in some studies [30–32].

Decompensated cirrhosis. In patients bleeding from varices a HVPG $\geq$20 mmHg measured within 48 h of admission was strongly associated with failure to control bleeding/early rebleeding, transfusion requirement, intensive care unit sty and mortality on follow-up [33], providing a rationale for the use of early TIPS in this population [34, 35].

In decompensated patients awaiting liver transplantation HVPG maintains an independent prognostic value with respect to MELD score [36]. In patients with severe alcoholic hepatitis a HVPG over 22 mmHg is associated with a higher risk of death [37].

3.3.4 Repeated Measurements of HVPG

Several studies and meta-analysis confirmed that a sufficient HVPG reduction, either spontaneous (i.e. in patients achieving abstinence from alcohol) or induced by pharmacological or interventional therapies, can prevent the first appearance and the recurrence of complications of portal hypertension in patients with cirrhosis [2]. This does not hold true only for variceal bleeding, but also for other complications such as ascites and spontaneous bacterial peritonitis. Clinical-hemodynamic studies clarified that a HVPG decrease below 12 mmHg is associated with a complete protection from variceal bleeding [38, 39]; in patients not achieving this ideal threshold, a decrease of at least 20% vs. pre-treatment value markedly decreases the risk of bleeding [38, 40] and the risk of other complications [41, 42], and improves survival [40]. Therefore, patients achieving these hemodynamic targets are termed "responders". On the other hand, the lack of hemodynamic response is associated with higher risk of variceal bleeding or rebleeding [40].

To ascertain whether HVPG is sufficiently decreased on pharmacological therapy (e.g. with non-selective beta-blockers), two measurements were typically needed (one before starting treatment and one on treatment). Two different studies proposed a simplified testing, based on the administration of i.v. propranolol during the baseline assessment and the measurement of the HVPG change to this acute challenge [43, 44]. On this acute i.v. propranolol test a 10% decrease in HVPG is associated with good outcomes in the follow-up, and defines acute HVPG responders [43, 44].

References

1. Tsochatzis EA, Bosch J, Burroughs AK. Liver cirrhosis. Lancet. 2014;383:1749–61.
2. Garcia-Tsao G, Abraldes JG, Berzigotti A, Bosch J. Portal hypertensive bleeding in cirrhosis: risk stratification, diagnosis, and management: 2016 practice guidance by the American Association for the study of liver diseases. Hepatology. 2017;65:310–35.
3. Bosch J, Abraldes JG, Berzigotti A, Garcia-Pagan JC. The clinical use of HVPG measurements in chronic liver disease. Nat Rev Gastroenterol Hepatol. 2009;6:573–82.

4. Groszmann RJ, Glickman M, Blei AT, Storer E, Conn HO. Wedged and free hepatic venous pressure measured with a balloon catheter. Gastroenterology. 1979;76:253–8.
5. Groszmann RJ, Wongcharatrawee S. The hepatic venous pressure gradient: anything worth doing should be done right. Hepatology. 2004;39:280–2.
6. Zipprich A, Winkler M, Seufferlein T, Dollinger MM. Comparison of balloon vs. straight catheter for the measurement of portal hypertension. Aliment Pharmacol Ther. 2010;32:1351–6.
7. Brass P, Hellmich M, Kolodziej L, Schick G, Smith AF. Ultrasound guidance versus anatomical landmarks for internal jugular vein catheterization. Cochrane Database Syst Rev. 2015;1:CD006962.
8. Steinlauf AF, Garcia-Tsao G, Zakko MF, Dickey K, Gupta T, Groszmann RJ. Low-dose midazolam sedation: an option for patients undergoing serial hepatic venous pressure measurements. Hepatology. 1999;29:1070–3.
9. Casu S, Berzigotti A, Abraldes JG, Baringo MA, Rocabert L, Hernandez-Gea V, Garcia-Pagan JC, et al. A prospective observational study on tolerance and satisfaction to hepatic haemodynamic procedures. Liver Int. 2015;35:695–703.
10. La Mura V, Abraldes JG, Berzigotti A, Erice E, Flores-Arroyo A, Garcia-Pagan JC, Bosch J. Right atrial pressure is not adequate to calculate portal pressure gradient in cirrhosis: a clinical-hemodynamic correlation study. Hepatology. 2010;51:2108–16.
11. Hari A, Nair HK, De Gottardi A, Baumgartner I, Dufour JF, Berzigotti A. Diagnostic hepatic haemodynamic techniques: safety and radiation exposure. Liver Int. 2017;37:148–54.
12. Kalambokis G, Manousou P, Vibhakorn S, Marelli L, Cholongitas E, Senzolo M, Patch D, et al. Transjugular liver biopsy—indications, adequacy, quality of specimens, and complications—a systematic review. J Hepatol. 2007;47:284–94.
13. Carrion JA, Navasa M, Bosch J, Bruguera M, Gilabert R, Forns X. Transient elastography for diagnosis of advanced fibrosis and portal hypertension in patients with hepatitis C recurrence after liver transplantation. Liver Transpl. 2006;12:1791–8.
14. Blasco A, Forns X, Carrion JA, Garcia-Pagan JC, Gilabert R, Rimola A, Miquel R, et al. Hepatic venous pressure gradient identifies patients at risk of severe hepatitis C recurrence after liver transplantation. Hepatology. 2006;43:492–9.
15. Nagula S, Jain D, Groszmann RJ, Garcia-Tsao G. Histological-hemodynamic correlation in cirrhosis a histological classification of the severity of cirrhosis. J Hepatol. 2006,44.111–7.
16. Sethasine S, Jain D, Groszmann RJ, Garcia-Tsao G. Quantitative histological-hemodynamic correlations in cirrhosis. Hepatology. 2012;55:1146–53.
17. Krogsgaard K, Christensen E, Gluud C, Henriksen JH, Christoffersen P. Variables predicting elevated portal pressure in alcoholic liver disease. Results of a multivariate analysis. Scand J Gastroenterol. 1987;22:82–6.
18. Rincon D, Ripoll C, Lo Iacono O, Salcedo M, Catalina MV, Alvarez E, Nunez O, et al. Antiviral therapy decreases hepatic venous pressure gradient in patients with chronic hepatitis C and advanced fibrosis. Am J Gastroenterol. 2006;101:2269–74.
19. Roberts S, Gordon A, McLean C, Pedersen J, Bowden S, Thomson K, Angus P. Effect of sustained viral response on hepatic venous pressure gradient in hepatitis C-related cirrhosis. Clin Gastroenterol Hepatol. 2007;5:932–7.
20. Burroughs AK, Groszmann R, Bosch J, Grace N, Garcia-Tsao G, Patch D, Garcia-Pagan JC, et al. Assessment of therapeutic benefit of antiviral therapy in chronic hepatitis C: is hepatic venous pressure gradient a better end point? Gut. 2002;50:425–7.
21. Gluud C, Brok J, Gong Y, Koretz RL. Hepatology may have problems with putative surrogate outcome measures. J Hepatol. 2007;46:734–42.
22. Groszmann RJ, Garcia-Tsao G, Bosch J, Grace ND, Burroughs AK, Planas R, Escorsell A, et al. Beta-blockers to prevent gastroesophageal varices in patients with cirrhosis. N Engl J Med. 2005;353:2254–61.
23. Ripoll C, Groszmann R, Garcia-Tsao G, Grace N, Burroughs A, Planas R, Escorsell A, et al. Hepatic venous pressure gradient predicts clinical decompensation in patients with compensated cirrhosis. Gastroenterology. 2007;133:481–8.

24. Ripoll C, Groszmann RJ, Garcia-Tsao G, Bosch J, Grace N, Burroughs A, Planas R, et al. Hepatic venous pressure gradient predicts development of hepatocellular carcinoma independently of severity of cirrhosis. J Hepatol. 2009;50:923–8.
25. Bruix J, Castells A, Bosch J, Feu F, Fuster J, Garcia-Pagan JC, Visa J, et al. Surgical resection of hepatocellular carcinoma in cirrhotic patients: prognostic value of preoperative portal pressure. Gastroenterology. 1996;111:1018–22.
26. Berzigotti A, Reig M, Abraldes JG, Bosch J, Bruix J. Portal hypertension and the outcome of surgery for hepatocellular carcinoma in compensated cirrhosis: a systematic review and meta-analysis. Hepatology. 2015;61:526–36.
27. Bruix J, Reig M, Sherman M. Evidence-based diagnosis, staging, and treatment of patients with hepatocellular carcinoma. Gastroenterology. 2016;150:835–53.
28. Garcia-Tsao G, Groszmann RJ, Fisher RL, Conn HO, Atterbury CE, Glickman M. Portal pressure, presence of gastroesophageal varices and variceal bleeding. Hepatology. 1985;5:419–24.
29. Casado M, Bosch J, Garcia-Pagan JC, Bru C, Banares R, Bandi JC, Escorsell A, et al. Clinical events after transjugular intrahepatic portosystemic shunt: correlation with hemodynamic findings. Gastroenterology. 1998;114:1296–303.
30. Merkel C, Bolognesi M, Bellon S, Zuin R, Noventa F, Finucci G, Sacerdoti D, et al. Prognostic usefulness of hepatic vein catheterization in patients with cirrhosis and esophageal varices. Gastroenterology. 1992;102:973–9.
31. Berzigotti A, Rossi V, Tiani C, Pierpaoli L, Zappoli P, Riili A, Serra C, et al. Prognostic value of a single HVPG measurement and Doppler-ultrasound evaluation in patients with cirrhosis and portal hypertension. J Gastroenterol. 2011;46:687–95.
32. Stanley AJ, Robinson I, Forrest EH, Jones AL, Hayes PC. Haemodynamic parameters predicting variceal haemorrhage and survival in alcoholic cirrhosis. QJM. 1998;91:19–25.
33. Moitinho E, Escorsell A, Bandi JC, Salmeron JM, Garcia-Pagan JC, Rodes J, Bosch J. Prognostic value of early measurements of portal pressure in acute variceal bleeding. Gastroenterology. 1999;117:626–31.
34. Garcia-Pagan JC, Caca K, Bureau C, Laleman W, Appenrodt B, Luca A, Abraldes JG, et al. Early use of TIPS in patients with cirrhosis and variceal bleeding. N Engl J Med. 2010;362:2370–9.
35. Monescillo A, Martinez-Lagares F, Ruiz-del-Arbol L, Sierra A, Guevara C, Jimenez E, Marrero JM, et al. Influence of portal hypertension and its early decompression by TIPS placement on the outcome of variceal bleeding. Hepatology. 2004;40:793–801.
36. Ripoll C, Banares R, Rincon D, Catalina MV, Lo Iacono O, Salcedo M, Clemente G, et al. Influence of hepatic venous pressure gradient on the prediction of survival of patients with cirrhosis in the MELD era. Hepatology. 2005;42:793–801.
37. Rincon D, Lo Iacono O, Ripoll C, Gomez-Camarero J, Salcedo M, Catalina MV, Hernando A, et al. Prognostic value of hepatic venous pressure gradient for in-hospital mortality of patients with severe acute alcoholic hepatitis. Aliment Pharmacol Ther. 2007;25:841–8.
38. Feu F, Garcia-Pagan JC, Bosch J, Luca A, Teres J, Escorsell A, Rodes J. Relation between portal pressure response to pharmacotherapy and risk of recurrent variceal haemorrhage in patients with cirrhosis. Lancet. 1995;346:1056–9.
39. Vorobioff J, Groszmann RJ, Picabea E, Gamen M, Villavicencio R, Bordato J, Morel I, et al. Prognostic value of hepatic venous pressure gradient measurements in alcoholic cirrhosis: a 10-year prospective study. Gastroenterology. 1996;111:701–9.
40. D'Amico G, Garcia-Pagan JC, Luca A, Bosch J. Hepatic vein pressure gradient reduction and prevention of variceal bleeding in cirrhosis: a systematic review. Gastroenterology. 2006;131:1611–24.
41. Abraldes JG, Tarantino I, Turnes J, Garcia-Pagan JC, Rodes J, Bosch J. Hemodynamic response to pharmacological treatment of portal hypertension and long-term prognosis of cirrhosis. Hepatology. 2003;37:902–8.
42. Turnes J, Garcia-Pagan JC, Abraldes JG, Hernandez-Guerra M, Dell'Era A, Bosch J. Pharmacological reduction of portal pressure and long-term risk of first variceal bleeding in patients with cirrhosis. Am J Gastroenterol. 2006;101:506–12.

43. La Mura V, Abraldes JG, Raffa S, Retto O, Berzigotti A, Garcia-Pagan JC, Bosch J. Prognostic value of acute hemodynamic response to i.v. propranolol in patients with cirrhosis and portal hypertension. J Hepatol. 2009;51:279–87.
44. Villanueva C, Aracil C, Colomo A, Hernandez-Gea V, Lopez-Balaguer JM, Alvarez-Urturi C, Torras X, et al. Acute hemodynamic response to beta-blockers and prediction of long-term outcome in primary prophylaxis of variceal bleeding. Gastroenterology. 2009;137:119–28.

Endoscopy

4

Alessandra Dell'Era and Roberto de Franchis

4.1 Introduction

Bleeding from portal-hypertension related sources is one of the most severe complications of liver cirrhosis, and still carries a 6-week mortality of 10% or higher. Over the last 50 years, gastrointestinal endoscopy has increasingly been used both to diagnose and to treat bleeding from ruptured esophageal and gastric varices. In addition, endoscopic classifications of portal hypertension related lesions have been developed to help stratifying the bleeding risk of patients. In this chapter, the endoscopic methods used to diagnose these lesions will be described, and the results of studies aimed at stratifying patients into risk classes for bleeding will be analyzed.

4.2 Endoscopy—Technique

4.2.1 Esophago-Gastro-Duodenoscopy

Upper gastrointestinal (GI) endoscopy is the gold standard for the diagnosis of portal hypertension-related lesions, [namely esophageal varices (EV), gastric varices (GV), portal hypertensive gastropathy (PHG)], of gastric vascular ectasia (GVE) and for the visualization of red color signs on varices.

Esophago-gastro-duodenoscopy (EGD) may be performed under light sedation, if the conditions of the patient allow for it (e.g. portosystemic encephalopathy is a relative contraindication). It must include the careful examination of the entire upper GI tract (oropharyngeal region, esophagus, stomach and duodenum).

A. Dell'Era, M.D., Ph.D. • R. de Franchis, M.D. (✉)
University of Milan, Milan, Italy
e-mail: roberto.defranchis@unimi.it

In order to standardize the procedure, reduce the errors (i.e. misinterpret esophageal folds as varices and vice versa) and interobserver variability in the diagnosis and classification of **esophageal varices**, some rules must be followed:

– the evaluation must be done at the end of the upper GI endoscopy, during the withdrawal of the endoscope, and after removing as much air as possible from the stomach. This is important as the presence of air in the stomach may reduce the blood flow from the stomach to the esophagus and thus reduce variceal size.
– the esophagus must be distended with air as much as possible before assessing the size of the varices. This maneuver flattens the esophageal folds reducing the risk of misinterpretation. Other criteria to differentiate esophageal folds from varices are the color (white or pink for esophageal folds, more often bluish for esophageal varices), and the shape (linear in the first case, and often tortuous in the second). Varices should be classified according to the esophageal lumen occupancy [1] into grade 1 (small varices that occupy less than 1/3 of the lumen), grade 2 (medium varices occupying 1/3 to 2/3 of the lumen) and grade 3 (large varices occupying more than 2/3 of the lumen) (Fig. 4.1).
– in describing esophageal varices the following features must be recorded [2]:
    location of the varices in the esophagus (more commonly in the middle and distal esophagus, but sometimes with extension to the cervical esophagus).
    number of variceal trunks.
    color (blue or white).
    size of esophageal varices (see above).

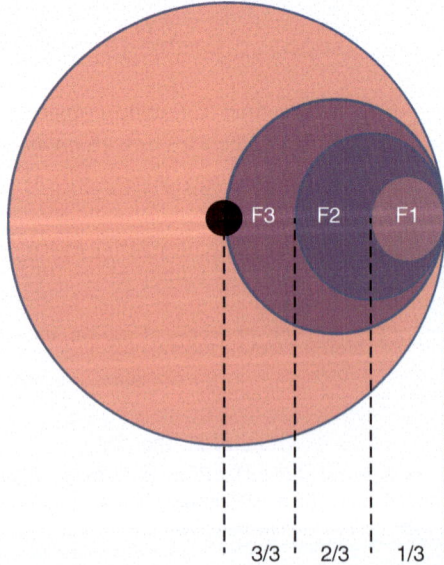

Fig. 4.1 Size of varices as classified by the Italian Liver Cirrhosis Project (Ref. 1) Modified from de Franchis R and Dell'Era A Eds. Variceal Hemorrhage; Springer, New York 2014, p 49

presence of red color signs. Four types of red color signs have been described and classified: *red wale markings* (red streaks on the variceal surface which represent dilated venules overlying the variceal wall), *cherry red spots* (small circular dots less than 2 mm diameter), *hematocystic spots* (single, large, raised red lesion similar to a blister full of blood) and *diffuse redness* (red area over one or more varices).

A validated classification must be used. The most used classifications are that of the Japanese Research Society for Portal Hypertension [2] and that of the Italian Liver Cirrhosis Project Classification (ILCP) [1].

Besides identifying and classifying esophageal varices, EGDS also allows the identification of other portal hypertension related lesions in the stomach and the duodenum. **Gastric varices** must be sought for by performing careful visualization of the stomach at full distension, taking care to visualize also the fundic and cardial region by the retroversion maneuver. The location, the size and the presence of red color signs on gastric varices must be evaluated and recorded, since all these signs have an impact on the bleeding risk [3, 4]. The location of gastric varices and their association with EV has a meaning for their correlation to the bleeding risk and for the choice of treatment in case of bleeding [3] (see below). A careful examination of the duodenum must also be performed to identify **ectopic varices**.

EGD may also identify **portal hypertensive gastropathy** (PHG), gastric (antral) vascular ectasia [G(A)VE] and portal hypertensive enteropathy of the duodenum. Several classifications of PHG exist [5–7] but the one of the North Italian Endoscopic Club (NIEC) was validated [8]. According to the NIEC classification elementary lesions of PHG consist in:

- mosaic-like pattern: small, polygonal areas surrounded by a whitish-yellow, depressed border. When the areola is uniformly pink the pattern is defined mild, moderate when the center is red, and severe if the areola is uniformly red.
- red-point lesions: defined as small, flat, 1-mm-wide, punctate, red lesions.
- cherry-red spots: red, 2-mm-wide, round lesions which protrude slightly into the gastric lumen.
- black-brown spots defined as irregularly shaped flat black or brown spots from intramucosal hemorrhage that remain after endoscopic irrigation.

PHG is defined as mild when only a mosaic-like pattern is present, and severe when red-point lesions, cherry red spots, or black-brown spots are present.

GAVE is a completely different entity, which can be found both in cirrhosis and in other diseases such as scleroderma, and should be differentiated from PHG. In fact, GAVE must be treated differently from PHG, since, contrary to the latter, it does not respond to a reduction of portal hypertension [9]. GAVE is characterized by red patches or spots in either a diffuse or linear array in the antrum of the stomach (because of this appearance, it is commonly referred to as "watermelon stomach") [10].

4.2.2 Videocapsule Endoscopy

Videocapsule endoscopy (VCE) is a less invasive method compared to upper GI endoscopy. A dedicated capsule, different form the one designed to study the small intestine, was developed to visualize the esophageal region. The largest study performed to evaluate the role of VCE in screening and surveillance of esophageal varices compared VCE with upper GI endoscopy used as the gold standard. This was a non-inferiority study and the assumption was that equivalence would be demonstrated if a difference in sensitivity between EGDS and VCE of 10% or less was found [11]. VCE had a positive predictive value of 92%, negative predictive value of 77%, LR+ 7, LR− 0.18 but the difference in sensitivity was 16% in favor of upper GI endoscopy, and did not meet the assumption for equivalence. Few studies have assessed the diagnostic accuracy of VCE in diagnosing and grading PHG, with variable results (concordance ranging between 69% [12] and 90.6% [13].

In view of the above results, it is unlikely that esophageal capsule endoscopy will be routinely used as an alternative to EGDS in the future.

4.2.3 Endoscopy and Risk of Bleeding: Esophageal Varices

It is known that the risk of bleeding is related to the size of varices [14]. It is therefore logical to use the variceal appearance at endoscopy as a criterion to identify patients at risk of bleeding. Indeed, since more than 50 years ago, even before flexible endoscopy came around, attempts have been made at classifying varices into risk classes for bleeding.

In 1966, Dagradi et al. [15] published an endoscopic classification in which varices were divided into five classes of increasing risk for bleeding, based mainly on their size. In Dagradi's study, the size of varices was estimated by comparison with the 10 mm internal diameter of the Eder-Hufford esophagoscope the Authors used (Table 4.1).

In the 1980s, further attempts at classifying esophageal varices were made: in 1980, the Japanese Research Society for Portal Hypertension [2] published a new classification, in which endoscopic features such as size, color, location and longitudinal extent of varices were considered, together with the presence of red wale markings, cherry-red spots and hematocystic spots overlying the varices and with diffuse redness and esophagitis.

This classification was used in 1981 in the first attempt at quantifying the risk of variceal hemorrhage based on the endoscopic features of varices: Beppu et al. [16] conducted a retrospective study of 172 cirrhotic patients with varices, 90 of whom had had a previous variceal bleed. The relationship of various endoscopic features of varices with previous bleeding was analyzed by discriminant analysis: previous bleeding was strongly related to size, blue color of varices, presence of cherry red spots, hematocystic spots, red wale markings on the variceal surface and esophagitis. Based on the results of the discriminant analysis, a variceal scoring system was developed to quantitatively express the predictability of bleeding (Table 4.2). The variceal score ranged between >+1.14 and <−1.14, and allowed the stratification of

Table 4.1 Dagradi's classification of esophageal varices

Grade of varices	Endoscopic features	Behavior
1	Color: blue or red Diameter: <2 mm Shape: linear or sigmoid	Appear by compression of the esophageal wall with the tip of the esophagoscope; not appreciably elevated in a relaxed esophagus
2	Color: bluish Diameter: 2–3 mm Shape: mildly tortuous or straight	Discernibly elevated above the surface of the relaxed esophagus, without compression by the tip of the instrument
3	Color: bluish Diameter: 3–4 mm Shape: straight or tortuous	Prominently elevated, isolated distribution around the wall of the esophagus; good mucosal cover
4	Color: bluish Diameter: >4 mm Shape: tortuous	Completely surround the esophageal lumen and almost meet in the mid-lumen; closely packed around the wall; may or may not have a good mucosal cover
5	Color: blue-gray with small cherry-red varices overlying them Shape: grape-like	Occlude the lumen of the esophagoscope. overlying mucosa is markedly thinned

patients into six risk classes, in which the occurrence of previous episodes of bleeding ranged from 0% to 100%.

In 1982, the endoscopic evaluation of varices was used for the first time by Paquet to select patients for a trial of prophylactic endoscopic sclerotherapy [17]. In that study, Paquet's own classification was used, which was similar to Dagradi's classification but divided varices in four risk classes instead of five.

None of the above classifications was independently validated; in addition, the reproducibility and interobserver agreement in the assessment of the individual variceal features had not been evaluated. For the Japanese classification, this gap was filled in 1987 by the Italian Liver Cirrhosis Project (ILCP) [1], which evaluated the reliability of endoscopy in the assessment of the individual variceal features of the classification. In the ILCP study a semi quantitative rating system was used to evaluate by kappa statistics the interobserver agreement between endoscopists in classifying the various features of varices. The agreement was fair to good for location, size (Fig. 4.2), and lumen occupancy of varices, presence of blue color, presence and extension of red color signs and hematocystic spot.

In 1988, the North Italian Endoscopic Club (NIEC) published a prospective multicenter study [18] in 321 patients with cirrhosis and varices but with no previous bleeding, in which a comprehensive analysis of the clinical features of the patients and of the endoscopic appearances of their varices was made to attempt at identifying the patients at highest risk for bleeding. Varices were classified endoscopically as suggested by the Japanese Research Society for Portal Hypertension [2]. Patients were followed for a median of 23 months, during which 85 patients (26.5%) bled. When the patients of this study were stratified into risk classes according to Beppu's variceal score, it was found that this score grossly overestimated the bleeding risk (Table 4.2).

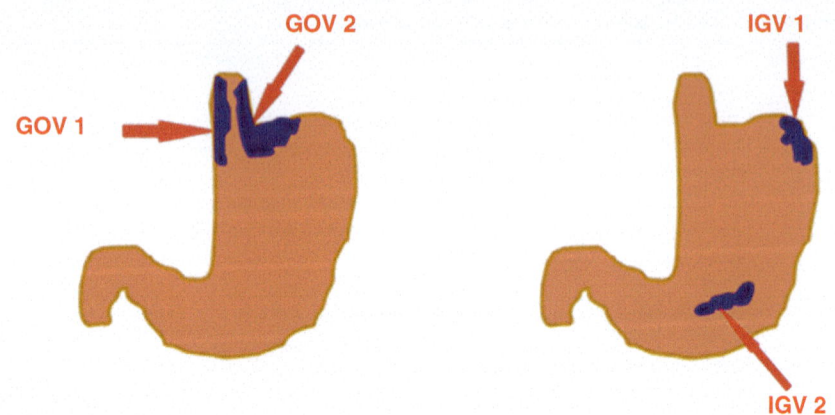

Fig. 4.2 Sarin's classification of gastric varices (Ref. 3) GOV 1: Gastro-oesophageal Varices, Type 1: GOV 2: Gastro-oesophageal Varices, Type 2: IGV: Isolated Gastric Varices, Type 1; IGV 2: Isolated Gastric Varices, Type 2

Table 4.2 Beppu's variceal score, rate of previous bleeding in Beppu's study population; n° of bleeds and 2-year rate of bleeding in the NIEC study population

Risk class	Value	Rate of previous bleeding in Beppu's study population (%)	N° who bled/total in the NIEC study population	2-year rate of bleeding in the NIEC study population (%)
1	>+1.14	0	7/61	9.2
2	0.38–1.14	20.6	35/146	22.1
3	<0.38–0.0	40.0	6/12	33.3
4	0.0 to >−0.38	64.5	13/50	29.0
5	−0.38 to >−1.14	90.1	11/25	41.0
6	<−1.14	100.0	13/23	51.7

From: N Engl J Med. NIEC Prediction of the first variceal hemorrhage in patients with cirrhosis of the liver and esophageal varices. A prospective multicenter study;319:986 Copyright © 1988 Massachusetts Medical Society. Reprinted with permission

A multiple regression analysis (Cox's model) of the NIEC study population was then carried out, identifying the Child-Pugh class, size of the varices, and presence of red wale markings on the varices as independent prognostic factors for first variceal bleeding. A prognostic index based on these variables (the NIEC index) was developed according to the formula:

$$NIEC\ Index = \left\{ \begin{array}{c} (0.6450 \times Child\ class) + (0.4365 \times Variceal\ size) \\ + (0.3193 \times Red\ wale\ markings) \end{array} \right\} \times 10$$

The NIEC Index ranges from <20 to >40 points, and can be used to stratify patients into classes of increasing bleeding risk. The index was prospectively

validated in an independent series of patients, with excellent results. A pocket
chart for calculation of the risk of bleeding in individual patients at the bedside
was developed by plotting the estimated 1 year probabilities of bleeding as a function of all the possible combinations of the three variables (Table 4.3). The table
shows that the probability of bleeding increases from 6% for Child's A patients
with small varices and no red signs, to 56% for Child's C patients with large varices and red signs. The table underscores the prognostic importance of the red
color signs; in fact, across Child's classes and variceal sizes, the presence of red
wale markings on the variceal surface nearly doubles the 1-year risk of variceal
hemorrhage.

The main limitation of the NIEC index is that, although the risk of bleeding
increases steadily from class 1 to class 6 (Table 4.4), about one fifth of the
patients who actually bled belonged to the two lowest-risk classes, and only
about 40% of the bleeds occurred in patients belonging to the two highest-risk
classes.

After the publication of the NIEC study, several other investigators addressed
the issue of predicting variceal hemorrhage by using endoscopic parameters alone
or in combination with other variables (Table 4.5). However, none of the other
prognostic scores proposed supplanted the use of the NIEC index in clinical
practice.

Table 4.3 Estimated 1-year percentage probability of bleeding as a function of all possible
combinations of the three variables of the NIEC index

Child class	A			B			C		
Size (F) of varices	F1	F2	F3	F1	F2	F3	F1	F2	F3
Red color sign									
Absent	6	10	16	10	16	24	14	25	36
Present	10	18	28	17	26	40	26	38	56

Based on data from: N Engl J Med. NIEC Prediction of the first variceal hemorrhage in patients
with cirrhosis of the liver and esophageal varices. A prospective multicenter study;319:988;
Copyright © 1988 Massachusetts Medical Society. Reprinted with permission

Table 4.4 Distribution of variceal bleeds among risk classes of the NIEC index

Risk class-risk level	NIEC index value	No who bled/total (%)	% of total bleeds
1—low	<20.0	6/73 (9.5)	22.2
2—low	20.0–25.0	12/76 (15.7)	
3—medium	25.1–30.0	14/63 (22.2)	39.6
4—medium	30.1–35.0	18/56 (32.1)	
5—high	35.1–40.0	24/48 (50.0)	38.2
6—high	>40.0	7/11 (63.6)	

From: N Engl J Med. NIEC Prediction of the first variceal hemorrhage in patients with cirrhosis of
the liver and esophageal varices. A prospective multicenter study;319:988 Copyright © 1988
Massachusetts Medical Society. Reprinted with permission

Table 4.5 Studies evaluating the role of endoscopic parameters as independent predictors of variceal hemorrhage

Author	Year	Ref. N°	Endoscopic parameters	Other parameters
Kleber et al.	1991	[19]	Gastric fundal varices, size of esophageal varices, presence of red signs on varices	Alcoholic etiology of cirrhosis
Siringo et al.	1994	[20]	Variceal size, cherry-red spots	Serum bilirubin, congestion index of the portal vein
Zoli	1996	[21]	Size of esophageal varices, gastric varices, congestive gastropathy	
Nevens	1998	[22]	NIEC score + measurement of variceal pressure by an endoscopic pressure-sensitive gauge	

4.2.4 Endoscopy and Risk of Bleeding: Gastric Varices

Gastric varices are the second most common source of portal hypertension-related bleeding in patients with cirrhosis [3]. The most widely used classification of gastric varices is the Sarin classification [3]. According to this classification, varices are categorized into four types: type 1 and 2 Gastroesophageal varices (GOV 1 and GOV 2), and type 1 and 2 isolated gastric varices (IGV 1 and IGV 2). GOV1 extend 2–5 cm below the gastroesophageal junction, in continuity with esophageal varices; GOV2 are fundal varices in continuity with esophageal varices; IGV1 occur in the fundus of the stomach in the absence of esophageal varices, whereas IGV2 occur in the gastric body, antrum, or pylorus. In Sarin's original study, gastric varices occurred in 25.9% of patients, with GOV 1, GOV 2, IGV 1 and IGV 2 accounting for 15.9%, 5.5%, 1.6% and 3.9% respectively. The propensity to bleed of the different types of gastric varices is variable, being high in fundal varices (GOV 2 and IGV 1) and low for the other two types. In 1997, Kim et al. [4] published a study aimed at identifying risk factor for bleeding from gastric fundal varices. They enrolled 117 patients with gastric fundal varices and no previous bleeds. During a median follow up of 15 months, 34 patients (29%) bled from fundal varices, with no difference between GOV 2 and IGV1 in terms of incidence of bleeding. Multivariate analysis identified the Child-Pugh class, the size of varices and the presence of red signs on varices as independent risk factors for gastric variceal bleeding. Based on the results of this analysis, Kim et al. [4] developed a prognostic index, which was used to produce a pocket chart for calculating the estimated 1 year probabilities of bleeding as a function of all the possible combinations of the three variables.

4.2.5 Endoscopy and Risk of Bleeding: Portal Hypertensive Gastropathy

In addition to esophageal and gastric varices, mucosal changes caused by portal hypertension can also cause gastrointestinal bleeding. These mucosal changes often involve the stomach (portal hypertensive gastropathy, PHG) and less frequently the small bowel (portal hypertensive enteropathy) or the colon (portal hypertensive colopathy). PHG may be the source of chronic or, more rarely, acute GI bleeding, while the incidence and clinical importance of bleeding from portal hypertensive enteropathy or colopathy are ill defined. Even for PHG there is much controversy, regarding its reported prevalence, which ranges between 7% and 98% in the different studies, as well as the rate of PHG-related acute bleeds, which range between 2.7% and 44.6%, and also the evolution of PHG after endoscopic treatment of esophageal varices. These differences, at least in part, depend on the existence of different PHG classifications (Table 4.6). All three classifications listed in Table 4.6 distinguish between a mild and a severe form of portal hypertensive gastropathy. The reproducibility of the NIEC classification of PHG was validated [8] and the classification was used in a large multicenter study of the natural history of the condition [23]. During a mean of 18 months of follow-up, gastropathy was stable in 29% of patients, deteriorated in 23%, improved in 23%, and fluctuated with time in 25%. Acute bleeding from PHG occurred in 2.5%, chronic bleeding in 12% of patients. No correlation was found between the grade of gastropathy and the risk of acute or chronic bleeding from PHG.

Table 4.6 Most used classifications of portal hypertensive gastropathy

Author, year	Ref. N°	Elementary lesions	Mild PHG	Severe PHG
McCormack et al. (1985)	[5]	1. Scarlatina type rash 2. Superficial reddening (striped appearance) 3. Fine white reticular pattern separating areas of raised edematous mucosa (snake skin) 4. Discrete red spots (analogous to cherry red spots in esophagus) 5. Diffuse hemorrhagic gastritis	Scarlatina type rash Striped appearance Snake skin	Discrete red spots Diffuse hemorrhagic gastritis
Spina et al. [NIEC] (1994)	[6]	1. Mosaic-pattern: Presence of small polygonal areas surrounded by a whitish-yellow depressed border 2. Red point lesions (1 mm in diameter, flat) 3. Cherry-red spots (2 mm, slight protrusion) 4. Black-brown spots (irregularly shaped, persistently present after washing)	Mosaic pattern	Red point lesions Cherry-red spots Black-brown spots
Sarin (1996) [Baveno II]	[7]	1. Mosaic like pattern Mild 1 p.; severe 2 p 2. Red markings Isolated 1 p; confluent 2 p 3. GAVE Absent 0 p; confluent 2 p	≤3 points	≥4 points

References

1. Italian Liver Cirrhosis Project. Reliability of endoscopy in the assessment of variceal features. J Hepatol. 1987;4:93–8.
2. Japanese Research Society for Portal Hypertension. The general rules for recording endoscopic findings on esophageal varices. Jpn J Surg. 1980;10:84–7.
3. Sarin SK, Lahoti D, Saxena SP, Murthy NS, Makwana UK. Prevalence, classification and natural history of gastric varices: a long-term follow-up study in 568 portal hypertension patients. Hepatology. 1992;16:1343–9.
4. Kim T, Shijo H, Kokawa H, Tokumitsu I, Kubara K, Ota K, et al. Risk factors for hemorrhage from gastric fundal varices. Hepatology. 1997;25:307–12.
5. McCormack TT, Sims J, Eyre-Brook I, Kennedy H, Goepel J, Johnson AJ, Triger DR. Gastric lesions in portal hypertension:inflammatory gastritis or congestive gastropathy? Gut. 1985;26:1226–32.
6. Spina GP, Arcidiacono R, Bosch J, Pagliaro L, Burroughs AK, Santambrogio R, Rossi A. Gastric endoscopic features in portal hypertension: final report of a consensus conference, Milan, Italy, September 19, 1992. J Hepatol. 1994;21:461–7.
7. Sarin SK. Diagnostic issues: portal hypertensive gastropathy and gastric varices. In: de Franchis R, editor. Portal hypertension II. Proceedings of the second Baveno international consensus workshop on definitions, methodology and therapeutic strategies. Oxford: Blackwell; 1996. p. 30–55.
8. Carpinelli L, Primignani M, Preatoni P, Angeli P, Battaglia G, Beretta L, et al. Portal hypertensive gastropathy: reproducibility of a classification, prevalence of elementary lesions, sensitivity and specificity in the diagnosis of cirrhosis of the liver. A NIEC multicentre study. New Italian Endoscopic Club. Ital J Gastroenterol Hepatol. 1997;29:533–40.
9. Kamath PS, Lacerda M, Ahlquist DA, McKusick MA, Andrews JC, Nagorney DA. Gastric mucosal responses to intrahepatic portosystemic shunting in patients with cirrhosis. Gastroenterology. 2000;118:905–11.
10. Jabbari M, Cherry R, Lough JO, et al. Gastric antral vascular ectasia: the watermelon stomach Gastroenterology. 1984;87:1165 70.
11. de Franchis R, Eisen GM, Laine L, et al. Oesophageal capsule endoscopy for screening and surveillance of oesophageal varices in patients with portal hypertension. Hepatology. 2008;47:1595–603.
12. Aoyama T, Oka S, Aikata H, Nakano M, Watari I, Naeshiro N, Yoshida S, Tanaka S, Chayama K. Is small-bowel capsule endoscopy effective for diagnosis of esophagogastric lesions related to portal hypertension? J Gastroenterol Hepatol. 2014;29:511–6.
13. Eisen GM, Eliakim R, Zaman A, Schwartz J, Faigel D, Rondonotti E, Villa F, Weizman E, Yassin K, deFranchis R. The accuracy of PillCam ESO capsule endoscopy versus conventional upper endoscopy for the diagnosis of esophageal varices: a prospective three-center pilot study. Endoscopy. 2006;38:31–5.
14. Lebrec D, De Fleury P, Rueff B, Nahum H, Benhamou JP. Portal hypertension, size of esophageal varices, and risk of gastrointestinal bleeding in alcoholic cirrhosis. Gastroenterology. 1980;79:1139–44.
15. Dagradi AE, Stempien SJ, Owens LK. Bleeding esophagogastric varices. An endoscopic study of 50 cases. Arch Surg. 1966;92:944–7.
16. Beppu K, Inokuchi K, Koyanagi N, Nakayama S, Sakata H, Kitano S, et al. Prediction of variceal haemorrhage by esophageal endoscopy. Gastrointest Endosc. 1981;27:213–8.
17. Paquet KJ. Prophylactic endoscopic sclerosing treatment of the esophageal wall in varices—a prospective controlled randomized trial. Endoscopy. 1982;14:4–5.
18. North Italian Endoscopic Club for the Study and Treatment of Esophageal Varices. Prediction of the first variceal hemorrhage in patients with cirrhosis of the liver and esophageal varices. A prospective multicenter study. N Engl J Med. 1988;319:983–9.

19. Kleber G, Sauerbruch T, Ansari H, Paumgartner G. Prediction of variceal hemorrhage in cirrhosis: a prospective follow-up study. Gastroenterology. 1991;100:1332–7.
20. Siringo S, Bolondi L, Gaiani S, Sofia S, Zironi G, Rigamonti A, et al. Timing of the first variceal hemorrhage in cirrhotic patients: prospective evaluation of Doppler flowmetry, endoscopy and clinical parameters. Hepatology. 1994;20:66–73.
21. Zoli M, Merkel C, Magalotti D, Marchesini G, Gatta A, Pisi E. Evaluation of a new endoscopic index to predict first bleeding from the upper gastrointestinal tract in patients with cirrhosis. Hepatology. 1996;24:1047–52.
22. Nevens F, Bustami R, Scheys I, Lesaffre E, Fevery J. Variceal pressure is a factor predicting the risk of a first variceal bleeding: a prospective cohort study in cirrhotic patients. Hepatology. 1998;27:15–9.
23. Primignani M, Carpinelli L, Preatoni P, Battaglia G, Carta A, Prada A, et al. Natural history of portal hypertensive gastropathy in patients with liver cirrhosis. Gastroenterology. 2000;119:181–7.

Part II

Non-Invasive Diagnostic Methods

Non-invasive Serum Markers of Fibrosis

5

Thomas Pembroke and Giada Sebastiani

5.1 Introduction

Liver fibrosis occurs when a chronic injury of any etiology leads to excessive accumulation of extracellular matrix proteins in the hepatic parenchyma. Staging of liver fibrosis and subsequent identification of patients with liver cirrhosis and portal hypertension is pivotal for the management and prognostication of chronic liver diseases of any etiology. Liver biopsy and the measurement of hepatic venous pressure gradient through transjugular catheterization of hepatic vein have long been the gold standard of reference to diagnose hepatic cirrhosis and for detection of clinically significant portal hypertension, respectively. However, due to their cost and invasiveness, recent years have seen the development and implementation of non-invasive serum biomarkers. Some serum fibrosis biomarkers present with high accuracy for diagnosis of liver cirrhosis and monitoring of its related complications. Moreover, they demonstrate prognostic value to predict clinical outcomes deriving from portal hypertension complications. Serum fibrosis biomarkers have been gradually incorporated into clinical guidelines and are progressively becoming first-line diagnostic tests for liver cirrhosis, with significant reduction in the need for liver biopsy. We here provide an update on pathophysiological rationale on the diagnostic and prognostic application of serum fibrosis biomarkers and on their accuracy in clinical scenarios related to liver cirrhosis and its complications.

T. Pembroke
Royal Victoria Hospital, McGill University Health Centre, Montreal, QC, Canada

School of Medicine, Cardiff University, Cardiff, UK

G. Sebastiani (✉)
Royal Victoria Hospital, McGill University Health Centre, Montreal, QC, Canada
e-mail: giada.sebastiani@mcgill.ca

© Springer International Publishing AG, part of Springer Nature 2018   63
A. Berzigotti, J. Bosch (eds.), *Diagnostic Methods for Cirrhosis and Portal Hypertension*, https://doi.org/10.1007/978-3-319-72628-1_5

5.2   Liver Cirrhosis: The Importance of Being Diagnosed and Staged

Chronic liver diseases are a major cause of morbidity and mortality worldwide, affecting 360 per 100,000 persons and ranking as the 12th leading cause of overall mortality [1]. The main etiologies include nonalcoholic fatty liver disease (NAFLD), chronic viral hepatitis and alcoholic liver disease (ALD). The development and accumulation of liver fibrosis is the hallmark of a progressive disease eventually leading to cirrhosis and its end-stage complications, including liver failure and hepatocellular carcinoma (HCC) [2]. Once liver cirrhosis is established, healthcare costs raise dramatically, with estimated direct costs, such as drug and hospitalization, of $2.5 billion per year, and indirect costs, including loss of work productivity and reduction in health-related quality of life, of $10.6 billion [3].

Hepatic cirrhosis represents the most advanced stage of any chronic liver disease characterized by accumulating fibrosis. The natural course of cirrhosis progressively involves an increase in portal pressure and worsening of hepatocellular function, which ultimately leads to the development of the complications defining the transition to a decompensated disease. Garcia-Tsao et al. have defined cirrhosis as a dynamic entity, better characterized as a disease spectrum rather than a single stage disease [4]. In this view, the natural history of cirrhosis involves an early asymptomatic stage or "compensated", which over time progresses to a symptomatic or "decompensated" stage, identified by the presence of clinically evident complications from portal hypertension such as ascites, spontaneous bacterial peritonitis, variceal bleeding, encephalopathy or hepatorenal syndrome. Furthermore, two distinct stages can be differentiated in the compensated phase of cirrhosis. The first stage is characterized by the absence of esophageal varices and hepatic venous portal gradient (HVPG) <10 mmHg, and is associated with a mortality of less than 1%. The second stage is characterized by the presence of varices and HVPG ≥10 mmHg, and is associated with a mortality of 3.4% per year. Not only do patients with liver cirrhosis have increased overall mortality as compared to those with earlier fibrosis stages, but the prognosis of a cirrhotic patient also depends heavily on the disease stage [5]. More specifically, a HVPG ≥10 mmHg (stage 2 cirrhosis) defines clinically significant portal hypertension and is predictive of hepatic decompensation (Fig. 5.1). End-stage liver complications mainly occur in patients with clinically significant portal hypertension [4, 6].

Early identification and staging of liver cirrhosis is pivotal for initiation of surveillance protocols for prevention of HCC and esophageal varices and specific treatment interventions for such devastating complications. Recognition of patients at risk for worse prognosis is of paramount importance for risk stratification, optimization of healthcare resources, counseling about urgent need for treatment interventions and referral for liver transplantation, when appropriate. Unfortunately, in 20–63% of cirrhotic patients, the diagnosis is only made upon first presentation of its end-stage complications, which continue to accumulate, recur more frequently and ultimately shorten life expectancy [4, 7].

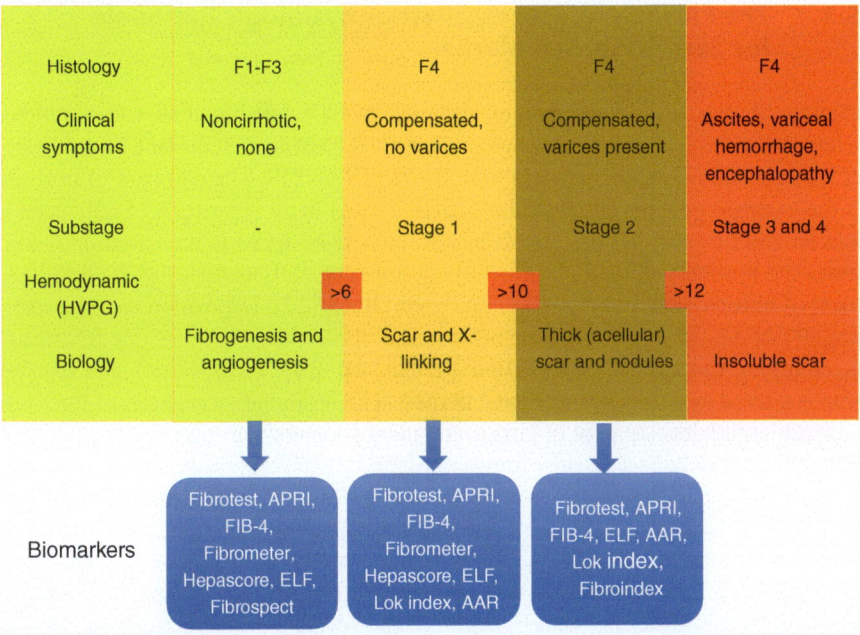

Fig. 5.1 Classification of chronic liver disease based on histological, clinical, hemodynamic, and biological parameters. Serum fibrosis biomarkers validated for each fibrosis stage are reported

Liver biopsy has long been the gold standard to diagnose liver cirrhosis. However, liver biopsy is unfeasible as serial monitoring tool for prognostication because of its invasiveness, cost, sampling error [8]. The measurement of HVPG is the gold standard for detection of clinically significant portal hypertension and for staging cirrhosis [4]. The procedure occurs through transjugular catheterization of hepatic vein; thus, it is also invasive and unfeasible as screening prognostic tool for such a prevalent disease. Finally, upper endoscopy is the gold standard to diagnose and grade esophageal varices [9]. However, a generalized screening program of periodical upper endoscopy in cirrhotic patients carries high costs and may result in low compliance since the procedure is invasive and may be poorly accepted by the patients, if repeatedly required. For these reasons, a non-invasive approach for selection of patients who may be at a higher risk of bearing esophageal varices, especially those at risk of rupture, would be highly beneficial and cost-effective.

When considering the number of people affected by liver cirrhosis globally, invasive tools like liver biopsy, measurement of HVPG and endoscopy can be viewed as a diagnostic and prognostic bottleneck for implementation of screening strategies for cirrhosis. During the past two decades, research efforts have been focused on identification and validation of serum fibrosis biomarkers capable of providing a non-invasive diagnosis of cirrhosis and prognostic assessment. We here provide an update on pathophysiological rationale and clinical application of serum fibrosis biomarkers for diagnostic and prognostic evaluation of liver cirrhosis.

5.3 The Fibrogenic Process: Pathophysiologic Rationale for Serum Fibrosis Markers

Hepatic fibrosis is a wound healing response to liver inflammation which can be related to multiple etiologies. In healthy liver, the basement membrane of the space of Disse predominantly composes of collagens IV and VI. The hallmark of fibrosis is the extension of this extracellular matrix (ECM), with deposition of collagens I and III and fibronectin [10]. In advanced fibrosis, the ECM is increased up to six times the normal volume [11]. Cirrhosis is histologically defined by the development of fibrous septa linking individual portal tracts [12]. Deposition and remodelling of fibrotic tissue is a dynamic process and fibrosis may be reversible following acute injury. In chronic inflammation, the balance of ECM deposition and regression is altered to result in progressive fibrosis. The regenerative capacity of the liver means that the development of cirrhosis typically occurs over years. It is clear that individuals may be fast or slow fibrosis progressors in response to injury and both genetic and environmental factors influence the rate of progression [11, 13]. In advanced cirrhosis, morphological changes to the liver impinges upon parenchymal perfusion resulting in focal ischaemia and progressive loss of hepatocytes. This process has been termed parenchymal extinction, and is a non-reversible phase of severe cirrhosis associated with liver failure and severe portal hypertension [14].

Hepatic stellate cells (HSC) are the key effector cells that orchestrate deposition of ECM in health and in response to inflammation. HSC reside in the subendothelial space between the hepatocytes and endothelial cells and are thus able to respond to stimuli from hepatocytes, liver sinusoidal endothelial cells and Kupffer cells, in addition to locally and systemically secreted cytokines and chemokines [15]. HSC activation can be initiated by lipid peroxidases and other products released from damaged hepatocytes through multiple pathways. The best characterised pathways include platelet derived growth factor (PDGF) signalling through the Ras-MAPK pathway and intracellular influx of calcium [16], and Akt activation by JNK phosphorylation [17]. HSC activation is associated with a shift to a myofibroblast phenotype with cellular contraction and priming for fibrogenesis [18]. HSC proliferation perpetuates the fibrogenic response to inflammatory signalling, including transforming growth factor α (TGFα) and epidermal growth factor (EGF) which are both secreted by and stimulate mitogenesis of HSCs [19, 20]. In addition, vascular endothelial growth factor (VEGF) receptors are expressed upon HSCs allowing further proliferation in response to angiogenesis [21]. Following inflammatory activation and proliferation, HSCs are primed to secrete fibril-forming collagens I and III and hyaluronan. TGFβ is the most potent fibrogenic cytokine in the liver and induces HSC transformation to myofibroblasts and ECM secretion [22, 23]. Leptin, a key adipokine, may induce fibrogenesis in NAFLD directly and through a number of pathways including TGFβ secretion by Kupffer cells [24, 25]. Activated HSCs secrete chemokines activating Kupffer cells, NK cells, T cells and macrophages and dendritic cells which in turn stimulate HSC through secretion of TNFα and other inflammatory cytokines to result in further inflammatory/fibrogenic feedback [26].

The initial toxic insult to the liver or the ensuing inflammatory response causes damage to hepatocytes. Hepatocyte damage and apoptosis induces release of the enzymes alanine transaminase, aspartate transaminase and γGT into the systemic circulation, which can be routinely measured by hospital biochemistry. Hepatic function is reduced in advanced liver damage and can most readily be measured by the ability of the liver to maintain a normal coagulation profile or production of albumin. Bilirubin is not processed and excreted effectively in liver injury and serum levels will rise as a result. In advanced cirrhosis, portal hypertension develops and it is hypothesised that the congested spleen hypertrophies [27]. Thrombocytopenia may reflect splenic pooling of platelets in portal hypertension or hepatic synthetic function and reduced thrombopoietin excretion [28].

Based on the pathophysiologic rationale described above, serum biomarkers can be broadly divided in two main classes: direct or indirect. Direct markers include two groups of molecules: (1) fragments of the liver matrix components, such as hyaluronan and products of collagen synthesis or degradation, produced by HSCs during the fibrotic process; (2) molecules regulating the mechanisms and cross-talks in fibrogenesis. Direct biomarkers reflect the metabolism of hepatic ECM and they have the potential of assessing dynamics of liver fibrogenesis. A limitation to the widespread use of direct fibrosis markers could be that they are not routinely available in all clinical settings. Indirect fibrosis markers are biochemical parameters measurable in the peripheral blood that are routinely performed in patients with liver disease. Those include molecules are synthesized, regulated or excreted by the liver, such as platelets, cholesterol, bilirubin, transaminases, albumin (Fig. 5.2). Table 5.1 depicts an overview of the main fibrosis biomarkers.

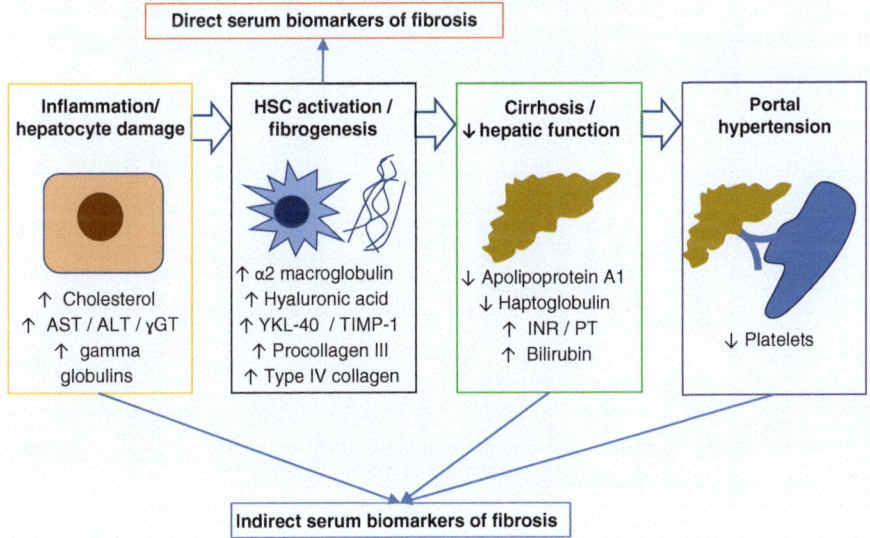

Fig. 5.2 Pathophysiologic rationale for serum fibrosis biomarkers

Table 5.1 Comparison of the main characteristics of the most studied serum fibrosis biomarkers for cirrhosis

	Hyaluronan	Fibrotest	Fibrometer	Hepascore	ELF	APRI	FIB4
Parameters	Hyaluronic acid	γGT, total bilirubin, haptoglobin, α-2 macroglobulin, apolipo-protein A1, age, gender	Platelets, prothrombin index, AST, a_2-macroglobulin, hyaluronan, urea, age	Age, gender, bilirubin, γGT, hyaluronan, a_2-macroglobulin	Age, TIMP-1, hyaluronan, procollagen type III	AST, platelets	Age, ALT, AST, platelets
Validated etiologies	HCV, NAFLD, ALD	HCV, HBV, NAFLD, ALD	HCV, NAFLD ALD	HCV, HBV, NAFLD, ALD	HCV, NAFLD, ALD	HCV, HBV, NAFLD, ALD	HCV, HBV, NAFLD, ALD
Limitations	Not routine test, cost	Not routine test, cost	Not routine test, cost	Not routine test, cost	Not routine test, cost	High rates of unclassified patients	High rates of unclassified patients
Risk factors for error	Systemic inflammatory states	Gilbert's syndrome, extrahepatic cholestasis, hemolytic anemia, systemic inflammatory states	Autoimmune thrombocytopenia, systemic inflammatory states	Gilbert's syndrome, extrahepatic cholestasis, systemic inflammatory states	Systemic inflammatory states	Autoimmune thrombocytopenia, acute transaminitis	Autoimmune thrombocytopenia, acute transaminitis

ALD alcoholic liver disease, *AUC* area under the receiving operating characteristic curve, *ELF* enhanced liver fibrosis, *HBV* hepatitis B virus, *HCV* hepatitis C virus, *MMP* metalloproteinase, *NAFLD* nonalcoholic fatty liver disease, *NA* not available, *TIMP* tissue inhibitor of metalloproteinase

5.4   Direct Serum Markers of Fibrosis (Class I Biomarkers) and Patented Tests

Direct markers for liver fibrosis are fragments and molecules correlated to the fibro-genetic pathophysiology, specifically to deposition and removal of ECM. Levels of direct fibrosis markers into the peripheral blood are reflective of the two main events of ECM metabolism: fibrogenesis and fibrolysis. The use of these biomarkers to diagnose liver cirrhosis is hypothesis-driven, however they are usually parameters that are not routinely determined in clinical practice. The performance of direct fibrosis biomarkers for the diagnosis of cirrhosis is depicted in Table 5.2.

Direct biomarkers include a number of molecules involved in the ECM metabolism, such as enzymes, collagen and its fragments, glycoproteins and inhibitors of metalloproteinases, glycosaminoglicans, cytokines. The most investigated biomarkers include hyaluronan, procollagen III, Type IV collagen, chitinase-3-like-1 human cartilage glycoprotein-39 (YKL-40), metalloproteinase 2 (MMP-2) and tissue inhibitor of metalloproteinase 1 (TIMP-1).

Hyaluronic acid is a glycosaminoglycan synthesized in HSCs and degraded by the liver sinusoidal cells [42]. The increase of its serum concentration indicates a dysfunction of the sinusoidal endothelial cells and reflects increased fibrogenesis [43]. Hyaluronan is the most investigated among the direct markers for liver fibrosis and it has been validated in chronic hepatitis C and B, ALD and NAFLD. The reported area under the curve (AUC) varies from 0.89 to 0.92.

Procollagen type III amino-terminal peptide and type IV collagen are elevated in chronic liver diseases and correlate with transaminase levels in patients with active hepatitis and with serum bilirubin levels in those with cirrhosis [44, 45]. These biomarkers have been validated mostly in chronic hepatitis C.

YKL-40 is a 39-kDa glycoprotein involved in remodeling of the ECM. YKL-40 has been tested in patients with chronic hepatitis C, showing an AUC of 0.80 for cirrhosis [29]. A limitation of YKL-40 is its ubiquitous presence, therefore it cannot be considered a liver-specific marker.

The matrix metalloproteinases and the tissues inhibitors of metalloproteinases are molecules actively involved in the control of ECM degradation. However, only few among them exhibit a potential as biomarkers for liver fibrosis. MMP-2 is secreted by activated HSCs and is involved in the degradation of fibrotic matrix. One study reported an excellent AUC of 0.97 for the detection of liver cirrhosis [31]. Serum levels of TIMP-1 and TIMP-2 correlate with the histological activity index and with fibrosis, respectively [46]. One study attributed to TIMP-1 a sensitivity of 100% for the detection of cirrhosis [31].

Direct markers for liver fibrogenesis have also been proposed as combination panels to increase the diagnostic performance of the single parameters. Among the panels of non-invasive direct markers, one of the most validated is the Enhanced Liver Fibrosis (ELF) test, combining age, hyaluronan, type III collagen and TIMP-1. This patented test has been validated in chronic hepatitis C, NAFLD and ALD [38]. Another combination panel, named Fibrometer, uses age, platelets, prothrombin index, AST, α-2-macroglobulin, hyaluronan and urea. Fibrometer has been

Table 5.2 Performance of direct and patented serum fibrosis biomarkers to diagnose liver cirrhosis

Index	Etiology	AUC	Cut-off	Sensitivity	Specificity
Hyaluronic acid [29, 30]	HCV/NAFLD/ALD	0.89–0.92/0.92/0.80–0.93	50–184/42/60	79.2–100/NA/NA	80–89.4/NA/NA
Procollagen III [29, 30]	HCV	0.79	0.995	77	66
Type IV Collagen [29, 30]	HCV	0.80	6.55	60	61
MMP-2 [31]	HCV	0.97	1500–320	74–83	96–100
TIMP-1 [31]	HCV	0.90	950–85	100	56–75
YKL-40 [29, 30]	HCV	0.80	284.8	80	77
Fibrometer [32–34]	HCV/NAFLD/ALD	0.91/0.90/0.85–0.94	0.754	94.1/NA/NA	87.6/NA/NA
Hepascore [33, 35–37]	HCV/HBV/NAFLD/ALD	0.85–0.94/0.82–0.9 /0.91/0.76–0.92	0.80–0.84/0.52–0.90/0.7/0.97	60–100/56–87/87/90	74–97/75–92/89/87
ELF score [32, 38]	HCV/NAFLD/ALD	0.77/0.87–0.99/0.94	0.063/0.375/0.431	95/89/93	29/96/100
Fibrotest [32, 33, 39–41]	HCV/HBV/NAFLD/ALD	0.71–0.87/0.76/0.84/0.79–0.95	0.75	50–87/55.6/NA/91–100	70–92.9/96.3/NA/66–93

ALD alcoholic liver disease, *AUC* area under the receiving operating characteristic curve, *ELF* enhanced liver fibrosis, *HBV* hepatitis B virus, *HCV* hepatitis C virus, *MMP* metalloproteinase, *NAFLD* nonalcoholic fatty liver disease, *NA* not available, *TIMP* tissue inhibitor of metalloproteinase

validated in chronic hepatitis C and NAFLD [32]. Another model, named Hepascore, combines bilirubin, γGT, hyaluronan, α-2-macroglobulin, age, and sex, and it has been validated in hepatitis C and ALD [35]. Fibrotest-Fibrosure is a patented panel of non-invasive fibrosis markers incorporating γGT, total bilirubin, haptoglobin, α-2 macroglobulin, apolipoprotein A1, age and gender [39]. Among the patented tests, Fibrotest-Fibrosure is the most validated one in various etiologies of liver diseases [47]. Interestingly, approximately one third of those studies are independent from the group of researchers who commercialized the test.

5.5   Indirect Serum Markers of Fibrosis (Class II Biomarkers)

Indirect biomarkers assess fibrosis through surrogates of inflammation, reduced liver function in cirrhosis and portal hypertension. Markers of inflammation encompass factors released from apoptotic or stressed hepatocytes, including the hepatic enzymes, aspartate aminotransferase, alanine aminotransferase and γGT. In addition, gamma globulins are markers of inflammation and frequently elevated in cirrhosis. These biomarkers are cheap and rapidly available upon routine clinic appointments. The indirect biomarkers developed in the first decade of the twenty-first century focused upon chronic hepatitis C infection. Interferon-based eradication therapy at that time had variable response rates (40–80%) and most patients suffering significant adverse effects of treatment [48]. A major challenge within clinical practice in hepatitis C was to select patients most at risk of subsequent complications, who would most benefit from receiving interferon therapy. The aim of early studies developing indirect biomarkers was to identify these individuals without resorting to liver biopsy. These biomarkers have been applied to other chronic liver diseases, which have also been the focus of new models of indirect biomarkers. The performance for cirrhosis of these biomarkers is described in Table 5.3.

One of the first serum biomarkers for fibrosis to be described was ALT in a retrospective cohort of hepatitis C patients by Pradat et al. in 2002 [49]. In this study 99% of patients with a persistently elevated ALT had a METAVIR fibrosis score of at F1. Conversely, 65% of those with a persistently normal ALT had F1 fibrosis (positive predictive value [PPV] 99%, negative predictive value [NPV] 35%). By setting a ALT threshold of 2.25 times the upper limit of normal (ULN) the sensitivity and specificity increased to 72% and 74%, respectively.

Indirect biomarkers have been subsequently used in combination to increase the diagnostic accuracy of scoring systems. The AST/ALT ratio (AAR) is a long standing and easily available marker reflecting hepatocyte stress and apoptosis [50]. An AAR >1 predicts cirrhosis in hepatitis C and NAFLD, with a PPV of up to 93% [50, 51]. The BARD score adapted AAR for NAFLD by designating points for AAR ≥0.8, elevated BMI and presence of diabetes to increase the accuracy of predicting F3-4 fibrosis [52].

Thrombocytopenia is a common hematological disorder in liver disease which independently correlates with the severity of fibrosis and cirrhosis [69]. The AST/ platelets ratio index (APRI) is based on the following formula: (AST/ULN) * (100/

Table 5.3 Performance of direct and patented serum fibrosis biomarkers to diagnose liver cirrhosis

Index	Etiology	AUC	Cut-off	Sensitivity	Specificity
ALT [49]	HCV	0.815	2.25 × ULN	72%	74%
AST/ALT ratio [50, 51]	HCV		≥1	77.8%	96.9%
	NAFLD	0.83	0.8	74%	78%
BARD [52]	NAFLD	0.81	2		
APRI [53–57]	HCV/	0.83	1.0	76%	72%
	HBV/	0.86	1.4	79%	83%
	ALD/	0.79	1.0		
	NALFD	0.73	1.0	21.4%	89.9%
Lok index [58]	HCV	0.906	0.5	53%	95%
Fibroindex [59]	HCV	0.62–0.83	2.25	35.8%	97.4%
Forns' index [60–62]	HCV	0.78–0.86	0.69	30%	95%
	HBV	0.888	0.69	32.5%	94.87%
	ALD	0.38	0.69		
FIB-4 [51, 54, 62–65]	HCV/HIV	0.73	≥3.25	23%	96.6%
	HCV	0.91	≥3.25	37.6%	98.2%
	HBV	0.79	≥3.25		
	NAFLD	0.802	≥2.67	33%	98%
	ALD	0.8	≥3.25		
FibroQ test [66, 67]	Chronic viral hepatitis	0.791	>2.6	64.9%	100%
NALFD FS [68]	NAFLD	0.82	≥0.676	51%	98%

ALD alcoholic liver disease, *AUC* area under the receiving operating characteristic curve, *ELF* enhanced liver fibrosis, *HBV* hepatitis B virus, *HCV* hepatitis C virus, *MMP* metalloproteinase, *NAFLD* nonalcoholic fatty liver disease, *NAFLD FS* NAFLD fibrosis score, *NA* not available, *TIMP* tissue inhibitor of metalloproteinase

Platelets). In the initial study in hepatitis C, a cut-off of 1.5 gave an AUC of 0.8 for 0.89 for cirrhosis [69]. Multiple studies have demonstrated the value of APRI in HCV infection and a meta-analysis by Lin et al. found a cut-off of 0.7 gave the greatest sensitivity and specificity (77% and 72% respectively) [53]. The predictive value of APRI was reduced in HCV/HIV co-infected individuals in this meta-analysis. In post liver transplant HCV infection, APRI is highly diagnostic of significant liver fibrosis [70]. APRI has also been used to examine fibrosis in chronic HBV, alcoholic liver disease and NAFLD (Table 5.3) [54–57]. APRI was found to have low sensitivity in alcoholic liver disease (13%) [55]. A further study by Loaeza-del-Castillo found that APRI did not have diagnostic value in autoimmune hepatitis (AUC 0.53) [71].

The Lok index incorporates ALT and INR to the APRI, resulting in greater diagnostic accuracy in HCV [58]. The Fibro Index combines platelet count with AST and gamma globulin to predict fibrosis in chronic HCV infection [59]. Although Fibro Index was shown to have a robust AUC (0.81) in the initial Japanese study, this was not borne out in subsequent French validation study (AUC 0.62) [72]. The Forns index was developed in 2002 using a chronic HCV infected cohort [60]. It combines patient age with platelet count, serum cholesterol and γ glutamyl transferase (GGT) without using serum transferases. The Forn's index was found to be more accurate at predicting mild fibrosis from ≥F2 fibrosis however, if was less accurate at distinguishing F2 from cirrhosis. Forn's index predicts cirrhosis with high accuracy in chronic HBV infection [61] but less reliably in alcoholic liver disease (Table 5.3) [62]. The lower predictive value in alcoholic liver disease reflects the significant elevations in GGT during active drinking and in early disease.

The FIB-4 incorporates age, platelet count AST and ALT and was developed to predict fibrosis in HCV/HIV co-infection [63]. Further studies have demonstrated its utility in HCV and HBV mono-infections and alcoholic liver disease [62, 64, 65]. FIB-4 has been used to accurately predict cirrhosis in NAFLD but with a lower cut-off value than in viral hepatitis and ALD (AUC 0.802, cut-off ≥2.67 v ≥ 3.25) [54]. FIB-4 had a better performance in NAFLD in two studies compared to other non-patented scores including AAR, APRI and the NAFLD Fibrosis score [51, 54]. FibroQ test combines age, AST, ALT and platelets but with the addition of pro-thrombin time [66]. A FibroQ test score of ≤0.783 had a NPV of 100% for excluding cirrhosis in a predominantly chronic hepatitis C. The FibroQ was more accurate than APRI, AAR, APRI and Lok's score in predicting significant fibrosis in a similar study by the same group, however, it is much less validated than those tests [66, 67].

The NAFLD Fibrosis Score (NAFLD FS), developed by Angulo and colleagues, is the first serum biomarker specifically designed to address the growing global burden of fatty liver disease [68]. The NAFLD FS is calculated from body mass index, age, glycaemic status (diabetes or hyperglycaemia), platelets, albumin and the AST/ALT ratio. A high cut-off (0.676) was used to accurately predict advanced fibrosis in 82–90% of individuals studied [68].

These studies of non-direct biomarkers have shown promise as an early screening tool for cirrhosis, particularly as they rely on parameters routinely measured in the outpatient setting, thus not adding additional cost to the assessment of patients.

5.6 Algorithms Combining Serum Fibrosis Biomarkers

Liver fibrosis biomarkers have also been combined in diagnostic algorithms. This strategy is aimed at improving the performance of a single test and at reducing the number of liver biopsies necessary for a correct classification. Combination algorithms of fibrosis biomarkers have been recommended by recent guidelines of the European Association for the Study of the Liver (EASL) about non-invasive assessment of liver fibrosis [73]. The guidelines state that, although these algorithms are more effective in detecting significant fibrosis than individual tests, they do not increase diagnostic accuracy for cirrhosis. However, given the important clinical implications that follow the diagnosis of cirrhosis, it is justified to confirm a diagnosis of cirrhosis by two concordant but unrelated tests.

A diagnostic algorithm for cirrhosis can give the following responses: (1) presence/absence of cirrhosis, which indicates the need for a specific screening for esophageal varices and HCC; (2) liver biopsy needed to correctly stage hepatic fibrosis. Table 5.4 summarizes several diagnostic algorithms combining liver fibrosis markers.

Table 5.4 Combination algorithms of non-invasive methods for liver fibrosis proposed in chronic hepatitis C

Algorithm's name	Etiology	Type	Non-invasive methods adopted	AUC for F4	Saved liver biopsies (%)
SAFE biopsy [74, 75]	HCV, HBV	Stepwise	APRI, Fibrotest	0.87–0.92	74.8–93.4
Fibropaca algorithm [76]	HCV	Synchronous	APRI, Fibrotest, Forns' index	0.85	76.2–81.3
Angers algorithms [77]	HCV	Synchronous	Fibrotest, Fibrometer	0.917	89.7
Bourliere's algorithm [78]	HCV	Stepwise	APRI, Hepascore	91–96% (accuracy)	33–45

APRI AST-to-platelets ratio index, *AUC* area under the receiving operating characteristic curve, *HBV* hepatitis B virus, *HCV* hepatitis C virus

The Sequential Algorithm for Fibrosis Evaluation (SAFE) biopsy, combining sequentially APRI and Fibrotest, is the most validated combination algorithm of fibrosis biomarkers. Stepwise algorithm modeling was based on the predictive values of the single markers and led to a save in liver biopsies of 74.8–93.4% [74].

A stepwise algorithm combining Hepascore, a patented test, and APRI was also proposed [35, 78]. The authors reported a high diagnostic accuracy (91%) with 45% saved liver biopsies to diagnose significant fibrosis.

The Fibropaca algorithm combines APRI, Fibrotest and Forns' index in a synchronous fashion. It showed a good performance for cirrhosis while saving about 80% for the diagnosis of cirrhosis. In a study by one of us, SAFE biopsy and Fibropaca algorithm were applied to 1013 HCV cases. Fibropaca algorithm and SAFE biopsy showed a similar accuracy but the latter saved more liver biopsies and allowed to perform a minor number of Fibrotest, with a consequent saving in terms of costs [79].

The Angers' algorithm consists of a combination of Fibrometer and Fibrotest, which can save 44.8% liver biopsies with an overall accuracy of 95.3% [80].

The EASL guidelines recommend to combine a fibrosis biomarker with transient elastography for best diagnostic performance. Two of such algorithms have been proposed, the Bordeaux algorithm combining transient elastography and Fibrotest, and the synchronous combination of transient elastography and Fibrometer. The Bordeaux algorithm demonstrated an excellent AUC of 0.95 for the diagnosis of liver cirrhosis and saved 78.8% liver biopsies [81]. The latter algorithm led to an overall diagnostic accuracy of 86.7% while no liver biopsy was required [77].

Overall, combination algorithms can significantly improve the diagnostic accuracy of the single fibrosis biomarker and they can safely reduce the number of liver biopsies needed. The choice of the fibrosis biomarker or combination algorithm to be used in clinical practice can rely on the following considerations: (1) local availability; (2) validation in the specific etiology of liver disease; (3) patient's comorbidities which may affect the result; (4) physician's choice based on what he feels more comfortable with.

5.7   Monitoring of Liver Disease Complications

Complications of liver cirrhosis, including esophageal varices, ascites and hepatic encephalopathy, occur when portal hypertension develops. The measurement of HVPG is the gold standard of reference to diagnose portal hypertension. However, it is invasive and limited to highly specialized centers where transjugular liver biopsy is available. Moreover, measurement of HVPG are unfeasible for serial monitoring because of invasiveness, cost, waiting times at radiologic facilities. Several studies have searched for non-invasive methods able to predict clinically significant portal hypertension (HVPG >10 mmHg) and/or presence of esophageal varices. Table 5.5 summarizes the main tests that have been investigated under this scope.

In 1999, a study of patients undergoing primary variceal screening during liver transplant evaluation found a platelet count <88,000 was the only factor associated with large esophageal or gastric varices in univariate or multivariate analyses [82]. A larger multicenter study of cirrhotic patients, not confined to those undergoing transplantation assessment, confirmed a similar cut-off for clinically significant varices [83]. In the same study indirect biomarkers that incorporated platelet count (APRI, Forns' index, Lok index, FIB-4, Fibroindex) or the AAR did not have improved positive predictive performance compared to platelets alone. However, a Lok's score below 1.5 had the highest NPV, 96%, for significant esophageal varices [83]. Berzigotti and colleagues developed an indirect score specifically for the prediction of clinically significant portal hypertension based upon albumin, INR and

Table 5.5 Performance of patented serum fibrosis biomarkers to predict HVPG ≥10 mmHg and/or esophageal varices

	Endpoint	AUC	Cut-off	Sensitivity	Specificity
Platelets [82, 83]	Large EV	0.66	89,000	54%	78%
AST/ALT ratio [83]	Large EV	0.61	1.1	68%	53%
APRI [83]	Large EV	0.6	1.5	54%	63%
FIB-4 [83]	Large EV	0.63	4.3	68%	57%
Lok index [83]	Large EV	0.71	1.5	74%	63%
Forn's index [83]	Large EV	0.61	8.8	62%	60%
Fibroindex [83]	Large EV	0.55	2.5	59%	50%
Berzigotti score [84]	HPVG ≥10	0.805	>0.06	93%	61%
	Any grade varices	0.795	>−1.02	93%	37%
Hyaluronic acid [85, 86]	Medium/large EV	0.86–0.92	207	94	77.8
Type IV collagen [87]	Any grade EV	0.78	NA	NA	NA
PIIINP [86]	HVPG >10 mmHg	0.74	NA	NA	NA
TIMP-1 [86]	HVPG >10 mmHg	0.85	NA	NA	NA
ELF score [86]	HVPG >10 mmHg	0.88	NA	NA	NA
Fibrotest [88, 89]	Large EV	0.77/0.78	0.75–0.80	77–92	21–61

ALD alcoholic liver disease, *AUC* area under the receiving operating characteristic curve, *ELF* enhanced liver fibrosis, *EV* esophageal varices, *NAFLD* nonalcoholic fatty liver disease, *NA* not available, *PIIINP* procollagen III, *TIMP* tissue inhibitor of metalloproteinase

ALT [84]. A separate model incorporating the presence or absence of spider angiomas, INR and ALT was used to predict the presence of varices of any grade. This model was more accurate at predicting clinically significant portal hypertension (93% sensitivity and 61% specificity) than varices.

Among direct fibrosis markers, type IV collagen, Fibrotest and hyaluronic acid have been investigated as non-invasive tests to predict presence of esophageal varices. Ascites and serum hyaluronic acid level higher than 207 predicted presence of medium or large esophageal varices with an AUC of 0.92 [85]. In patients with alcoholic cirrhosis, type IV collagen had a 0.78 AUC for predicting esophageal varices [87]. In a study of 160 patients with various etiologies of liver cirrhosis, Sandahl et al. found that ELF marker had higher diagnostic accuracy to predict HVPG >10 mmHg than procollagen type III, hyaluronic acid, and TIMP-1. A combination of macrophage activation marker sCD163 and ELF achieved the highest diagnostic performance, with an AUC of 0.90 [86].

Finally, Fibrotest showed a high negative predictive value of 86% to exclude the presence of large esophageal varices in cirrhotic patients [88]. At present, the Baveno VI consensus conference in portal hypertension states that patients with a liver stiffness <20 kPa and with a platelet count >150,000 have a very low risk of having varices requiring treatment, and can avoid screening endoscopy [9].

5.8 Prognostic Value of Non-invasive Methods for Liver Fibrosis

The stage of liver fibrosis is pivotal not only for management of the patient, including need for specific interventions and initiation of screening for HCC and esophageal varices, but also to establish his long-term prognosis. It is well known that patients with mild fibrosis at diagnosis have a low risk of developing cirrhosis over the subsequent 20 years, while those with septal fibrosis will develop cirrhosis in 8–10 years [90]. Moreover, end-stage complications occur in patients with advanced fibrosis stages. Given that the degree of liver fibrosis predicts liver-related complications and survival, prompt identification of those at risk of bad prognosis may promote early interventions and counselling about liver transplantation.

Liver biopsy or HVPG measurement are unfeasible for serial monitoring and surrogate end-point marker tool because of invasiveness and cost. The role of non-invasive methods for liver fibrosis in predicting clinical outcomes has been investigated. AAR is one of the earliest biomarkers to correlate with clinical outcomes, demonstrating similar prognostic value for 1-year mortality in hepatitis C as MELD score >9 and Child Pugh score >7 [50]. Fibrotest displayed a significant correlation with clinical outcomes, with a 5-year prognostic value similar to that of liver biopsy for the prediction of cirrhosis decompensation and survival in patients with chronic hepatitis C and ALD [62, 91]. Hyaluronic acid has also been significantly associated with mortality in patients with chronic hepatitis C [92]. In a cohort of 1457 patients with chronic hepatitis C, Vergniol et al. found that Fibrotest predicts all-causes death, liver-related death, and liver transplantation during a 5-year follow-up period, with an AUC of 0.80 and 0.82, respectively [93]. On the same line, a recent study of 3927 patients with chronic hepatitis C showed that Fibrotest predicted 10 years occurrence of severe liver-related complications, HCC, variceal bleeding and hepatic failure [94]. Changes in liver fibrosis tests overtime have been found to have a strong association with prognosis [95]. In a recent study of 360 patients, Fibrometer showed a high prognostic value to predict clinical outcomes in patients with NAFLD [96]. In a cohort of 218 patients with ALD followed for over 10 years Fibrotest, Fibrometer and Hepascore were highly predictive of mortality (AUC 0.77–0.8), similarly to histologic fibrosis staging (AUC 0.77). These direct biomarkers significantly outperformed the prognostic value of Child's Pugh classification and FIB4, APRI and Forns' index [62]. The prognostic performance of direct and indirect serum biomarkers is good and can predict patients most at risk of decompensation and mortality over long term follow up. Patients with biomarker scores beyond the cut-off for poor prognosis should be closely monitored for complications and considered for liver transplantation.

Conclusion

Over the last two decades the use of serum biomarkers in cirrhosis has evolved considerably. Direct and indirect biomarkers of cirrhosis, combined scores and algorithms of these tests have been demonstrated and validated to be highly accurate at the prediction of cirrhosis in large cohorts of patients. These tests are established in clinical guidelines as the first investigations for cirrhosis and have been applied to the diagnosis of portal hypertension and for long-term prognosis. Patient acceptability, safety, low cost and ease of use in the outpatient environment are key factors in the success of biomarkers as first line tools in daily clinical practice.

The limitations of serum biomarkers of cirrhosis predominantly reflect their relatively poor accuracy at predicting mild and moderate fibrosis. The clinical performance of these tests may further be reduced by variations in normal ranges and poor inter-laboratory standardization of routine assays. All studies to date have used liver biopsy as the reference for liver fibrosis. There is however, even with larger biopsy samples, a risk of sampling and reporting errors. In the future, more global assessment of liver fibrosis by approaches such as magnetic resonance elastography may reduce this sampling error [97]. Biomarkers have been predominantly developed to investigate fibrosis in chronic hepatitis C infection and to a lesser extent fatty liver disease. Whilst these scores may be transferred to hepatitis B and ALD, there is a paucity of evidence, or even evidence against the value of using biomarkers in autoimmune hepatitis, primary sclerosing cholangitis and primary biliary cholangitis. Finally, the effectiveness of biomarkers to predict complications requires further validation, particularly beyond the presence of clinically significant portal hypertension, including the development of ascites, spontaneous bacterial peritonitis, variceal hemorrhage and HCC.

From these limitations, further studies are needed focused upon reducing the "grey area" of these tests and algorithms. In addition, the role of biomarkers in prognostication for decompensation and HCC development needs to be fully defined, particularly in viral hepatitis cirrhosis following viral suppression or eradication. Studies investigating the role of biomarkers in autoimmune and cholestatic liver diseases are warranted.

Notwithstanding these limitations, there is currently a huge growing global burden of liver disease, predominantly driven by NAFLD. In this developing clinical environment, it is essential that serum biomarkers of cirrhosis are placed at the center of clinical evaluation by non-specialists to ensure rapid triage and appropriate referral. Biomarkers may be further exploited by gastroenterologists and hepatologists to avoid liver biopsy, initiate variceal screening and prognosticate. In addition, it is likely that, in the near future, serum biomarkers, together with other non-invasive methods, will help the selection of patients for new NAFLD medications currently in phase 3 trials.

References

1. Roulot D, Costes JL, Buyck JF, et al. Transient elastography as a screening tool for liver fibrosis and cirrhosis in a community-based population aged over 45 years. Gut. 2011;60:977–84.
2. Friedman SL. Mechanisms of hepatic fibrogenesis. Gastroenterology. 2008;134:1655–69.
3. Neff GW, Duncan CW, Schiff ER. The current economic burden of cirrhosis. Gastroenterol Hepatol (N Y). 2011;7:661–71.
4. Garcia-Tsao G, Friedman S, Iredale J, Pinzani M. Now there are many (stages) where before there was one: in search of a pathophysiological classification of cirrhosis. Hepatology. 2010;51:1445–9.
5. Dulai PS, Singh S, Patel J, et al. Increased risk of mortality by fibrosis stage in nonalcoholic fatty liver disease: systematic review and meta-analysis. Hepatology. 2017;65:1557–65.
6. D'Amico G, Garcia-Tsao G, Pagliaro L. Natural history and prognostic indicators of survival in cirrhosis: a systematic review of 118 studies. J Hepatol. 2006;44:217–31.
7. Durand F, Valla D. Assessment of prognosis of cirrhosis. Semin Liver Dis. 2008;28:110–22.
8. Rockey DC, Caldwell SH, Goodman ZD, Nelson RC, Smith AD, American Association for the Study of Liver D. Liver biopsy. Hepatology. 2009;49:1017–44.
9. de Franchis R, Baveno VIF. Expanding consensus in portal hypertension: report of the Baveno VI consensus workshop: stratifying risk and individualizing care for portal hypertension. J Hepatol. 2015;63:743–52.
10. Lee UE, Friedman SL. Mechanisms of hepatic fibrogenesis. Best Pract Res Clin Gastroenterol. 2011;25:195–206.
11. Bataller R, Brenner DA. Liver fibrosis. J Clin Invest. 2005;115:209–18.
12. Ishak K, Baptista A, Bianchi L, et al. Histological grading and staging of chronic hepatitis. J Hepatol. 1995;22:696–9.
13. Bataller R, North KE, Brenner DA. Genetic polymorphisms and the progression of liver fibrosis: a critical appraisal. Hepatology. 2003;37:493–503.
14. Anstee QM, Wright M, Goldin R, Thursz MR. Parenchymal extinction: coagulation and hepatic fibrogenesis. Clin Liver Dis. 2009;13:117–26.
15. Tsuchida T, Friedman SL. Mechanisms of hepatic stellate cell activation. Nat Rev Gastroenterol Hepatol. 2017;14:397–411.
16. Failli P, Ruocco C, De Franco R, et al. The mitogenic effect of platelet-derived growth factor in human hepatic stellate cells requires calcium influx. Am J Phys. 1995;269:C1133–9.
17. Kluwe J, Pradere JP, Gwak GY, et al. Modulation of hepatic fibrosis by c-Jun-N-terminal kinase inhibition. Gastroenterology. 2010;138:347–59.
18. Gressner AM. Transdifferentiation of hepatic stellate cells (Ito cells) to myofibroblasts: a key event in hepatic fibrogenesis. Kidney Int Suppl. 1996;54:S39–45.

19. Meyer DH, Bachem MG, Gressner AM. Modulation of hepatic lipocyte proteoglycan synthesis and proliferation by Kupffer cell-derived transforming growth factors type beta 1 and type alpha. Biochem Biophys Res Commun. 1990;171:1122–9.
20. Win KM, Charlotte F, Mallat A, et al. Mitogenic effect of transforming growth factor-beta 1 on human Ito cells in culture: evidence for mediation by endogenous platelet-derived growth factor. Hepatology. 1993;18:137–45.
21. Yoshiji H, Kuriyama S, Yoshii J, et al. Vascular endothelial growth factor and receptor interaction is a prerequisite for murine hepatic fibrogenesis. Gut. 2003;52:1347–54.
22. Kinoshita K, Iimuro Y, Fujimoto J, et al. Targeted and regulable expression of transgenes in hepatic stellate cells and myofibroblasts in culture and in vivo using an adenoviral Cre/loxP system to antagonise hepatic fibrosis. Gut. 2007;56:396–404.
23. Breitkopf K, Godoy P, Ciuclan L, Singer MV, Dooley S. TGF-beta/Smad signaling in the injured liver. Z Gastroenterol. 2006;44:57–66.
24. Saxena NK, Ikeda K, Rockey DC, Friedman SL, Anania FA. Leptin in hepatic fibrosis: evidence for increased collagen production in stellate cells and lean littermates of ob/ob mice. Hepatology. 2002;35:762–71.
25. Wang J, Leclercq I, Brymora JM, et al. Kupffer cells mediate leptin-induced liver fibrosis. Gastroenterology. 2009;137:713–23.
26. Seki E, Schwabe RF. Hepatic inflammation and fibrosis: functional links and key pathways. Hepatology. 2015;61:1066–79.
27. Peck-Radosavljevic M. Thrombocytopenia in chronic liver disease. Liver Int. 2016;37:778–93.
28. Qian S, Fu F, Li W, Chen Q, de Sauvage FJ. Primary role of the liver in thrombopoietin production shown by tissue-specific knockout. Blood. 1998;92:2189–91.
29. Saitou Y, Shiraki K, Yamanaka Y, et al. Noninvasive estimation of liver fibrosis and response to interferon therapy by a serum fibrogenesis marker, YKL-40, in patients with HCV-associated liver disease. World J Gastroenterol. 2005;11:476–81.
30. Sebastiani G, Gkouvatsos K, Plebani M. Non-invasive assessment of liver fibrosis: it is time for laboratory medicine. Clin Chem Lab Med. 2011;49:13–32.
31. Boeker KH, Haberkorn CI, Michels D, Flemming P, Manns MP, Lichtinghagen R. Diagnostic potential of circulating TIMP-1 and MMP-2 as markers of liver fibrosis in patients with chronic hepatitis C. Clin Chim Acta. 2002;316:71–81.
32. Cales P, Oberti F, Michalak S, et al. A novel panel of blood markers to assess the degree of liver fibrosis. Hepatology. 2005;42:1373–81.
33. Leroy V, Hilleret MN, Sturm N, et al. Prospective comparison of six non-invasive scores for the diagnosis of liver fibrosis in chronic hepatitis C. J Hepatol. 2007;46:775–82.
34. Leroy V, Sturm N, Faure P, et al. Prospective evaluation of FibroTest(R), FibroMeter(R), and HepaScore(R) for staging liver fibrosis in chronic hepatitis B: comparison with hepatitis C. J Hepatol. 2014;61:28–34.
35. Adams LA, Bulsara M, Rossi E, et al. Hepascore: an accurate validated predictor of liver fibrosis in chronic hepatitis C infection. Clin Chem. 2005;51:1867–73.
36. Becker L, Salameh W, Sferruzza A, et al. Validation of hepascore, compared with simple indices of fibrosis, in patients with chronic hepatitis C virus infection in United States. Clin Gastroenterol Hepatol. 2009;7:696–701.
37. Huang Y, Adams LA, Joseph J, Bulsara MK, Jeffrey GP. The ability of Hepascore to predict liver fibrosis in chronic liver disease: a meta-analysis. Liver Int. 2017;37:121–31.
38. Rosenberg WM, Voelker M, Thiel R, et al. Serum markers detect the presence of liver fibrosis: a cohort study. Gastroenterology. 2004;127:1704–13.
39. Imbert-Bismut F, Ratziu V, Pieroni L, Charlotte F, Benhamou Y, Poynard T. Biochemical markers of liver fibrosis in patients with hepatitis C virus infection: a prospective study. Lancet. 2001;357:1069–75.
40. Sebastiani G, Vario A, Guido M, et al. Stepwise combination algorithms of non-invasive markers to diagnose significant fibrosis in chronic hepatitis C. J Hepatol. 2006;44:686–93.
41. Shaheen AA, Wan AF, Myers RP. FibroTest and FibroScan for the prediction of hepatitis C-related fibrosis: a systematic review of diagnostic test accuracy. Am J Gastroenterol. 2007;102:2589–600.

42. McGary CT, Raja RH, Weigel PH. Endocytosis of hyaluronic acid by rat liver endothelial cells. Evidence for receptor recycling. Biochem J. 1989;257:875–84.
43. Guechot J, Laudat A, Loria A, Serfaty L, Poupon R, Giboudeau J. Diagnostic accuracy of hyaluronan and type III procollagen amino-terminal peptide serum assays as markers of liver fibrosis in chronic viral hepatitis C evaluated by ROC curve analysis. Clin Chem. 1996;42:558–63.
44. Montalto G, Soresi M, Aragona F, et al. Procollagen III and laminin in chronic viral hepatopathies. Presse Med. 1996;25:59–62.
45. Misaki M, Shima T, Yano Y, et al. Basement membrane-related and type III procollagen-related antigens in serum of patients with chronic viral liver disease. Clin Chem. 1990;36:522–4.
46. Walsh KM, Timms P, Campbell S, MacSween RN, Morris AJ. Plasma levels of matrix metalloproteinase-2 (MMP-2) and tissue inhibitors of metalloproteinases -1 and -2 (TIMP-1 and TIMP-2) as noninvasive markers of liver disease in chronic hepatitis C: comparison using ROC analysis. Dig Dis Sci. 1999;44:624–30.
47. Sebastiani G, Alberti A. Non invasive fibrosis biomarkers reduce but not substitute the need for liver biopsy. World J Gastroenterol. 2006;12:3682–94.
48. Dusheiko G. Side effects of alpha interferon in chronic hepatitis C. Hepatology. 1997;26: 112S–21S.
49. Pradat P, Alberti A, Poynard T, et al. Predictive value of ALT levels for histologic findings in chronic hepatitis C: a European collaborative study. Hepatology. 2002;36:973–7.
50. Giannini E, Risso D, Botta F, et al. Validity and clinical utility of the aspartate aminotransferase-alanine aminotransferase ratio in assessing disease severity and prognosis in patients with hepatitis C virus-related chronic liver disease. Arch Intern Med. 2003;163:218–24.
51. McPherson S, Stewart SF, Henderson E, Burt AD, Day CP. Simple non-invasive fibrosis scoring systems can reliably exclude advanced fibrosis in patients with non-alcoholic fatty liver disease. Gut. 2010;59:1265–9.
52. Harrison SA, Oliver D, Arnold HL, Gogia S, Neuschwander-Tetri BA. Development and validation of a simple NAFLD clinical scoring system for identifying patients without advanced disease. Gut. 2008;57:1441–7.
53. Lin ZH, Xin YN, Dong QJ, et al. Performance of the aspartate aminotransferase-to-platelet ratio index for the staging of hepatitis C-related fibrosis: an updated meta-analysis. Hepatology. 2011;53:726–36.
54. Shah AG, Lydecker A, Murray K, et al. Comparison of noninvasive markers of fibrosis in patients with nonalcoholic fatty liver disease. Clin Gastroenterol Hepatol. 2009;7:1104–12.
55. Lieber CS, Weiss DG, Morgan TR, Paronetto F. Aspartate aminotransferase to platelet ratio index in patients with alcoholic liver fibrosis. Am J Gastroenterol. 2006;101:1500–8.
56. Fujii H, Enomoto M, Fukushima W, et al. Noninvasive laboratory tests proposed for predicting cirrhosis in patients with chronic hepatitis C are also useful in patients with non-alcoholic steatohepatitis. J Gastroenterol. 2009;44:608–14.
57. Shin WG, Park SH, Jang MK, et al. Aspartate aminotransferase to platelet ratio index (APRI) can predict liver fibrosis in chronic hepatitis B. Dig Liver Dis. 2008;40:267–74.
58. Lok AS, Ghany MG, Goodman ZD, et al. Predicting cirrhosis in patients with hepatitis C based on standard laboratory tests: results of the HALT-C cohort. Hepatology. 2005;42:282–92.
59. Koda M, Matunaga Y, Kawakami M, Kishimoto Y, Suou T, Murawaki Y. FibroIndex, a practical index for predicting significant fibrosis in patients with chronic hepatitis C. Hepatology. 2007;45:297–306.
60. Forns X, Ampurdanes S, Llovet JM, et al. Identification of chronic hepatitis C patients without hepatic fibrosis by a simple predictive model. Hepatology. 2002;36:986–92.
61. Zhou K, Gao CF, Zhao YP, et al. Simpler score of routine laboratory tests predicts liver fibrosis in patients with chronic hepatitis B. J Gastroenterol Hepatol. 2010;25:1569–77.
62. Naveau S, Gaude G, Asnacios A, et al. Diagnostic and prognostic values of noninvasive biomarkers of fibrosis in patients with alcoholic liver disease. Hepatology. 2009;49:97–105.
63. Sterling RK, Lissen E, Clumeck N, et al. Development of a simple noninvasive index to predict significant fibrosis in patients with HIV/HCV coinfection. Hepatology. 2006;43:1317–25.

64. Vallet-Pichard A, Mallet V, Nalpas B, et al. FIB-4: an inexpensive and accurate marker of fibrosis in HCV infection. Comparison with liver biopsy and fibrotest. Hepatology. 2007;46:32–6.
65. Mallet V, Dhalluin-Venier V, Roussin C, et al. The accuracy of the FIB-4 index for the diagnosis of mild fibrosis in chronic hepatitis B. Aliment Pharmacol Ther. 2009;29:409–15.
66. Hsieh YY, Tung SY, Lee IL, et al. FibroQ: an easy and useful noninvasive test for predicting liver fibrosis in patients with chronic viral hepatitis. Chang Gung Med J. 2009;32:614–22.
67. Hsieh YY, Tung SY, Lee K, et al. Routine blood tests to predict liver fibrosis in chronic hepatitis C. World J Gastroenterol. 2012;18:746–53.
68. Angulo P, Hui JM, Marchesini G, et al. The NAFLD fibrosis score: a noninvasive system that identifies liver fibrosis in patients with NAFLD. Hepatology. 2007;45:846–54.
69. Wai CT, Greenson JK, Fontana RJ, et al. A simple noninvasive index can predict both significant fibrosis and cirrhosis in patients with chronic hepatitis C. Hepatology. 2003;38:518–26.
70. Toniutto P, Fabris C, Bitetto D, et al. Role of AST to platelet ratio index in the detection of liver fibrosis in patients with recurrent hepatitis C after liver transplantation. J Gastroenterol Hepatol. 2007;22:1904–8.
71. Loaeza-del-Castillo A, Paz-Pineda F, Oviedo-Cardenas E, Sanchez-Avila F, Vargas-Vorackova FAST. To platelet ratio index (APRI) for the noninvasive evaluation of liver fibrosis. Ann Hepatol. 2008;7:350–7.
72. Halfon P, Penaranda G, Renou C, Bourliere M. External validation of FibroIndex. Hepatology. 2007;46:280–1. author reply 1–2
73. European Association for Study of L, Asociacion Latinoamericana para el Estudio del H. EASL-ALEH Clinical Practice Guidelines: non-invasive tests for evaluation of liver disease severity and prognosis. J Hepatol. 2015;63:237–64.
74. Sebastiani G, Halfon P, Castera L, et al. SAFE biopsy: a validated method for large-scale staging of liver fibrosis in chronic hepatitis C. Hepatology. 2009;49:1821–7.
75. Sebastiani G, Vario A, Guido M, Alberti A. Sequential algorithms combining non-invasive markers and biopsy for the assessment of liver fibrosis in chronic hepatitis B. World J Gastroenterol. 2007;13:525–31.
76. Bourliere M, Penaranda G, Renou C, et al. Validation and comparison of indexes for fibrosis and cirrhosis prediction in chronic hepatitis C patients: proposal for a pragmatic approach classification without liver biopsies. J Viral Hepat. 2006;13:659–70.
77. Boursier J, de Ledinghen V, Zarski JP, et al. Comparison of 8 diagnostic algorithms for liver fibrosis in hepatitis C: new algorithms are more precise and entirely non-invasive. Hepatology. 2012;55:58–67.
78. Bourliere M, Penaranda G, Ouzan D, et al. Optimized stepwise combination algorithms of non-invasive liver fibrosis scores including Hepascore in hepatitis C virus patients. Aliment Pharmacol Ther. 2008;28:458–67.
79. Sebastiani G, Halfon P, Castera L, et al. Comparison of three algorithms of non-invasive markers of fibrosis in chronic hepatitis C. Aliment Pharmacol Ther. 2012;35:92–104.
80. Boursier J, Cales P. Combination of fibrosis tests: sequential or synchronous? Hepatology. 2009;50:656–7. author reply 7
81. Castera L, Sebastiani G, Le Bail B, de Ledinghen V, Couzigou P, Alberti A. Prospective comparison of two algorithms combining non-invasive methods for staging liver fibrosis in chronic hepatitis C. J Hepatol. 2010;52:191–8.
82. Zaman A, Hapke R, Flora K, Rosen HR, Benner K. Factors predicting the presence of esophageal or gastric varices in patients with advanced liver disease. Am J Gastroenterol. 1999;94:3292–6.
83. Sebastiani G, Tempesta D, Fattovich G, et al. Prediction of oesophageal varices in hepatic cirrhosis by simple serum non-invasive markers: results of a multicenter, large-scale study. J Hepatol. 2010;53:630–8.
84. Berzigotti A, Gilabert R, Abraldes JG, et al. Noninvasive prediction of clinically significant portal hypertension and esophageal varices in patients with compensated liver cirrhosis. Am J Gastroenterol. 2008;103:1159–67.

85. Galal GM, Amin NF, Abdel Hafeez HA, El-Baz MA. Can serum fibrosis markers predict medium/large oesophageal varices in patients with liver cirrhosis? Arab J Gastroenterol. 2011;12:62–7.
86. Sandahl TD, McGrail R, Moller HJ, et al. The macrophage activation marker sCD163 combined with markers of the Enhanced Liver Fibrosis (ELF) score predicts clinically significant portal hypertension in patients with cirrhosis. Aliment Pharmacol Ther. 2016;43:1222–31.
87. Mamori S, Searashi Y, Matsushima M, et al. Serum type IV collagen level is predictive for esophageal varices in patients with severe alcoholic disease. World J Gastroenterol. 2008;14:2044–8.
88. Thabut D, Trabut JB, Massard J, et al. Non-invasive diagnosis of large oesophageal varices with FibroTest in patients with cirrhosis: a preliminary retrospective study. Liver Int. 2006;26:271–8.
89. Castera L, Le Bail B, Roudot-Thoraval F, et al. Early detection in routine clinical practice of cirrhosis and oesophageal varices in chronic hepatitis C: comparison of transient elastography (FibroScan) with standard laboratory tests and non-invasive scores. J Hepatol. 2009;50:59–68.
90. Yano M, Kumada H, Kage M, et al. The long-term pathological evolution of chronic hepatitis C. Hepatology. 1996;23:1334–40.
91. Ngo Y, Munteanu M, Messous D, et al. A prospective analysis of the prognostic value of biomarkers (FibroTest) in patients with chronic hepatitis C. Clin Chem. 2006;52:1887–96.
92. Nunes D, Fleming C, Offner G, et al. Noninvasive markers of liver fibrosis are highly predictive of liver-related death in a cohort of HCV-infected individuals with and without HIV infection. Am J Gastroenterol. 2010;105:1346–53.
93. Vergniol J, Foucher J, Terrebonne E, et al. Non-invasive tests for fibrosis and liver stiffness predict 5-year outcomes of patients with chronic hepatitis C. Gastroenterology. 2011;140:1970–9.
94. Poynard T, Vergniol J, Ngo Y, et al. Staging chronic hepatitis C in seven categories using fibrosis biomarker (FibroTest) and transient elastography (FibroScan). J Hepatol. 2014;61:994–1003.
95. Vergniol J, Boursier J, Coutzac C, et al. Evolution of noninvasive tests of liver fibrosis is associated with prognosis in patients with chronic hepatitis C. Hepatology. 2014;60:65–76.
96. Boursier J, Vergniol J, Guillet A, et al. Diagnostic accuracy and prognostic significance of blood fibrosis tests and liver stiffness measurement by FibroScan in non-alcoholic fatty liver disease. J Hepatol. 2016;65:570–8.
97. Singh S, Venkatesh SK, Loomba R, et al. Magnetic resonance elastography for staging liver fibrosis in non-alcoholic fatty liver disease: a diagnostic accuracy systematic review and individual participant data pooled analysis. Eur Radiol. 2016;26:1431–40.

Ultrasound Elastography: General and Technical Overview

6

Veronica Salvatore and Fabio Piscaglia

6.1 Introduction

The technical improvements of ultrasonography experienced only a few completely revolutionary steps, which took place approximately every 10 years: ultrasonography started from mono-dimensional imaging around 1970 (the so-called A-mode). It moved to bi-dimensional imaging around 1980 (the conventional B-mode). Later functional imaging was introduced: at first Doppler was marketed in the late '80s, contrast enhanced ultrasound in 1999 and finally the assessment of tissue consistence with elastography started in 2003 but fully developed between 2010 and 2016. Altogether, technological advancement brought from the visualization of structures to their virtual palpation.

Elastography allows the evaluation of biomechanical proprieties of tissues, namely elasticity and viscosity, although at present these two components cannot be clearly separated. All elastography ultrasound information are based on the properties of body soft tissue to oppose themselves to a deformation induced by a force, due to their intrinsic stiffness [1]. Given this background, the main application of elastography to liver diseases has been the assessment of the degree of fibrous tissue deposition, categorized in fibrosis stages of chronic liver disease. Actually, the assessment of the tissue consistency, or as universally termed for ultrasound elastography of tissue stiffness, reflects not only the proportion of fibrous tissue deposited in the normal liver parenchyma, but also other conditions which might increase the perceived stiffness. In particular, any increase in fluid (which is incompressibile) content within the liver, which is wrapped by a poorly distensible fibrous capsule, the Glisson's capsule, tend to contribute to increase the overall organ stiffness.

V. Salvatore • F. Piscaglia (✉)
Department of Medical and Surgical Sciences, University of Bologna, Azienda Ospedaliero-Universitaria S.Orsola Malpighi di Bologna, Bologna, Italy
e-mail: veronica.salvatore@unibo.it; fabio.piscaglia@unibo.it

© Springer International Publishing AG, part of Springer Nature 2018   83
A. Berzigotti, J. Bosch (eds.), *Diagnostic Methods for Cirrhosis and Portal Hypertension*, https://doi.org/10.1007/978-3-319-72628-1_6

Therefore, conditions such as elevated inflammatory activity of hepatitis (which induces tissue edema) regardless of its etiology, cardiac failure, biliary obstruction, etc., tend to increase liver stiffness since all of them increase the fluid liver content. However, apart from the occurrence of these conditions, which tend to overincrease liver stiffness, the main determinant of the increase in liver stiffness remains the amount of fibrotic scarring, which is why stiffness assessment by ultrasound has been rapidly adopted in the evaluation of patients with chronic liver disease.

The first reports about ultrasound elastography date back to 1991 when Ophir and colleagues tried to calculate the deformation of tissues subjected to external compression using ultrasound [2]. They assumed that the applied force was uniform and consequently the elastic modulus (or Young modulus) was inversely related to the measured deformation, which correlates with its stiffness.

There are, however, several quantities for measuring the stiffness of materials, all of which arise from the generalized Hooke's law, stating that the force applied to deform a solid is proportional to its rate of extension. The main quantities to our interests for measuring stiffness are the following ones (adapted from https://en.wikipedia.org/wiki/Shear_modulus), which expand beyond the elasticity (Young's) modulus E alone:

- the *Young's modulus E*, which describes the material's strain (i.e. rate of change in size, expressing deformation) response to uniaxial stress in the direction of this stress (like pulling on the ends of a wire or putting a weight on top of a column, with the wire getting longer and the column losing height),
- the *Poisson's ratio ν*, which describes the response in the directions orthogonal to this uniaxial stress (the wire getting thinner and the column thicker),
- the *bulk modulus K*, which describes the material's response to (uniform) hydrostatic pressure (like the pressure at the bottom of the ocean or a deep swimming pool),
- the *shear modulus G*, which describes the material's response to shear stress (like cutting it with dull scissors).

These moduli are not independent: simplifying and assuming that incompressible and isotropic tissues are measured they can be connected via the equations

$$E = 2(1+v)G = 3G = 3\rho c_s^2$$

where v is the Poisson's ratio of soft tissue, assumed near 0.5 in case of incompressible medium, ρ the tissue density and c_s the propagation speed. Thus, the Young's modulus is assumed to be three times of the shear modulus G, which corresponds to the product of tissue density and shear wave speed velocity. Consequently, measuring shear wave speed velocity by ultrasound (c_s) and assuming a standard shear modulus G for soft tissues, it is possible to estimate the density of that specific portion of soft tissue (i.e. its stiffness).

In connection to the unit of measure it is worth to remind that Young's modulus is the ratio of stress (which has units of pressure) to strain (which is dimensionless, as it corresponds to a percent change in size), and hence Young's modulus has units of pressure. Its international standard unit is therefore the Pascal (Pa or N/m^2 or kg·m^{-1}·s^{-2}). Therefore also G, the shear modulus is measured in Pascal, making the kiloPascal the common unit of measure for soft body tissue stiffness in ultrasound elastography, although more correctly stiffness can be expressed also through the measured shear wave speed velocity, since this is the truly measured unit (see below in a following subheadings).

To better understand the different roles of the different quantities for measuring the stiffness of materials, which turn into different ultrasound elastography methods, and to exemplify the shear waves (which do not represent all types of ultrasound elastography measurements), it must be remarked that isotropic and homogenous elastic tissue are crossed by two main wave components when submitted to an external force: primary waves are longitudinal to the direction of the principal wave (S, parallel to the applied force = F, Fig. 6.1, inspired from https://en.wikipedia.org/wiki/Shear_stress) and in fact arise from the force vector component perpendicular to the material cross section on which it acts. They are constituted by alternate compressions and rarefactions which tend to travel at around 1500 m/s in soft tissue and for long distance (across the entire tissue). Secondary or shear waves are defined as the component of stress coplanar with a material cross section in respect to the applied force (Fig. 6.1), therefore they are perpendicular to the direction of the principal wave. They attenuate very rapidly (usually within 10 mm from the point where they were generated) and their velocity is in the range 1–10 m/s, slower than longitudinal waves. This makes G lower (1–100 kPa) and hence larger the difference between tissues [3]. For these reasons, transversal (shear) waves appeared of particular interest for stiffness quantification.

The speed (c_L) of the primary (longitudinal) waves may be expressed as

$$c_L = \sqrt{K / \rho}$$

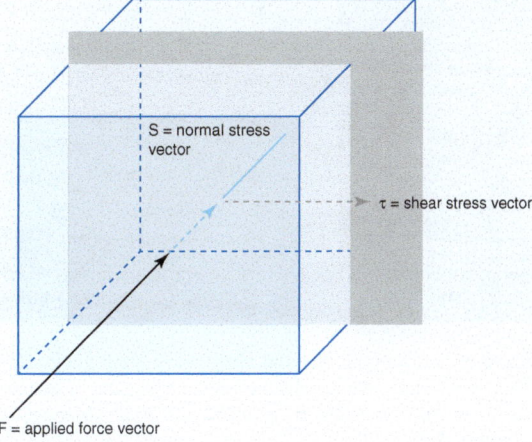

Fig. 6.1 Graphic representation of shear stress vector (Tau) that is on the same plane (coplanar) with the material cross section, thus perpendicular to the vector of the applied force. The normal stress vector is aligned (parallel) to that of the applied force. The speed of the longitudinal and of shear waves are related with the tissue density and express its stiffness

S = normal stress vector

τ = shear stress vector

F = applied force vector

where ρ is the density of the material and K the bulk modulus. In the same way, the speed (c_s) of the secondary (transversal) waves may be expressed as

$$c_s = \sqrt{G / \rho}$$

where G is the shear modulus. Thus, the speed of the longitudinal and of shear waves are related with the tissue density and express its stiffness. Measuring the waves speed and assuming standard K or G values for soft tissues, it becomes possible to estimate the tissue density or stiffness.

In other words, shear can be defined as a change in shape without change in volume in response to a pair of equal forces that act in opposite directions (one that tends to deform and the opposite that resists to deformation; without the opposite force resisting to deformation the tissue would simply move away). After the brief impulse has terminated, the tissue where the force was applied returns to its original shape, while shear waves propagate transversely across the adjacent layers [4].

According to the methods of generation and/or of type of measured waves, quantitative ultrasound elastography methods are categorized into three main classes [1]:

1. transient elastography
2. point shear wave elastography (pSWE) (Fig. 6.2)
3. bidimensional shear wave elastography (2D-SWE) (Fig. 6.3).

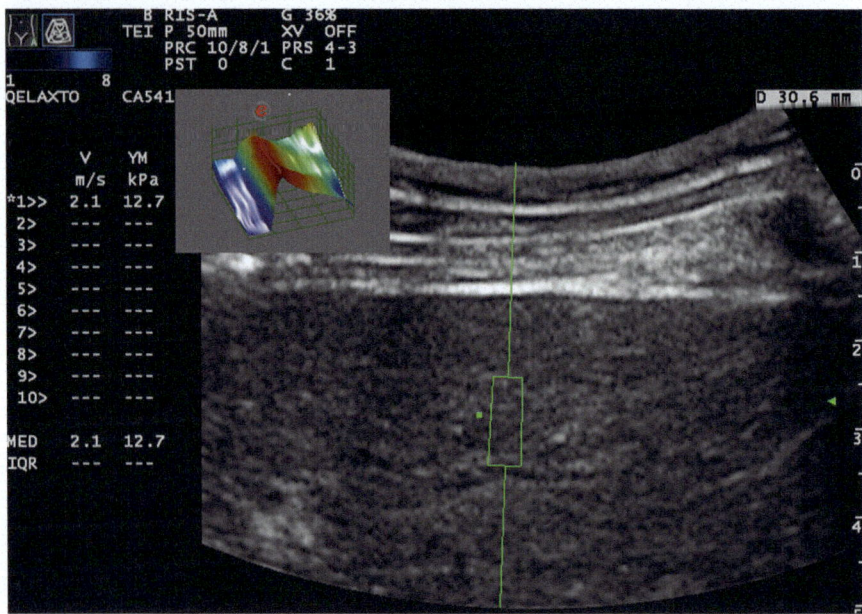

Fig. 6.2 An example of point shear-wave elastography (Esaote, Italy). The Region of Interest (ROI) can be moved freely by the operator. The dot indicates the focus point. On the left side of the screen measurements are given in kPa and in m/s. Median value and interquartile range (IQR) are also provided

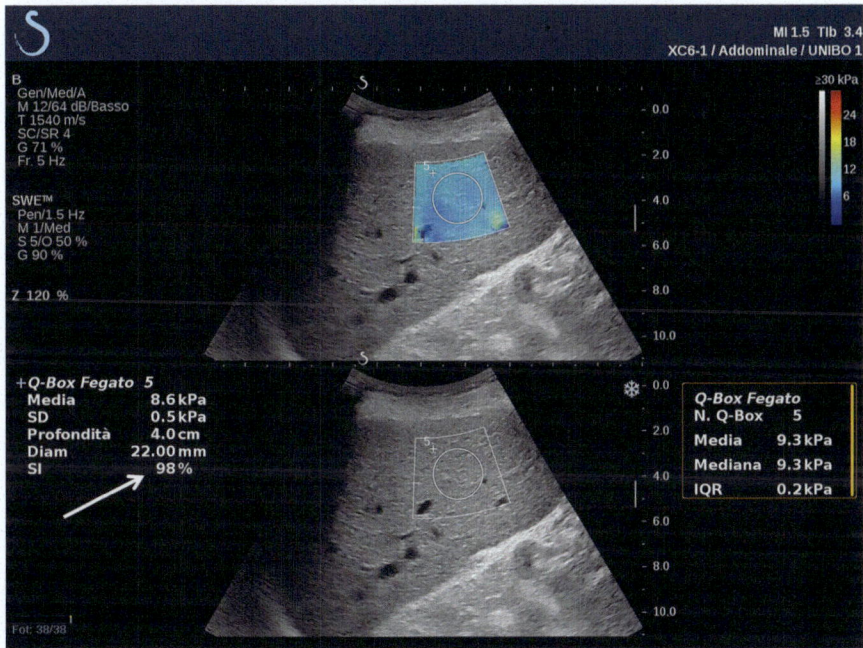

Fig. 6.3 An example of two-dimensional elastography (Aixplorer, Supersonic, France). The upper part shows the different elasticity in colors. Values related to the single image are shown in the left part, including the Stability Index (SI) (arrow) that is an indicator of homogeneity and temporal stability. To the contrary, cumulative values are reported in the right part: number of measurements, mean, median and interquartile range (IQR). Finally in the lower part of the screen, conventional B-mode is displayed

It's worth to point out that other methods exist for assessing tissue deformation when subjected to a force. When this assessment evaluates the relative deformation of a portion of tissue compared to the deformability of another portion, both subjected to the same external (ultrasound transducers rhythmically moved) or internal (force of heart beats) pressure, information about tissue stiffness is provided. These information is not quantitative and, due to the easier access of more superficial structures to the pressure of the transducers (e.g. thyroid, breast, prostate), than the liver, this technique is mostly utilized for tissue characterization of focal lesions embedded in superficial organs, rather than for absolute judgment of tissue stiffness. These techniques go under the definition of "Strain Imaging" and a color overlay indicated the degree of relative stiffness. They provide a semiquantitative assessment of tissue stiffness (ratio of different relative strains) and not a quantitative assessment. Since Strain elastography, sometimes also termed "real-time elastography" was the first method able to provide elastography information concurrently with conventional B-mode ultrasound imaging, its semiquantitative information was tested for liver stiffness assessment, but with insufficient success particularly in comparison to the shear wave elastography methods in Western patients [5] (differently from some Japanese initial reports) [6]. Therefore, they were never widely used in Western countries for liver fibrous staging and hence are no further described here. The present chapter will instead proceed with the illustration of the shear wave ultrasound technologies, since shearwave elastography provides quantitative measurements (shear wave speed, transformed into kPa) and has been extremely successful in hepatology.

6.2   Transient Elastography—Fibroscan (Echosens, France)

The first commercially available elastography technique goes under the name of Transient Elastography marketed as Fibroscan© (manufactured by Echosens™, France). The mechanical shear wave are generated by a servo-controlled vibrator, namely a piston, that acts as emitter and receiver. In the "reflection mode", the low-frequency elastic wave is sent by a single element transducer [7]. The 50 Hz centre frequency has been chosen because it combines the combination of lower diffraction effects and lower attenuation. Indeed, attenuation is directly related to frequency.

Compression waves are not directly quantified because too fast to be measured by ultrasound, whereas shear speed is slower. It can be calculated through the evaluation of displacement of radio-frequency lines within the tissue. The resultant parametric image is the so-called "shear wave propagation map", or SWPM, that derives from correlation between successive radio-frequency lines observed along a fixed ultrasound beam axis. The shear wave speed is estimated using a time of flight (TOF) algorithm by computing the slope of the peak displacement values observed on the SWPM, that is a graphic representation of the strain as a function of depth and time [8]. As for all shear wave elastography methods, stiffer the tissue, faster the wave propagation. The relative displacement of the piston-like vibrator is also taken into account. Finally, under the assumption of homogeneity, linearity and isotropy, elasticity is calculated using the above mentioned formula $E = 3\rho V$ [8].

Results are provided in kPa and the software takes into account any acquisition to automatically calculate median value and interquartile range (IQR) of multiple measurements. If the linear regression coefficient of a shear velocity estimate is below 0.85, the software automatically rejects the measurement and defines that measurement as non-valid (in fact the rate of valid, or successful, measurements and the IQR of the valid values are finally considered to define the degree of reliability of a liver stiffness assessment).

Differently from other elastographic methods, Fibroscan is a self-standing device unable to produce concurrent conventional B-mode images and its unique registered application is the liver. A prior B-mode examination of the hepatic tissue is not absolutely required, but might be useful or warranted to exclude the presence of large lesions or of any other abnormality that can affect elastography measurement. However, an idea of tissue morphology is provided by M-mode and A-mode, that are mono-dimensional ultrasound methods.

A relatively large volume (3 cm^3, 100 times more than a liver biopsy) is evaluated. Three probes are available: M-probe (conventional probe for adults), XL probe (for obese patients) and S probe (paediatric). The depth of measurement depends on the probe. The M-probe measures from 25 to 65 mm (since the ultrasound beam focus at slightly deeper than 20 mm, making more superficial information inadequate). The XL probe is designed for obese patients, whose intercostal wall thickness is expected to be greater than in non-obese subjects, thus making the liver located deeper from the transducer. This probe starts measuring stiffness at a 35 mm of depth in order to ensure measuring the liver parenchyma rather than the subcutaneous fat. Conversely, the paediatric (S-) probe measures from 15 mm. The frequency differs in the various probe, too: 5 MHz in the conventional and the paediatric probes and 2.5 MHz in the XL probe, since it is designed to collect information from deeper parts of the body [9]. Since the information is collected involving longitudinal waves, whose pressure and speed are altered in case of significant change in the crossed structures, the presence of interlaying ascites, between the intercostal wall and the liver, prevents collecting adequate information and is an obvious limit, except for some cases of small amount of fluid.

In order to provide a correct emission of the push pulse generating longitudinal waves and consequent shear waves and correct acquisitions of shear waves speed, the piston at the top of the transducer is to be pushed against the intercostal space skin exactly perpendicularly and with an adequate pressure. The adequacy of the pressure (that has to be not too strong not too light) is displayed on the screen and the push pulse is to be generated only when the push level is in the green range.

As of 2017, the Transient Elastography technique has become embedded also in one conventional ultrasound scanner following a commercial agreement with a manufacturer, but the method remains the same. This means that only the A-mode for elastography acquisition is displayed on the screen, without any concurrent display of the conventional B-mode real time modality, when the operator attempts elastography measurements. However, the combination may facilitate preliminary liver assessment with ultrasonography.

6.3   Point Shear Wave Elastography

Point shear wave elastography (pSWE) measures the speed of shear waves, that are perpendicular to longitudinal waves generated by a "push pulse" sent by the probe (i.e. Acoustic Radiation Force Impulse—ARFI) in a region of Excitation (ROE). A portion of the longitudinal waves generated by ARFI is intra-converted to shear waves through the absorption of acoustic energy [10]. The propagation time T is obtained by comparing the waveform profile of the displacement through time at different lateral positions. This is done within a short distance from the excitation line, usually 5–10 mm, a distance after which the shear waves tend to disappear. This region is commonly indicated by a small box, named Region of Interest (ROI), usually 5 mm wide × 10 mm long (Fig. 6.2). Being therefore this region quite small it was assumed to the measurement in a single point of the liver and therefore this elastography modality was named "point shear wave velocity" (pSWE) by EFSUMB in its 2013 first guidelines set [11]. Then, shear wave speed is calculated as the ratio between the distance and the propagation time. In this way, the elastic modulus E is obtained without estimating stress whilst the equation relies in the assumption, once more, of a linear, isotropic, incompressible and homogeneous material [12].

It is to be noted that an adequate contact between the probe and the skin is mandatory in order to generate a sufficient force for excitation propagating within the body for a sufficient distance. For the same reason, a big heterogeneity of acoustic properties of the material avoids the generation of shear waves.

One of the main advantages is that it can be performed with ultrasound equipments that can concurrently produce the conventional gray scale B-mode images. The pSWE ROI can be freely moved in any portion of the field of view up to 8 cm in depth (Fig. 6.2) within the usual conventional B-mode display modality. Therefore, the stiffness is obtained in well-defined regions, so that large fibrotic scars, focal lesions or vessels inside the liver can be accurately avoided as well as the most superficial regions, close to the Glisson's capsule. This method allows also easy measurement of the spleen stiffness, since the measurement box is easily put in the target region within the splenic parenchyma.

The first manufacturer that offered this kind of elastography was Siemens (under the name of ARFI virtual touch quantification VTq) but so far it has become available on Esaote, GE, Hitachi, Philips and Samsung devices, too.

Although working with the same theoretical principle, the different pSWE provided by the various manufacturers produced up to moderately different stiffness value when investigating the same liver [13]. This is due to different hardware (including both the equipment and the transducers) and different software to generate the shear wave and to measure its speed. Thus a recommendation is made that when this technology (pSWE) is utilized, the operator includes in report the stiffness value but also the equipment used to acquire it (and possibly the transducers and software version). This can be done briefly adopting a pSWE.XXX description (where the three letters stay for the manufacturers, e.g. pSWE.SIE for Siemens, pSWE.ESA for Esaote or pSWE.PHI for Philips and so on).

6.4   Two-Dimensional Shear-Wave Elastography

This approach shows elastography over a bidimensional region, usually at least of 3 × 2 cm. The Aixplorer Supersonic Imagine system (France) uses a multifocal zone configuration in which each next focal zone is interrogated a bit deeper than the previous in rapid succession, leading to a longitudinal pressure with Mach cone shape generating lateral shear-waves. Concurrently, the system acquires raw radiofrequency data along the same scan at a very high frame rate, up to 5000 frames/s. The resulting ROI, whose size can be adjusted, displays 2D-SWE findings in colours (or more rarely in gray scale) and in can be overlaid on the B-mode gray scale conventional image or displayed separately, side-by-side. Beside a visual judgment of the elastogram, different ROI (usually round-shaped) can be placed at desired locations to obtain statistical quantities such as mean, standard deviations, minimum and maximum values of the shear-wave speed (Fig. 6.3). Generally, red refers to stiffer regions, blue to softer regions are green and yellow to intermediate stiffness. It is worth to remark that the range of the scale can be modified by the operator in real time in most equipments. Consequently, the visual assessment of the distribution of color must take into consideration the upper limit of the scale in order to avoid misinterpretation. The shear wave speed is calculated using the above mentioned formula of the Young's modulus. The mean stiffness value of the circular ROI is displayed together with the standard deviations. When multiple acquisitions are taken the final value has to be expressed as median and Interquartile Range of the various mean values. On Supersonic devices 3D-SWE can be also implemented by using a 3D probe that contain mechanically swept 1D transducer array.

So far, besides Aixplorer Supersonic Imagine, 2-D shear wave elastography is available also on Toshiba, GE, Philips and Mindray equipments, products that are broadly similar in the way the stiffness is displayed on the screen but differ with respect to the details of the methods to produce the elastography information and the sampling rate. Among peculiarities, the motion of the excitation sources through the tissue, caused by rapid changes in beam focus, generates shear waves from the whole longitudinal axis in the Aixplorer equipment whereas multiple pushing beams are sent simultaneously in a comb-like pattern in the GE equipment.

Recently most equipments providing 2D SWE introduced also quality control measures, to verify that the shear wave speed is homogeneous over various parts of the color elastogram box. This allows to include in the final calculation only measures that are expected to provide reliable data, devoid of or with limited artifacts, but the choice whether to keep the measurement or not is left to the operator (together with the location where the circular ROI is set).

The evaluation of data reliability in the Toshiba equipment is possible using the propagation mode, that is the visualization of the arrival time contour of the shear waves: the intervals between lines is constant in absence of obstacles whereas a distortion of the contour lines indicates lower data reliability (Fig. 6.4).

One of the commonest artifact is a stiff area in the upper part of the ROI, probably due to the pressure of the probe that stiffens the superficial part. However, it is well recognizable so it can be easily rejected.

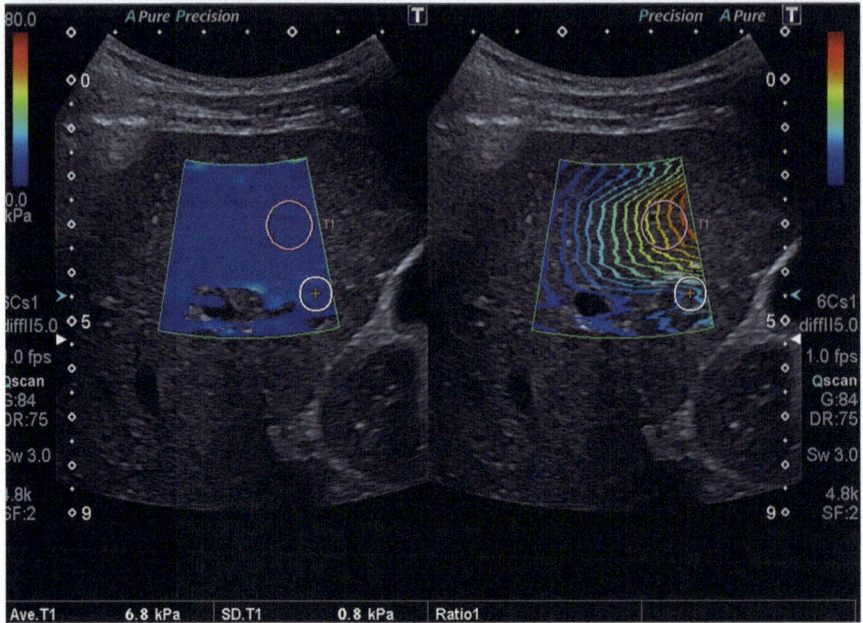

Fig. 6.4 An example of the propagation mode available on Toshiba (Toshiba Medical System Corporation, Japan) equipment. The visualization of the arrival time contour of the shear waves allows to take the measurement where lines are parallel, increasing data reliability

6.5 Kpa or m/s?

Whilst different technologies may share the same principle, the resulting values are different. Generally, values expressed in m/s can be expressed in kPa according to the formula:

value in kPa = 3 * (value in m/s).

However, cut off values obtained using a device cannot be universally adopted for defining liver fibrosis staging, for example, for all the machines [13] due to differences in each algorithm.

There is more than one reason to use m/s instead of kPa. Firstly, because m/s is the unit of shear wave speed and conversion to kPa using the above mentioned formula implies the assumptions of:

- tissue density always stable at 1000 kg/m³
- linear tissue response
- the elastic modulus is not affected by shear wave frequency
- the tissue in isotropic, that is that no variation occurs depending on direction
- there are any boundary that may affect the kind of wave and, thus, invalidate the relation between speed and elastic modulus [1].

Following all these reasons, in the USA, where elastography was approved only very recently, most equipments are arranged to provide stiffness in speed units, whereas in Europe stiffness is nearly invariably provided in kPa, since the first ultrasound elastography equipment providing a measure of stiffness, the Fibroscan©, which gained popularity and gave an imprinting to all followers creating a sort of mental standard for hepatologists, provides results only in kPa.

KPa is also the unit of G, the shear modulus, that is commonly used for MR elastography results, rather than Young's modulus. It is worth to remind that the numerical data for the two moduli are different. Thus, threshold emerged by MR elastography cannot be used for ultrasound elastography and vice versa and the relationship is in terms of three times (ultrasound elastography results are three times the values produced by MR elastography).

6.6   Examination Technique

Whatever the elastographic method, the examination technique is the same: the patient must be fasting since ≥ 2 h (at best 4–6 h) and placed in supine position with the right arm in maximum abduction in order to widen the intercostal spaces. Breathing is to be suspended for 2–5 s when the operator is ready for the measurements, in order to minimize breathing motion and to place the transducer in the correct position. The measurement is taken with a convex probe though a right intercostal space, usually in the right liver lobe, 1–2 cm under the liver capsule in full parenchyma, with only a light pressure applied with the transducers on the skin. The transducer has to be positioned at best in a way producing the insonation plane to be perpendicular to the skin and with good acoustic contact on the entire footprint. The examination site has been chosen to maximize the agreement with liver biopsy, usually performed intercostally in the right lobe, and to increase reproducibility. Focal lesions, large vessels and scars are to be avoided in the measurement region. Factors that may decrease reproducibility are high BMI, high interquartile range (IQR) values of the measurements, large waist circumference. Accuracy may also be affected by deep inspiration, recent meal intake (usually <2 h), inflammation, cholestasis, heart failure (all of which tend to increase stiffness values), drinking behavior, coffee or herbal tea consumption and antiviral treatment (which decrease liver stiffness without a corresponding decrease in liver fibrosis). The influence of the severity of liver steatosis remains questioned, although it was suggested that severe fatty infiltration tend to overestimate liver fibrosis, regardless of the methods utilized [14–19].

Conclusions

In conclusion, many different technologies share the name "elastography". However, everyone has its own peculiarities whose knowledge is mandatory to use them appropriately for fibrosis estimation. The distinction in strain elastography, transient elastography, point shear wave elastography or two dimensional shear wave elastography is relevant and should be included in the report together with the equipment utilized. In fact, results obtained with different equipment from different manufacturers (and possibly even from different models of the same manufacturer) are not identical.

References

1. Dietrich CF, Bamber J, Berzigotti A, et al. EFSUMB guidelines and recommendations on the clinical use of liver ultrasound elastography, update 2017 (long version). Ultraschall Med. 2017;38(4):e16–47. Epub 2017Apr 13
2. Ophir J, Céspedes I, Ponnekanti H, et al. Elastography: a quantitative method for imaging the elasticity of biological tissues. Ultrason Imaging. 1991;13(2):111–34.
3. Shiina T, Nightingale KR, Palmeri ML, et al. WFUMB guidelines and recommendations for clinical use of ultrasound elastography. Part 1: Basic principles and terminology. Ultrasound Med Biol. 2015;41(5):1126–47.
4. Taljanovic MS, Gimber LH, Becker GW, et al. Shear-wave elastography: basic physics and musculoskeletal applications. Radiographics. 2017;37(3):855–70.
5. Friedrich-Rust M, Schwart A, Ong M, et al. Real-time tissue elastography versus FibroScan for noninvasive assessment of liver fibrosis in chronic liver disease. Ultraschall Med. 2009;30:478–84.
6. Morikawa H, Fukuda K, Kobayashi S, et al. Real-time tissue elastography as a tool for the noninvasive assessment of liver stiffness in patients with chronic hepatitis C. J Gastroenterol. 2011;46(3):350–8.
7. Sandrin L, Tanter M, Catheline S, et al. Shear modulus imaging with 2-D transient elastography. IEEE Trans Ultrason Ferroelectr Freq Control. 2002;49(4):426–35.
8. Audière S, Angelini ED, Sandrin L, et al. Maximum likelihood estimation of shear wave speed in transient elastography. IEEE Trans Med Imaging. 2014;33(6):1338–49.
9. de Lédinghen V, Vergniol J, Foucher J, et al. Feasibility of liver transient elastography with FibroScan using a new probe for obese patients. Liver Int. 2010;30(7):1043–8.
10. Nightingale K. Acoustic radiation force impulse (ARFI) imaging: a review. Curr Med Imaging Rev. 2011;7(4):328–39.
11. Bamber J, Cosgrove D, Dietrich CF, et al. EFSUMB guidelines and recommendations on the clinical use of ultrasound elastography. Part 1: Basic principles and technology. Ultraschall Med. 2013;34(2):169–84.
12. Shiina T. JSUM ultrasound elastography practice guidelines: basics and terminology. J Med Ultrason (2001). 2013;40(4):309–23.
13. Piscaglia F, Salvatore V, Mulazzani L, et al. Differences in liver stiffness values obtained with new ultrasound elastography machines and Fibroscan: a comparative study. Dig Liver Dis. 2017;49(7):802–8. PII: S1590-8658(17)30246-3
14. Alferink LJM, Fittipaldi J, Kiefte-de Jong JC, et al. Coffee and herbal tea consumption is associated with lower liver stiffness in the general population: the Rotterdam study. J Hepatol. 2017;S0168-8278(17):30147–2.
15. Boursier J, Konaté A, Gorea G, et al. Reproducibility of liver stiffness measurement by ultrasonographic elastometry. Clin Gastroenterol Hepatol. 2008;6(11):1263–9.
16. Cordero-Ruiz P, Carmona-Soria I, Rodríguez-Téllez M, et al. Long-term follow-up of patients with chronic hepatitis C treated with α-interferon and ribavirin antiviral therapy: clinical and fibrosis impact of treatment response. Eur J Gastroenterol Hepatol. 2017;29(7):792–9.
17. Park SH, Kim SY, Suh CH, et al. What we need to know when performing and interpreting US elastography. Clin Mol Hepatol. 2016;22(3):406–14.
18. Petta S, Maida M, Macaluso FS, et al. The severity of steatosis influences liver stiffness measurement in patients with nonalcoholic fatty liver disease. Hepatology. 2015;262(4):1101–10.
19. Stevenson M, Lloyd-Jones M, Morgan MY, et al. Non-invasive diagnostic assessment tools for the detection of liver fibrosis in patients with suspected alcohol-related liver disease: a systematic review and economic evaluation. Health Technol Assess. 2012;16(4):1–174.

Liver Stiffness by Ultrasound Elastography

7

Laurent Castera

7.1 Introduction

Over the past decade, non-invasive methods have been increasingly validated and used for staging liver fibrosis. Among these methods, transient elastography (TE) (FibroScan™, Echosens, Paris, France), an ultrasound-based technique allowing to measure liver stiffness (LS), has reached an established role in clinical practice, and is now routinely used worldwide, particularly in viral hepatitis [1]. Given its excellent performance for diagnosing cirrhosis (with mean AUROC values above 0.90), TE use has been recommended as first line tool for prioritizing patients for HCV therapy, based on disease stage, by several international guidelines [2–4]. With the wide availability of TE, most patients are currently diagnosed at a very initial stage of cirrhosis, in which clinically significant portal hypertension (CSPH, defined by an hepatic venous gradient pressure (HVPG) ≥ 10 mmHg) or eosophageal varices (OV) are often absent. In order to better reflect the fact that the spectrum of severe fibrosis and cirrhosis is a continuum in asymptomatic patients, and that distinguishing between the two is often not possible on clinical grounds, the alternative term "compensated advanced chronic liver disease (cACLD)", defined by LS >10 kPa using TE, has been proposed by the Baveno VI consensus on PH [5]. In this new scenario, a large proportion of HVPG measurements and screening endoscopy may be unnecessary. Therefore, efforts should be directed at limiting these procedures to those patients at higher risk of CSPH and varices, so as to reducing healthcare cost and lessen patients' discomfort [6]. Alternative ultrasound-based elastography techniques, such as point shear wave elastography (pSWE), also known as acoustic radiation force impulse imaging (ARFI) and 2D-shearwave elastography (2D-SWE)

L. Castera, M.D., Ph.D.
Department of Hepatology, Hôpital Beaujon, Assistance Publique—Hôpitaux de Paris,
INSERM UMR 1149, CRI, University of Paris-VII, Clichy, France
e-mail: laurent.d.castera@gmail.com; laurent.castera@bjn.aphp.fr

© Springer International Publishing AG 2018, part of Springer Nature
A. Berzigotti, J. Bosch (eds.), *Diagnostic Methods for Cirrhosis and Portal Hypertension*, https://doi.org/10.1007/978-3-319-72628-1_7

have also been proposed [7]. This chapter is aimed at reviewing the role of LS measurement, using the different available ultrasound elastography techniques (TE, pSWE and 2D SWE), for the prediction and the follow-up of patients with portal hypertension (PH).

7.2   Currently Available Ultrasound Elastography Methods

7.2.1   Transient Elastography

TE was the first commercially available elastography method developed for the measurement of LS, using a dedicated device, which uses an amplitude modulation (A)-mode image for organ and measurement site localization. An ultrasound transducer probe is mounted on the axis of a vibrator, which induces an elastic shear wave that propagates through the tissue. Pulse-echo ultrasound acquisition is used to follow the propagation of the shear wave and to measure its velocity, which is directly related to tissue stiffness—the stiffer the tissue, the faster the shear wave propagates [8]. The examination is performed on the right lobe of the liver through the intercostal space. The measurement depth is between 25–65 mm using the M-probe (standard probe) and between 35–75 mm using the XL-probe. As suggested by the manufacturer, the median of ten successful acquisitions should be used for interpretation. Results are expressed in kilopascals (kPa), and range from 1.5 to 75 kPa with a normal value around 5 kPa [9].

Advantages of TE include a short procedure time (<5 min), immediate results, excellent inter- and intra-observer agreement, and the ability to perform the test at the bedside or in an outpatient clinic—it is not a difficult procedure to learn (Table 7.1). However, accurate results require careful interpretation of data, based on at least ten validated measurements and an interquartile range (IQR, reflects variations among measurements) of less than 30% of the median value (IQR/LSM ≤30%) [11]. It has been suggested that an even lower interquartile range should be used, especially in non-Asian patients with advanced fibrosis, but these criteria have not been independently validated [12].

7.2.2   Point and 2D Shear Wave Elastography

As compared with TE, pSWE/ARFI and 2D-SWE have the advantage of being integrated in conventional ultrasonography systems, enabling the additional performance of elastography with the same probes as those performing an abdominal ultrasound scan [10] (Table 7.1). The region of interest (ROI) for measurement can be positioned under B-mode ultrasound vision away from interfering structures such as vessels or the gallbladder. While using point SWE, a single acoustic impulse is used to induce a shear wave within a small ROI (approximately 1.0 × 0.5 cm). Multiple shear waves can be induced using acoustic impulses in 2D SWE, either as a single image or in real-time in a larger field of the liver (approximately 2 × 2 cm).

Table 7.1 Respective advantages and disadvantages of currently available ultrasound elastography methods (adapted from Ref. [10])

Method	Devices	Advantages	Disadvantages
Transient elastography	• FibroScan (Echosens, France)	• User friendly, rapid learning curve, bedside examination • Well-defined quality criteria • Good reproducibility • Most extensively evaluated • Good diagnostic accuracy for liver fibrosis staging • Excellent diagnostic accuracy for excluding liver cirrhosis • Prognostic value in cirrhosis	• Dedicated device is required • ROI cannot be selected • ROI is rather small • No B-mode orientation • Limited applicability (ascites, severe obesity) • Operator-related and patient-related variability
Point SWE	• VTQ using ARFI imaging (Siemens Healthcare, Germany) • ElastPQ (Philips Healthcare, Netherlands) • Shear Wave Measurement (Hitachi Aloka Medical, Japan)	• Integrated into a conventional ultrasound machine • ROI localization can be chosen under B-mode visualization • Good applicability (ascites, obesity) • Comparable diagnostic accuracy to transient elastography for the staging of liver fibrosis and diagnosis of cirrhosis	• Units in m/s only in some machines with narrow range of values • Quality criteria not well defined • Smaller ROI size than transient elastography • Size of ROI cannot be modified • Less well evaluated • No prognostic studies published
2D SWE	• ShearWave Elastography (SuperSonic Imagine, France) • Virtual Touch IQ (Siemens Healthcare, Germany) • Logiq E9 (GE Healthcare, UK) • Aplio 500 (Toshiba Medical Systems, UK)	• Integrated into a conventional ultrasound machine • ROI size larger than transient elastography and point SWE • ROI size can be modified • Real-time measurement possible • High range of values (2–150 kPa) • Good applicability (ascites, obesity) • Comparable diagnostic accuracy to transient elastography for the staging of liver fibrosis and diagnosis of cirrhosis	• Quality criteria not well defined • Less well evaluated • No prognostic studies published

The velocity can then be measured, selecting ROIs in any location within this measurement field. Depending on the company and technique, the size of the ROI is either fixed or can be chosen by the examiner. Measurement results can be displayed in m/s, kPa or both. The technique for shear wave induction, and the frequencies used, differ between companies and should be taken into account when interpreting the results. Also to date, no clear quality criteria for the performance and interpretation of ARFI and 2D SWE are recommended by the manufacturers.

7.2.3 Limitations of Ultrasound Elastography

High reproducibility has been reported for all elastography methods, with intra-observer and inter-observer agreement at >85% [10]. TE has been evaluated most intensively, leading to identification of substantial operator-related variability as well as patient-related variability. The main limitation of TE in clinical practice is its limited applicability (80%) (failure 4% and unreliable results 16%) in case of obesity and limited operator experience [13]. The limitation of high BMI using the M-probe has been improved with the development of the XL-probe, which measures deeper under the tissue. However, LS values with the XL-probe are lower than with the M-probe, which should be taken into account when interpreting the results [14]. Point SWE and 2D-SWE can be performed with one probe in all patients, independent of body weight, as the ROI can be positioned manually in different depths of the liver. As compared to TE, ascites is not a limitation for pSWE and 2D-SWE.

Whatever the elastography technique, LS values increase after meal intake [15]. Elastography should therefore be performed after fasting for at least 2 h. In addition, factors that increase tension within the Glisson's capsule also increase LS measured with the elastography methods, leading to an overestimation of liver fibrosis. Such factors include the following: necroinflammatory histological activity; alanine aminotransferase flare in acute or chronic hepatitis; elevated central venous pressure; cardiac failure and intrahepatic or extrahepatic cholestasis; and excessive alcohol intake [2].

In summary, these techniques need to be performed using a standardized protocol and with critically interpreted results, taking confounding factors into account.

7.3   Detection of Cirrhosis

7.3.1   Transient Elastography

The good performance of TE for detecting cirrhosis, evidenced initially in patients with chronic hepatitis C [16, 17], has been confirmed in other chronic liver diseases, including chronic hepatitis B, NAFLD as well as cholestatic liver diseases [18–32]. Several meta-analyses [33–37], based on several thousands of patients, have shown the excellent diagnostic accuracy of TE for cirrhosis with AUROCs of 0.93–0.96, sensitivities of 83–87%, specificities of 89–95% and cut-offs ranging from 13.0 to 15.6 kPa. It should be noted that TE is better at ruling out, rather than ruling in liver cirrhosis (with negative predictive value higher than 90%). Also different cut-offs have been proposed for different liver diseases, depending on the distribution of fibrosis stages in different cohorts, but no consensus has been reached. In that respect, it should be kept in mind that the cut-off choice must also consider the pre-test probability of cirrhosis in the target population (varying from <1% in the general population to 10–20% in tertiary referral centres). For example, it has been shown that in a population with a pre-test probability of 13.8%, cirrhosis probability at a cut-off <7 kPa ranged from 0–3%, whereas at a cut-off >17 kPa, cirrhosis probability was 72% [31]. Thus, observer experience, patient factors, disease aetiology, as well as pre-test probability of cirrhosis should be taken into account when LS values are interpreted.

7.3.2   pSWE and 2D SWE

pSWE performance has been evaluated in several meta-analyses reporting accuracies of 91–93% for diagnosing cirrhosis [38–40] and cut-offs ranging from 1.80–2.31 m/s. ARFI like TE is better at ruling out than ruling in liver cirrhosis. Another meta-analysis comparing ARFI with TE reported comparable sensitivities and specificities for the assessment of liver fibrosis [41]. As for 2D SWE, a meta-analysis, based on individual data in 1340 patients with chronic liver disease, reported diagnostic accuracies of 95% for cirrhosis with an optimal cut-off of 13.5 kPa [42]. Again, 2D SWE is also better at ruling out than ruling in liver cirrhosis. When comparing 2D SWE to TE in this meta-analysis, no significant difference was found between the two methods if the quality criteria of TE were respected. Finally, studies comparing TE, pSWE and 2D SWE in the same patient population reported comparable results for all three methods [43, 44].

7.4   Detection of Clinically Significant Portal Hypertension

7.4.1   Transient Elastography

There is substantial evidence indicating that LS using TE can be quite effective in detecting patients with a high risk of having (or not having) developed CSPH. First, a good correlation between LS values and HVPG has been shown more than 10 years ago, initially in patients with recurrence of hepatitis C infection after liver transplantation [45]. These findings have been confirmed by many studies in patients with advanced liver disease since [46–60]. Second, as shown in Table 7.2, the diagnostic performances of TE for the detection of CSPH in the setting of patients with compensated chronic liver disease/cirrhosis are good, with area under the ROC curve (AUROCs) ranging from 0.80 to 0.99. These excellent performances have been confirmed in a recent meta-analysis (based on 11 studies including 1451

Table 7.2 Diagnostic performance of TE for the detection of clinically significant portal hypertension (HVPG ≥10 mmHg)

Authors	Year	Study design	Patients (n)	Etiologies	Child A (%)	CSPH (%)	Cut-offs (kPa)	AUROC	Se (%)	Sp (%)
Vizzutti et al. [46]	2007	Retrospective	61	HCV	46	77	13.6	0.99	97	92
Lemoine et al. [48]	2008	Retrospective	44	HCV	100	77	20.5	0.76	63	70
			48	OH		83	34.9	0.94	90	88
Bureau et al. [47]	2008	Prospective	150	CLD	20	51	21.0	0.94	90	93
Sanchez-Condé et al. [49]	2011	Prospective	38	HIV-HCV	71	74	14.0	0.80	93	50
Llop et al. [50]	2012	Prospective	79	CLD	100	40	13.6/21.0	0.84	91/58	57/91
Reiberger et al. [52]	2012	Retrospective	502	CLD	NA	55	18.0	0.82	83	82
Colecchia et al. [51]	2012	Prospective	100	HCV	68	65	16.0/24.2	0.92	95/52	69/92
Berzigotti et al. [61]	2013	Prospective	117	CLD	88	67	13.6/21.1	0.88	91/65	56/92
			56	CLD	70	86	13.6/21.1	0.91	NA	NA
Hong et al. [55]	2013	Retrospective	59	OH-HBV	NA	NA	21.9	0.85	82	74
Augustin et al. [54]	2014	Prospective	40	CLD	100	65	25.0	NA	65	93
Cho et al. [58]	2015	Retrospective	219	OH	59	NA	NA	0.85	NA	NA
Zykus et al. [56]	2015	Prospective	107	CLD	64	73	17.4	0.95	88	87
Schwabl et al. [57]	2015	Retrospective	188	Viral-OH	NA	31	16.1	0.96	95	87
Kitson et al. [53]	2015	Prospective	95	CLD	91	74	29.0	0.90	72	100
Lee et al. [60]	2016	Retrospective	47	Viral-OH	60	83	19.7	0.75	74	83
Kumar et al. [59]	2017	Retrospective	326	NASH-OH	NA	85	21.6	0.74	79	67

patients) with a hierarchical summary AUROC of 0.90 and with sensitivity and specificity above 85% (sensitivity: 87.5%; 95% confidence interval [CI]: 75.8–93.9%; specificity: 85.3%; 95% CI: 76.9–90.9%) [62]. Nevertheless, the results of these studies (summarized in Table 7.2) deserve several comments: most of them have been conducted in European expert centers where HVPG is available with a likely referral bias and half of them were retrospective. Indeed, studied populations were mostly viral in terms of etiologies, with small sample size (<100 patients) and high prevalence of CSPH (51–86%) and some studies included patients with decompensated cirrhosis. These are limitations that are inherent to the HVPG technique and thus will be difficult to overcome but that hamper the applicability of these results to the target population of patients with early cirrhosis eligible for screening. Also proposed cut-offs for predicting CSPH vary from 13.6 to 34.9 kPa, making the optimal cut-off difficult to be defined. In the largest studied population (n = 502), Reiberger et al. [52] have shown that, at a cut-off of 18 kPa, TE was better at ruling in than ruling out CSPH (Positive and negative predictive values of 86% of 81%). Other authors [50] have proposed a dual cut-off strategy (<13.6 kPa with a 90% sensitivity for CSPH diagnosis and >21 kPa with a 90% specificity), allowing a correct stratification of presence/absence of CSPH in patients with compensated cirrhosis and potentially resectable hepatocellular carcinoma, reducing the need for invasive hemodynamic assessment in around 50% of patients. However, while the correlation is excellent for HVPG values between 5 and 10–12 mmHg (typical of cirrhosis without evident clinical manifestations related to portal hypertension), it hardly reaches statistical significance for values above 12 mmHg [46]. This is because, with the progression of cirrhosis, the mechanisms of portal hypertension (PH) become less and less dependent on the intrahepatic resistance to portal flow due to tissue fibrosis and progressively more dependent on extra-hepatic factors (i.e. hyperdynamic circulation, splanchnic vasodilatation) [63]. This observation sets a key limitation to the use of liver stiffness measurements as a non-invasive surrogate of HVPG beyond the prediction of clinically significant (HVPG ≥10 mmHg) and severe (HVPG ≥12 mmHg) PH, and, accordingly, TE of the liver is unlikely to be useful in monitoring the hemodynamic response to the administration of beta-blockers or disease progression in the decompensated phase. Finally, given the amount of published data, the Baveno VI consensus on PH agreed that values of LS by TE >20–25 kPa can be used to identify CSPH [5]. It should be kept in mind, however, that these cut-offs have been identified in patients with mostly viral hepatitis-related cirrhosis and need to be validated in other etiologies.

Last but not least, some authors have proposed in order to increase the diagnostic accuracy to combine LS with parameters associated with PH, such as platelet count or spleen diameter by ultrasound [61, 64]. Indeed, in a population of 117 patients with compensated cirrhosis, using LSPS (LSM-Spleen diameter to Platelet ratio Score) or PH risk score, more than 80% of patients were accurately classified for CSPH [61]. These results have been confirmed recently in a large multicenter retrospective cohort of 518 patients with cACLD [65] and could represent an attractive strategy for screening patients for CSPH.

7.4.2   pSWE and 2D SWE

There is a limited number of studies (n = 7) reporting on the performance of pSWE and 2D SWE, which are summarized in Table 7.3. In the three studies using pSWE [66–68], the diagnostic accuracy for CSPH was very good with AUROCs ranging from 0.82 to 0.90 and high applicability. As for 2D-SWE, the diagnostic performances were very good as well (AUROC 0.82–0.90). Two studies only compared 2D-SWE head to head with TE and with conflicting results: in one study [70], performance of 2D-SWE was better than that of TE whereas in the other [69] performance did not differ. Conversely, in both studies, applicability of 2D-SWE was significantly better than that of TE. More studies are therefore needed before any firm conclusion can be drawn.

7.5   Detection of Eosophageal Varices

7.5.1   Transient Elastography

The diagnostic accuracy of LS to predict the presence and size of OV has been the subject of more than 50 studies [73]. LS values are higher in patients with OV and tend to be higher in patients with large OV (LOV). However, LS is less accurate for the prediction of OV than for CSPH [74]. In a recent meta-analysis [75] (based on 18 studies and 3644 patients), the diagnostic performances of TE for predicting OV and LOV were not as good as for CSPH, with AUROCS of 0.84 and 0.78, respectively. Although the summary sensitivity for the prediction of the presence of OV and LOV was high (0.87 (95% CI: 0.80–0.92); 0.86 (95% CI: 0.71–0.94), respectively), specificity was much lower (0.53 (95% CI: 0.36–0.69); 0.59 (95% CI: 0.45–0.72), respectively) and less satisfactory. Finally, as mentioned before for CSPH, scores combining LS with platelet count and spleen diameter by ultrasound such as LSPS or the Varices Risk Score have been proposed [61, 64]. For instance, in 401 Korean patients with HBV cirrhosis, LSPS had a significantly better AUROC than TE alone for prediction of high-risk OV (0.95 vs. 0.88 in the training set, respectively, p < 0.001) [64]. At a cut-off <3.5, LSPS had a 94.0% negative predictive value and a 94.2% positive predictive value at a cut-off >5.5. Overall, upper GI endoscopy could be saved in 90.3% patients. In another study in 173 patients with compensated cirrhosis, Berzigotti et al. [61] have shown, using the Varices Risk Score, that only 3 of 70 with varices (4%; all with small varices) would have been missed if upper GI endoscopy was delayed. The performances of LSPS have also been confirmed externally [51, 61, 65, 76]. Some other authors have proposed the combination of LS and platelet count [54, 77], with good results for ruling out varices needing treatment (low false-negative rates using thresholds of LS <20–25 kPa plus platelet count >120–150 g/L). Similarly, in a large multicenter retrospective cohort of patients with cACLD, Abraldes et al. [65] have confirmed that both LSPS and a model combining TE and platelet count identified patients with very low risk (<5%) risk of varices needing treatment. Thus the Baveno VI consensus on PH

Table 7.3 Diagnostic performance of pSWE or 2D-SWE for the detection of clinically significant portal hypertension (HVPG $\geq$10 mmHg)

Authors	Year	Design	Patients (n)	Etiologies	CP A (%)	CSPH (%)	Cut-offs	AUROC	Se (%)	Sp (%)
pSWE										
Salzl et al. [66]	2014	Prospective	88	OH-Viral	17	66	TE 16.8 kPa	0.87	90	75
							ppSWE 2.6 m/s	0.85	71	87
Attia et al. [67]	2015	Prospective	78	CLD	27	90	pSWE 2.17 m/s	0.93	97	89
Takuma et al. [68]	2016	Prospective	60	Viral-OH	68	57	pSWE NA	0.83	NA	NA
2D-SWE										
Procopet et al. [69]	2015	Prospective	88/55[a]	CLD	100	49	TE 13.6/21.0 kPa	0.92	91/63	71/95
							2D-SWE 15.4 kPa	0.93	90	89
Elkrief et al. [70]	2015	Prospective	79	CLD	30	87	TE 65.3 kPa	0.78	52	100
							2D-SWE 24.5 kPa	0.87	81	88
Kim et al. [71]	2015	Prospective	115	CLD	49	84	2D-SWE 15.2 kPa	0.82	86	80
Jansen et al. [72]	2016	Prospective	158	CLD	63	NA	2D-SWE 24.5 kPa	0.86	69	80

[a]Compensated

proposed using the combination of LS and platelet count (i.e. platelet count >150 g/L and LSM <20 kPa) to identify patients with ACLD that could safely avoid screening endoscopy [5]. Interestingly, the performance of these criteria has been confirmed independently in various populations [65, 78–81] and all studies confirmed that about 20% of upper GI endoscopies could be safely avoided, missing less than 4% of patients with varices needing treatment. These recommendations represent a significant advance in the management of patients with cACLD and can be confidently applied in everyday practice. It should be kept in mind, however, that most patients in the studies on which these recommendations have been elaborated had viral hepatitis-related cACLD. Thus the proposed cut-offs for LS and platelet count may not apply to patients with other etiologies, such as cholestatic liver diseases. Finally, very recently some authors have proposed to expand the Baveno VI criteria: platelet count >110 g/L and LSM <25 kPa [82]. Overall, these Expanded-Baveno VI criteria would potentially spare a higher number of upper GI endoscopies (40% instead of 21% with Baveno VI criteria) with a risk of missing varices needing treatment of 1.6% (95% CI: 0.7–3.5%) in patients within the criteria and 0.6% (95% CI: 0.3–1.4%) in the overall population (n = 925 patients). These expanded criteria require additional validation before implementation.

7.5.2   pSWE and 2D SWE

There is a very limited number of studies (n = 5) reporting on the performance of pSWE and 2D SWE for detection of OV and LOV [66, 67, 70, 83, 84]. Generally, as for TE, LS values using pSWE and 2D SWE were higher in patients with varices than in those without varices, and increased in patients with large varices. However, validated cut-off values are not available yet. More data are needed before any firm conclusions can be drawn.

7.6   Follow-Up of Patients with Portal Hypertension

TE is a promising approach for predicting liver-related complications and mortality, with the first 'proof of concept' evidence coming from a retrospective study showing a correlation in patients with CLD between LS values and disease severity, including complications related to PH [20]. Several prospective studies [53, 85–89], as well as a meta-analysis [90], have confirmed these results since, showing the ability of baseline LS to predict clinical decompensation in patients with CLD. These studies, summarized in Table 7.4, deserve however several comments. Most of them only included small-to-medium size cohorts of patients (ranging from 95 to 577), mainly with viral hepatitis, short duration of follow-up (median ranging from 15 to 49 months), and heterogeneous rate of occurrence of complications (ranging from 3% to 41%). Nevertheless, LS had acceptable AUROCs for predicting complications (ranging from 0.72 to 0.93) with most common cut-off being around 21 kPa. Although it has been suggested that not only high baseline LS but also increase in

Table 7.4 Performance of TE for predicting complications related to portal hypertension in patients with cirrhosis

Reference	Year	Etiologies	Patients (n)	Follow-up (months)	Complications (%)	AUROC	Cut-offs (kPa)	Se (%)	Sp (%)
Decompensation									
Robic et al. [85]	2011	Mixed	100	24	41	0.84	21.1	100	41
Merchante et al. [86]	2012	HIV-HCV	239	20	13	0.72	40	NA	NA
Wang et al. [87]	2014	HCV/HBV	220	36.9	13	0.92	21.1	NA	NA
Kitson et al. [53]	2015	Mixed	95	15	29	0.73	34.5	75	70
Variceal bleeding									
Kim et al. [88]	2011	HBV	577	29	4	0.93	LSPS > 6.5	NA	NA
Merchante et al. [89]	2017	HIV-HCV	446	49	3	NA	21	NA	NA

LS (>1.5 kPa/year) over time was associated with a higher risk of death, liver transplantation, or hepatic complications within a 4-year period in patients with PBC [91], no data are available regarding PH-related complications.

Interestingly, LS is often markedly reduced in treated patients with chronic hepatitis C (including those with cACLD) who achieve a sustained virological response (SVR) [92, 93]. However, LS decrease does not accurately reflect changes in portal pressure and LS decrease should not be used as a surrogate of improvement of portal hypertension. On the other hand, the persistence of LS values ≥21 kPa in patients with SVR was almost invariably associated with the persistence of CSPH in a recent study [94], suggesting that these patients remain at risk of PH-related complications. Further studies are needed before any firm conclusion can be drawn.

Finally, in patients not requiring screening upper GI endoscopy according to non-invasive criteria on the first observation, Baveno VI recommended that these patients should undergo yearly LS measurement and platelet count determination to decide the optimum time for first endoscopy. This recommendation requires further validation.

Conclusions

Liver stiffness, using ultrasound elastography, has changed the clinical management of patients with compensated advanced chronic liver disease: it is now widely used in these patients as a non-invasive point-of-care tool to identify the presence of portal hypertension, its severity, and the risk of portal hypertension-related complications. Among the different available technique, transient elastography is by far the most validated one. More than 90% of patients with a liver stiffness >20–25 kPa will have clinically significant portal hypertension. Also upper GI endoscopy can be safely avoided by using the combination of liver stiffness and platelet count. when liver stiffness is <20 kPa and platelet count >150 g/L, varices needing treatment are very unlikely (<5% risk) to be present on endoscopy. Finally, liver stiffness can be used to predict clinical decompensation in patients with compensated advanced chronic liver disease.

References

1. Castera L. Noninvasive methods to assess liver disease in patients with hepatitis B or C. Gastroenterology. 2012;142:1293–302. e1294
2. EASL-ALEH Clinical Practice Guidelines. Non-invasive tests for evaluation of liver disease severity and prognosis. J Hepatol. 2015;63:237–64.
3. Dietrich CF, Bamber J, Berzigotti A, Bota S, Cantisani V, Castera L, Cosgrove D, et al. EFSUMB guidelines and recommendations on the clinical use of liver ultrasound elastography, update 2017 (short version). Ultraschall Med. 2017;38(4):377–94.
4. Ferraioli G, Filice C, Castera L, Choi BI, Sporea I, Wilson SR, Cosgrove D, et al. WFUMB guidelines and recommendations for clinical use of ultrasound elastography: Part 3. Liver. Ultrasound Med Biol. 2015;41:1161–79.
5. de Franchis R, Baveno VIF. Expanding consensus in portal hypertension: report of the Baveno VI Consensus Workshop: stratifying risk and individualizing care for portal hypertension. J Hepatol. 2015;63:743–52.

6. Berzigotti A, Bosch J, Boyer TD. Use of noninvasive markers of portal hypertension and timing of screening endoscopy for gastroesophageal varices in patients with chronic liver disease. Hepatology. 2014;59:729–31.
7. Berzigotti A, Castera L. Update on ultrasound imaging of liver fibrosis. J Hepatol. 2013;58:180–2.
8. Sandrin L, Fourquet B, Hasquenoph JM, Yon S, Fournier C, Mal F, Christidis C, et al. Transient elastography: a new noninvasive method for assessment of hepatic fibrosis. Ultrasound Med Biol. 2003;29:1705–13.
9. Roulot D, Czernichow S, Le Clesiau H, Costes JL, Vergnaud AC, Beaugrand M. Liver stiffness values in apparently healthy subjects: influence of gender and metabolic syndrome. J Hepatol. 2008;48:606–13.
10. Friedrich-Rust M, Poynard T, Castera L. Critical comparison of elastography methods to assess chronic liver disease. Nat Rev Gastroenterol Hepatol. 2016;13:402–11.
11. Castera L, Forns X, Alberti A. Non-invasive evaluation of liver fibrosis using transient elastography. J Hepatol. 2008;48:835–47.
12. Boursier J, Zarski JP, de Ledinghen V, Rousselet MC, Sturm N, Lebail B, Fouchard-Hubert I, et al. Determination of reliability criteria for liver stiffness evaluation by transient elastography. Hepatology. 2013;57:1182–91.
13. Castera L, Foucher J, Bernard PH, Carvalho F, Allaix D, Merrouche W, Couzigou P, et al. Pitfalls of liver stiffness measurement: a 5-year prospective study of 13,369 examinations. Hepatology. 2010;51:828–35.
14. Myers RP, Pomier-Layrargues G, Kirsch R, Pollett A, Duarte-Rojo A, Wong D, Beaton M, et al. Feasibility and diagnostic performance of the FibroScan XL probe for liver stiffness measurement in overweight and obese patients. Hepatology. 2012;55:199–208.
15. Arena U, Lupsor Platon M, Stasi C, Moscarella S, Assarat A, Bedogni G, Piazzolla V, et al. Liver stiffness is influenced by a standardized meal in patients with chronic hepatitis C virus at different stages of fibrotic evolution. Hepatology. 2013;58:65–72.
16. Castera L, Vergniol J, Foucher J, Le Bail B, Chanteloup E, Haaser M, Darriet M, et al. Prospective comparison of transient elastography, Fibrotest, APRI, and liver biopsy for the assessment of fibrosis in chronic hepatitis C. Gastroenterology. 2005;128:343–50.
17. Ziol M, Handra-Luca A, Kettaneh A, Christidis C, Mal F, Kazemi F, de Ledinghen V, et al. Noninvasive assessment of liver fibrosis by measurement of stiffness in patients with chronic hepatitis C. Hepatology. 2005;41:48–54.
18. Corpechot C, El Naggar A, Poujol-Robert A, Ziol M, Wendum D, Chazouilleres O, de Ledinghen V, et al. Assessment of biliary fibrosis by transient elastography in patients with PBC and PSC. Hepatology. 2006;43:1118–24.
19. Ganne-Carrie N, Ziol M, de Ledinghen V, Douvin C, Marcellin P, Castera L, Dhumeaux D, et al. Accuracy of liver stiffness measurement for the diagnosis of cirrhosis in patients with chronic liver diseases. Hepatology. 2006;44:1511–7.
20. Foucher J, Chanteloup E, Vergniol J, Castera L, Le Bail B, Adhoute X, Bertet J, et al. Diagnosis of cirrhosis by transient elastography (FibroScan): a prospective study. Gut. 2006;55:403–8.
21. Fraquelli M, Rigamonti C, Casazza G, Conte D, Donato MF, Ronchi G, Colombo M. Reproducibility of transient elastography in the evaluation of liver fibrosis in patients with chronic liver disease. Gut. 2007;56:968–73.
22. Coco B, Oliveri F, Maina AM, Ciccorossi P, Sacco R, Colombatto P, Bonino F, et al. Transient elastography: a new surrogate marker of liver fibrosis influenced by major changes of transaminases. J Viral Hepat. 2007;14:360–9.
23. Arena U, Vizzutti F, Abraldes JG, Corti G, Stasi C, Moscarella S, Milani S, et al. Reliability of transient elastography for the diagnosis of advanced fibrosis in chronic hepatitis C. Gut. 2008;57:1288–93.
24. Yoneda M, Yoneda M, Mawatari H, Fujita K, Endo H, Iida H, Nozaki Y, et al. Noninvasive assessment of liver fibrosis by measurement of stiffness in patients with nonalcoholic fatty liver disease (NAFLD). Dig Liver Dis. 2008;40:371–8.
25. Nobili V, Vizzutti F, Arena U, Abraldes JG, Marra F, Pietrobattista A, Fruhwirth R, et al. Accuracy and reproducibility of transient elastography for the diagnosis of fibrosis in pediatric nonalcoholic steatohepatitis. Hepatology. 2008;48:442–8.

26. Nahon P, Kettaneh A, Tengher-Barna I, Ziol M, de Ledinghen V, Douvin C, Marcellin P, et al. Assessment of liver fibrosis using transient elastography in patients with alcoholic liver disease. J Hepatol. 2008;49:1062–8.
27. Nguyen-Khac E, Chatelain D, Tramier B, Decrombecque C, Robert B, Joly JP, Brevet M, et al. Assessment of asymptomatic liver fibrosis in alcoholic patients using fibroscan: prospective comparison with 7 non-invasive laboratory tests. Aliment Pharmacol Ther. 2008;28:1188–98.
28. Marcellin P, Ziol M, Bedossa P, Douvin C, Poupon R, de Ledinghen V, Beaugrand M. Non-invasive assessment of liver fibrosis by stiffness measurement in patients with chronic hepatitis B. Liver Int. 2009;29:242–7.
29. Chan HL, Wong GL, Choi PC, Chan AW, Chim AM, Yiu KK, Chan FK, et al. Alanine aminotransferase-based algorithms of liver stiffness measurement by transient elastography (Fibroscan) for liver fibrosis in chronic hepatitis B. J Viral Hepat. 2009;16:36–44.
30. Wong VW, Vergniol J, Wong GL, Foucher J, Chan HL, Le Bail B, Choi PC, et al. Diagnosis of fibrosis and cirrhosis using liver stiffness measurement in nonalcoholic fatty liver disease. Hepatology. 2010;51:454–62.
31. Degos F, Perez P, Roche B, Mahmoudi A, Asselineau J, Voitot H, Bedossa P. Diagnostic accuracy of FibroScan and comparison to liver fibrosis biomarkers in chronic viral hepatitis: a multicenter prospective study (the FIBROSTIC study). J Hepatol. 2010;53:1013–21.
32. Zarski JP, Sturm N, Guechot J, Paris A, Zafrani ES, Asselah T, Boisson RC, et al. Comparison of nine blood tests and transient elastography for liver fibrosis in chronic hepatitis C: the ANRS HCEP-23 study. J Hepatol. 2012;56:55–62.
33. Chon YE, Choi EH, Song KJ, Park JY, Kim do Y, Han KH, Chon CY, et al. Performance of transient elastography for the staging of liver fibrosis in patients with chronic hepatitis B: a meta-analysis. PLoS One. 2012;7:e44930.
34. Friedrich-Rust M, Ong MF, Martens S, Sarrazin C, Bojunga J, Zeuzem S, Herrmann E. Performance of transient elastography for the staging of liver fibrosis: a meta-analysis. Gastroenterology. 2008;134:960–74.
35. Stebbing J, Farouk L, Panos G, Anderson M, Jiao LR, Mandalia S, Bower M, et al. A meta-analysis of transient elastography for the detection of hepatic fibrosis. J Clin Gastroenterol. 2010;44:214–9.
36. Talwalkar JA, Kurtz DM, Schoenleber SJ, West CP, Montori VM. Ultrasound-based transient elastography for the detection of hepatic fibrosis: systematic review and meta-analysis. Clin Gastroenterol Hepatol. 2007;5:1214–20.
37. Tsochatzis EA, Gurusamy KS, Ntaoula S, Cholongitas E, Davidson BR, Burroughs AK. Elastography for the diagnosis of severity of fibrosis in chronic liver disease: a meta-analysis of diagnostic accuracy. J Hepatol. 2011;54:650–9.
38. Friedrich-Rust M, Nierhoff J, Lupsor M, Sporea I, Fierbinteanu-Braticevici C, Strobel D, Takahashi H, et al. Performance of acoustic radiation force impulse imaging for the staging of liver fibrosis: a pooled meta-analysis. J Viral Hepat. 2012;19:e212–9.
39. Nierhoff J, Chavez Ortiz AA, Herrmann E, Zeuzem S, Friedrich-Rust M. The efficiency of acoustic radiation force impulse imaging for the staging of liver fibrosis: a meta-analysis. Eur Radiol. 2013;23:3040–53.
40. Hu X, Qiu L, Liu D, Qian L. Acoustic Radiation Force Impulse (ARFI) elastography for noninvasive evaluation of hepatic fibrosis in chronic hepatitis B and C patients: a systematic review and meta-analysis. Med Ultrason. 2017;19:23–31.
41. Bota S, Herkner H, Sporea I, Salzl P, Sirli R, Neghina AM, Peck-Radosavljevic M. Meta-analysis: ARFI elastography versus transient elastography for the evaluation of liver fibrosis. Liver Int. 2013;33:1138–47.
42. Herrmann E, de Lédinghen V, Cassinotto C, Chu WC, Leung VY, Ferraioli G, et al. Assessment of biopsy-proven liver fibrosis by two-dimensional shear wave elastography: An individual patient data-based meta-analysis. Hepatology. 2018;67(1):260–72.
43. Cassinotto C, Lapuyade B, Mouries A, Hiriart JB, Vergniol J, Gaye D, Castain C, et al. Non-invasive assessment of liver fibrosis with impulse elastography: comparison of supersonic shear imaging with ARFI and FibroScan(R). J Hepatol. 2014;61:550–7.

44. Gerber L, Kasper D, Fitting D, Knop V, Vermehren A, Sprinzl K, Hansmann ML, et al. Assessment of liver fibrosis with 2-D shear wave elastography in comparison to transient elastography and acoustic radiation force impulse imaging in patients with chronic liver disease. Ultrasound Med Biol. 2015;41:2350–9.
45. Carrion JA, Navasa M, Bosch J, Bruguera M, Gilabert R, Forns X. Transient elastography for diagnosis of advanced fibrosis and portal hypertension in patients with hepatitis C recurrence after liver transplantation. Liver Transpl. 2006;12:1791–8.
46. Vizzutti F, Arena U, Romanelli RG, Rega L, Foschi M, Colagrande S, Petrarca A, et al. Liver stiffness measurement predicts severe portal hypertension in patients with HCV-related cirrhosis. Hepatology. 2007;45:1290–7.
47. Bureau C, Metivier S, Peron JM, Selves J, Robic MA, Gourraud PA, Rouquet O, et al. Transient elastography accurately predicts presence of significant portal hypertension in patients with chronic liver disease. Aliment Pharmacol Ther. 2008;27:1261–8.
48. Lemoine M, Katsahian S, Ziol M, Nahon P, Ganne-Carrie N, Kazemi F, Grando-Lemaire V, et al. Liver stiffness measurement as a predictive tool of clinically significant portal hypertension in patients with compensated hepatitis C virus or alcohol-related cirrhosis. Aliment Pharmacol Ther. 2008;28:1102–10.
49. Sanchez-Conde M, Montes-Ramirez ML, Miralles P, Alvarez JM, Bellon JM, Ramirez M, Arribas JR, et al. Comparison of transient elastography and liver biopsy for the assessment of liver fibrosis in HIV/hepatitis C virus-coinfected patients and correlation with noninvasive serum markers. J Viral Hepat. 2010;17:280–6.
50. Llop E, Berzigotti A, Reig M, Erice E, Reverter E, Seijo S, Abraldes JG, et al. Assessment of portal hypertension by transient elastography in patients with compensated cirrhosis and potentially resectable liver tumors. J Hepatol. 2012;56:103–8.
51. Colecchia A, Montrone L, Scaioli E, Bacchi-Reggiani ML, Colli A, Casazza G, Schiumerini R, et al. Measurement of spleen stiffness to evaluate portal hypertension and the presence of esophageal varices in patients with HCV-related cirrhosis. Gastroenterology. 2012;143:646–54.
52. Reiberger T, Ferlitsch A, Payer BA, Pinter M, Schwabl P, Stift J, Trauner M, et al. Noninvasive screening for liver fibrosis and portal hypertension by transient elastography—a large single center experience. Wien Klin Wochenschr. 2012;124:395–402.
53. Kitson MT, Roberts SK, Colman JC, Paul E, Button P, Kemp W. Liver stiffness and the prediction of clinically significant portal hypertension and portal hypertensive complications. Scand J Gastroenterol. 2015;50:462–9.
54. Augustin S, Millan L, Gonzalez A, Martell M, Gelabert A, Segarra A, Serres X, et al. Detection of early portal hypertension with routine data and liver stiffness in patients with asymptomatic liver disease: a prospective study. J Hepatol. 2014;60:561–9.
55. Hong WK, Kim MY, Baik SK, Shin SY, Kim JM, Kang YS, Lim YL, et al. The usefulness of non-invasive liver stiffness measurements in predicting clinically significant portal hypertension in cirrhotic patients: Korean data. Clin Mol Hepatol. 2013;19:370–5.
56. Zykus R, Jonaitis L, Petrenkiene V, Pranculis A, Kupcinskas L. Liver and spleen transient elastography predicts portal hypertension in patients with chronic liver disease: a prospective cohort study. BMC Gastroenterol. 2015;15:183.
57. Schwabl P, Bota S, Salzl P, Mandorfer M, Payer BA, Ferlitsch A, Stift J, et al. New reliability criteria for transient elastography increase the number of accurate measurements for screening of cirrhosis and portal hypertension. Liver Int. 2015;35:381–90.
58. Cho EJ, Kim MY, Lee JH, Lee IY, Lim YL, Choi DH, Kim YJ, et al. Diagnostic and prognostic values of noninvasive predictors of portal hypertension in patients with alcoholic cirrhosis. PLoS One. 2015;10:e0133935.
59. Kumar A, Khan NM, Anikhindi SA, Sharma P, Bansal N, Singla V, Arora A. Correlation of transient elastography with hepatic venous pressure gradient in patients with cirrhotic portal hypertension: a study of 326 patients from India. World J Gastroenterol. 2017;23:687–96.
60. Lee CM, Jeong WK, Lim S, Kim Y, Kim J, Kim TY, Sohn JH. Diagnosis of clinically significant portal hypertension in patients with cirrhosis: splenic arterial resistive index versus liver stiffness measurement. Ultrasound Med Biol. 2016;42:1312–20.

61. Berzigotti A, Seijo S, Arena U, Abraldes JG, Vizzutti F, Garcia-Pagan JC, Pinzani M, et al. Elastography, spleen size, and platelet count identify portal hypertension in patients with compensated cirrhosis. Gastroenterology. 2013;144:102–11. e101
62. You MW, Kim KW, Pyo J, Huh J, Kim HJ, Lee SJ, Park SH. A meta-analysis for the diagnostic performance of transient elastography for clinically significant portal hypertension. Ultrasound Med Biol. 2017;43:59–68.
63. Reiberger T, Ferlitsch A, Payer BA, Pinter M, Homoncik M, Peck-Radosavljevic M. Nonselective beta-blockers improve the correlation of liver stiffness and portal pressure in advanced cirrhosis. J Gastroenterol. 2012;47:561–8.
64. Kim BK, Han KH, Park JY, Ahn SH, Kim JK, Paik YH, Lee KS, et al. A liver stiffness measurement-based, noninvasive prediction model for high-risk esophageal varices in B-viral liver cirrhosis. Am J Gastroenterol. 2010;105:1382–90.
65. Abraldes JG, Bureau C, Stefanescu H, Augustin S, Ney M, Blasco H, Procopet B, et al. Noninvasive tools and risk of clinically significant portal hypertension and varices in compensated cirrhosis: the "anticipate" study. Hepatology. 2016;64:2173–84.
66. Salzl P, Reiberger T, Ferlitsch M, Payer BA, Schwengerer B, Trauner M, Peck-Radosavljevic M, et al. Evaluation of portal hypertension and varices by acoustic radiation force impulse imaging of the liver compared to transient elastography and AST to platelet ratio index. Ultraschall Med. 2014;35:528–33.
67. Attia D, Schoenemeier B, Rodt T, Negm AA, Lenzen H, TO L, Manns M, et al. Evaluation of liver and spleen stiffness with acoustic radiation force impulse quantification elastography for diagnosing clinically significant portal hypertension. Ultraschall Med. 2015;36:603–10.
68. Takuma Y, Nouso K, Morimoto Y, Tomokuni J, Sahara A, Takabatake H, Matsueda K, et al. Portal hypertension in patients with liver cirrhosis: diagnostic accuracy of spleen stiffness. Radiology. 2016;279:609–19.
69. Procopet B, Berzigotti A, Abraldes JG, Turon F, Hernandez-Gea V, Garcia-Pagan JC, Bosch J. Real-time shear-wave elastography: applicability, reliability and accuracy for clinically significant portal hypertension. J Hepatol. 2015;62:1068–75.
70. Elkrief L, Rautou PE, Ronot M, Lambert S, Dioguardi Burgio M, Francoz C, Plessier A, et al. Prospective comparison of spleen and liver stiffness by using shear-wave and transient elastography for detection of portal hypertension in cirrhosis. Radiology. 2015;275:589–98.
71 Kim TY, Joong WK, Sohn JH, Kim J, Kim MY, Kim Y. Evaluation of portal hypertension by real-time shear wave elastography in cirrhotic patients. Liver Int. 2015;35:2416–24.
72. Jansen C, Bogs C, Verlinden W, Thiele M, Moller P, Gortzen J, Lehmann J, et al. Algorithm to rule out clinically significant portal hypertension combining shear-wave elastography of liver and spleen: a prospective multicentre study. Gut. 2016;65:1057–8.
73. Berzigotti A. Non-invasive evaluation of portal hypertension using ultrasound elastography. J Hepatol. 2017;67(2):399–411.
74. Castera L, Pinzani M, Bosch J. Non invasive evaluation of portal hypertension using transient elastography. J Hepatol. 2012;56:696–703.
75. Shi KQ, Fan YC, Pan ZZ, Lin XF, Liu WY, Chen YP, Zheng MH. Transient elastography: a meta-analysis of diagnostic accuracy in evaluation of portal hypertension in chronic liver disease. Liver Int. 2013;33:62–71.
76. Takuma Y, Nouso K, Morimoto Y, Tomokuni J, Sahara A, Toshikuni N, Takabatake H, et al. Measurement of spleen stiffness by acoustic radiation force impulse imaging identifies cirrhotic patients with esophageal varices. Gastroenterology. 2012;144:92–101.e2.
77. Ding NS, Nguyen T, Iser DM, Hong T, Flanagan E, Wong A, Luiz L, et al. Liver stiffness plus platelet count can be used to exclude high-risk oesophageal varices. Liver Int. 2016;36:240–5.
78. Marot A, Trepo E, Doerig C, Schoepfer A, Moreno C, Deltenre P. Liver stiffness and platelet count for identifying patients with compensated liver disease at low risk of variceal bleeding. Liver Int. 2017;37:707–16.
79. Jangouk P, Turco L, De Oliveira A, Schepis F, Villa E, Garcia-Tsao G. Validating, deconstructing and refining Baveno criteria for ruling out high-risk varices in patients with compensated cirrhosis. Liver Int. 2017;37:1177–83.

80. Maurice JB, Brodkin E, Arnold F, Navaratnam A, Paine H, Khawar S, Dhar A, et al. Validation of the Baveno VI criteria to identify low risk cirrhotic patients not requiring endoscopic surveillance for varices. J Hepatol. 2016;65:899–905.

81. Llop E, Lopez M, de la Revilla J, Fernandez N, Trapero M, Hernandez M, Fernandez C, et al. Validation of non invasive methods to predict the presence of gastroesophageal varices in a cohort of patients with compensated advanced chronic liver disease. J Gastroenterol Hepatol. 2017;32(11):1867–72.

82. Augustin S, Pons M, Maurice JB, Bureau C, Stefanescu H, Ney M, Blasco H, et al. Expanding the Baveno VI criteria for the screening of varices in patients with compensated advanced chronic liver disease. Hepatology. 2017;66(6):1980–8.

83. Kim TY, Kim TY, Kim Y, Lim S, Jeong WK, Sohn JH. Diagnostic performance of shear wave elastography for predicting esophageal varices in patients with compensated liver cirrhosis. J Ultrasound Med. 2016;35:1373–81.

84. Stefanescu H, Allegretti G, Salvatore V, Piscaglia F. Bidimensional shear wave ultrasound elastography with supersonic imaging to predict presence of oesophageal varices in cirrhosis. Liver Int. 2017;37(9):1405.

85. Robic MA, Procopet B, Metivier S, Peron JM, Selves J, Vinel JP, Bureau C. Liver stiffness accurately predicts portal hypertension related complications in patients with chronic liver disease: a prospective study. J Hepatol. 2011;55:1017–24.

86. Merchante N, Rivero-Juarez A, Tellez F, Merino D, Jose Rios-Villegas M, Marquez-Solero M, Omar M, et al. Liver stiffness predicts clinical outcome in human immunodeficiency virus/hepatitis C virus-coinfected patients with compensated liver cirrhosis. Hepatology. 2012;56:228–38.

87. Wang JH, Chuah SK, Lu SN, Hung CH, Kuo CM, Tai WC, Chiou SS. Baseline and serial liver stiffness measurement in prediction of portal hypertension progression for patients with compensated cirrhosis. Liver Int. 2014;34:1340–8.

88. Kim BK, Kim do Y, Han KH, Park JY, Kim JK, Paik YH, Lee KS, et al. Risk assessment of esophageal variceal bleeding in B-viral liver cirrhosis by a liver stiffness measurement-based model. Am J Gastroenterol. 2011;106:1654–62. 1730

89. Merchante N, Rivero-Juarez A, Tellez F, Merino D, Rios-Villegas MJ, Ojeda-Burgos G, Omar M, et al. Liver stiffness predicts variceal bleeding in HIV/HCV-coinfected patients with compensated cirrhosis. AIDS. 2017;31:493–500.

90. Singh S, Fujii LL, Murad MH, Wang Z, Asrani SK, Ehman RL, Kamath PS, et al. Liver stiffness is associated with risk of decompensation, liver cancer, and death in patients with chronic liver diseases: a systematic review and meta-analysis. Clin Gastroenterol Hepatol. 2013;11:1573–1584.e1–2. quiz e1588–9

91. Corpechot C, Gaouar F, El Naggar A, Kemgang A, Wendum D, Poupon R, Carrat F, et al. Baseline values and changes in liver stiffness measured by transient elastography are associated with severity of fibrosis and outcomes of patients with primary sclerosing cholangitis. Gastroenterology. 2014;146:970–9. quiz e915–6

92. Hezode C, Castera L, Roudot-Thoraval F, Bouvier-Alias M, Rosa I, Roulot D, Leroy V, et al. Liver stiffness diminishes with antiviral response in chronic hepatitis C. Aliment Pharmacol Ther. 2011;34:656–63.

93. Singh S, Facciorusso A, Loomba R, Falck-Ytter YT. Magnitude and kinetics of decrease in liver stiffness after antiviral therapy in patients with chronic hepatitis C: a systematic review and meta-analysis. Clin Gastroenterol Hepatol. 2017. https://doi.org/10.1016/j.cgh.2017.04.038.

94. Lens S, Alvarado E, Marino Z, Londono MC, LLop E, Martinez J, Fortea JI, et al. Effects of all-oral anti-viral therapy on HVPG and systemic hemodynamics in patients with hepatitis C virus-associated cirrhosis. Gastroenterology. 2017;153(5):1273–1283.e1.

Spleen Stiffness by Ultrasound Elastography

8

Antonio Colecchia, Federico Ravaioli, Giovanni Marasco, and Davide Festi

8.1 Introduction

Portal hypertension (PH) is a frequent complication of liver cirrhosis, contributing among other, to the development of ascites, esophageal varices (EV), variceal bleeding and hepatic encephalopathy. The measurement of the hepatic vein pressure gradient (HVPG) represents the accepted gold standard diagnostic procedure for PH assessment in patients with cirrhosis, even if it cannot be routinely used, being an invasive technique limited to specialized centers and requiring specific experience [1]. Thus, in the last decade there has been an increasing interest in identifying non-invasive methodologies able to safely and accurately predict the presence and degree of PH in order to ameliorate the management of cirrhotic patients. The first studies [2–5] used measurement of liver stiffness (LSM) by transient elastography (TE), documenting a good prediction for PH presence, as illustrated in another chapter of this book. However, LSM had a poor correlation with HVPG for values above 12 mmHg [4], which was suggested to be due to the fact that LSM cannot detect the increased portal blood inflow involved in the maintenance and aggravation of PH in advanced cirrhosis.

Splenomegaly, considered in the past to be a mere consequence of PH due to the increased portal pressure, has recently been suggested to have an active role in PH development; indeed, spleen parameters reflect not only the level of PH but also

A. Colecchia
Department of Medical and Surgical Sciences (DIMEC), University of Bologna, Gastroenterology Unit, S.Orsola-Malpighi Hospital, Bologna, Italy

Gastroenterology Unit, Verona University Hospital, Verona, Italy

F. Ravaioli • G. Marasco • D. Festi (✉)
Department of Medical and Surgical Sciences (DIMEC), University of Bologna, Gastroenterology Unit, S.Orsola-Malpighi Hospital, Bologna, Italy
e-mail: davide.festi@unibo.it

© Springer International Publishing AG, part of Springer Nature 2018
A. Berzigotti, J. Bosch (eds.), *Diagnostic Methods for Cirrhosis and Portal Hypertension*, https://doi.org/10.1007/978-3-319-72628-1_8

113

factors leading to increased splenic blood flow and hence to PH [6]. Data obtained in experimental PH rats showed that, in addition to passive congestion due to PH, splenomegaly was characterized structurally and functionally by enlargement and hyperactivation of the splenic lymphoid tissue as well as by increased angiogenesis and fibrogenesis [7]. Such hyperplasia, angiogenesis lead to increased splenic blood flow and contributes to the hyperdynamic splanchnic circulatory syndrome that characterizes the extra-hepatic abnormalities contributing to PH development.

Spleen parameters as predictors of liver complications such as EV were first proposed by Giannini et al. [8, 9] who suggested the clinical use of the combination of platelet count/spleen diameter ratio (Plt/Spl); further scores are represented by the LSPS score (liver stiffness-spleen size-to platelet ratio score) suggested and validated by Kim et al. [10] and the PH risk score proposed by Berzigotti et al. [11]. Spleen stiffness measurement (SSM) was then proposed by Stefanescu et al. [12] and Colecchia et al. [13, 14], both as a non-invasive marker of EV and PH and as a prognostic tool for evaluating the natural history of advanced chronic liver disease.

In this chapter we discuss both the clinical relevance of spleen stiffness measurement and the different ultrasonographic techniques that can be used.

8.2 Ultrasound Elastography for Measuring Spleen Stiffness

The use of elastography techniques is based on the study of tissue elastic and mechanical properties that can be measured by creating a distortion of the tissue, and subsequently in the evaluation of the response of the tissue to this distortion. The ultrasound evaluation consists in the analysis of the velocity of propagation of tissue distortion created by a shear wave, which is mainly influenced by changes in the tissue stiffness, as when fibrosis or congestion occurs. To date, there are several types of ultrasound elastography equipment, developed mainly for assessing liver fibrosis, whose technical aspects and clinical applications are discussed in another chapter of this book. Most methods and accuracy criteria used for liver elastography have also been used for SSM, even if they are not standardized as well as those for LSM. However, it is important to remember that it has been documented for LSM that it could be difficult to compare in terms of numerical thresholds the results obtained with different elastographic techniques [15], a limitation that also applies for SSM. In addition to the LSM methodological limitations, the SSM evaluation by elastography techniques is influenced mainly by spleen dimension [13]. Thus, SSM could face a higher failure rate than LSM, mainly when there is no splenomegaly.

8.2.1 Transient Elastography

Transient elastography is the most common technique used for the evaluation of spleen stiffness and it was first used assuming the same method and accuracy rules adopted for LSM [16] (M probe, patient lying supine or prone, fasting period of at least 6 h, success rate >60%, IQR <30% and at least ten valid measurements) [12,

13]. However, in contrast to LSM measurement, most authors recommend performing SSM with ultrasound assistance in order to better visualize the spleen parenchyma; furthermore, a spleen antero-posterior diameter of at least 4 cm [14] is necessary to perform a correct measurement. A possible limitation of SSM by TE is the ceiling effect due to the fact that the machine detects only values of SS up to 75 kPa, while in some patients SSM could reach values >75 kPa, that Fibroscan® cannot assess. To overcome this limitation, Calvaruso et al. [17] evaluated SSM with modified software ranging from 1.5 kPa to 150 kPa, showing a higher accuracy in predicting the presence of EV and a better correlation with portal pressure. However, despite this higher accuracy in the detection of PH, from a clinical point of view this is of limited relevance because patients with a SSM >75 kPa usually have obvious portal hypertension in the context of decompensated cirrhosis. An international multicenter study was recently started, aimed at evaluating the clinical accuracy of a new FibroScan device specifically dedicated to SSM [18]; the preliminary results showed a higher accuracy of the new device in evaluating PH and particularly in detecting large EV, compared to the conventional examination.

The average failure rate of SSM reported in the literature is around 15–20% (see Table 8.1); as already said, the use of US guidance may increase the frequency of valid examinations. The reported inter- and intra-observer agreement was very good to excellent, with intra-class correlation coefficients (ICC) of 0.89 and 0.94 respectively [19, 20].

8.2.2 Point Shear-Wave Elastography

Point shear-wave elastography (pSWE) is an elastographic technique that allows a quantitative assessment of parenchymal stiffness in an area directly chosen by the operator, in order to avoid sub-capsular areas or including vessels that could modify stiffness values; consequently, this technique can make SSM easier to perform in some patients. Furthermore, pSWE performance is not reduced, as is the case with TE, by the presence of ascites, obesity or narrow intercostal spaces [21, 22]. The overall feasibility of SSM by pSWE, as shown in Table 8.1, ranges from 85% to 100%, so it seems similar to that of LSM by TE, even if documented inter-observer (for expert operators it ranges from 0.68 to 0.98) and intra-observer agreement (ICC 0.60–0.98) was lower than for TE [23, 24].

8.2.3 Two-Dimensional Shear-Wave Elastography

Two-dimensional shear-wave elastography (2D-SWE) measurements are based on the principle that the shear wave velocities generated by a single ultrasound acoustic impulse can be measured in a two-dimensional area. SSM using 2D-SWE has been reported only in a few studies, as shown in Table 8.1. In general, feasibility ranges from 44% to 100%. To date, only the preliminary experience by Cassinotto et al. reported reproducibility data, showing an excellent intra-observer (ICC 0.96) and inter-observer (ICC 0.87) agreements by expert operators [25].

Table 8.1 Spleen stiffness measurement feasibility

Authors	Technique	Patients/controls	ICC/CCC Intra-observer	Inter-observer	Mean SSM Values	Affecting factors/NOTES	Feasibility
Goldschmidt et al. (2014) [20]	TE	Children: 62 CLD, 6 post-OLT, 31 HC	0.946	/	16.3 kPa (HC) 54.5 kPa (CLD)	SSM correlates with splenomegaly ($r^2 = 0.799$) Splenomegaly influences validity (90.5% vs 66.7%, *in normal spleen size*)	96%
Fraquelli et al. (2014) [19]	TE	132 viral CLD, 48 MD, 64 HC	/	0.89 (CLD) 0.9 (MD) 0.86 (HC)	37.1 kPa (CLD) 55.6 kPa (MD) 25.7 kPa (HC)	No systematic over-/under-estimation at Bland-Altman Plot	75–83% **98–100%** after 12–14 months
Lee et al. (2013) [92]	pSWE	202 HC, children	/	/	2.25 m/s	Mean SSM is age-related	99%
Takuma et al. (2013) [56]	pSWE	340 ACLD, 16 HC	0.98	0.98	2.16 m/s (HC) 3.36 m/s (ACLD)	/	95.5%
Ferraioli et al. (2014) [24]	pSWE	92 HC	Expert OP: 0.5 pre-, 0.72 after training Novice OP: 0.3 pre-, 0.39 after training	0.35 pre-, 0.69 after training	2.39–2.49 m/s	$CCC_{inter\text{-}obs}$ is higher when SS is measured at the lower pole Learning curve should be considered	87–94%
Karlas, Lindner, et al. (2014) [93]	pSWE	25 HC, 25 ACLD (Child A)	/	/	2.46 m/s (HC) 3.25 m/s (cirrhosis)	SSM increases with deep inspiration (3.46 m/s; 2.66 m/s) 10 measurements are sufficient (*instead of 20*)	/

Canas et al. (2015) [94]	pSWE	60 HC, **children**	/	/	2.17 m/s (convex probe) 2.15 m/s (linear probe)	SMM differs with age; significant difference between 2 groups: <1 year vs 1–14 years old	/
Balakrishnan et al. (2016) [95]	pSWE	177 ACLD	0.72	0.73	/	BMI >30, φ waist >105 cm did not affect SS; but spleen size does (φ < 12 cm)	94.3%
Kassym et al. (2016) [96]	pSWE	207 HC	/	/	LSM/SMM Ratio 4.72 (normal range 3–7)	SSM in females is higher than in males	/
Cassinotto, Charrie, et al. (2015) [25]	2D-SWE	401 ACLD	0.96	0.87	33.1 kPa	/	70.8%

2D-SWE 2-Dimensional Share Wave Elastography, *ACLD* Advanced Chronic Liver Disease, *CCC* Concordance Correlation Coefficient, *CLD* Chronic Liver Disease, *HC* Healthy Control, *ICC* Intraclass Correlation Coefficient, *LSM* Liver Stiffness Measurement, *MD* Myeloproliferative Disorder, *OLT* Orthotropic Liver Transplantation, *OP* operator, *pSWE* Point Share Wave Elastography, *SSM* Spleen Stiffness Measurement, *TE* Transient Elastography

8.3   Evaluation of Liver Fibrosis and Cirrhosis

One of the main objectives of the hepatologist managing patients with advanced chronic liver disease (ACLD) is to assess disease prognosis; liver fibrosis stages and in particular the presence of cirrhosis are known to be important aspects in that evaluation.

Up to about a decade ago, liver biopsy traditionally represented the "gold standard" for evaluating and staging the degree of hepatic fibrosis. Later, non-invasive methods were proposed as alternative or adjunctive diagnostic tools to liver biopsy; in particular, liver stiffness evaluation by elastographic techniques was introduced for evaluating liver fibrosis stage [26]. As intra-splenic pressure is closely correlated with portal pressure in cirrhosis, scientific attention has focused on the use of SSM, alone or in combination with LSM, in liver fibrosis staging.

Studies using TE showed that SS values were significantly higher in cirrhotic patients than in non-cirrhotic subjects [19, 27]. In a prospective study comparing liver biopsy (LB) with SSM, Fraquelli et al. [19] found good diagnostic estimates in predicting liver cirrhosis using a SSM cut-off of 46 kPa (AUROC 0.84; Sens 89%; Spec 78%).

Studies using by pSWE, [28–31] confirmed these results. Grgurevic et al. [28] showed that the SSM was substantially higher in patients with HBV or HCV-related ACLD than in healthy subject (2.73 m/s vs 1.86 m/s vs 1.3 m/s, respectively). Similar results were reached comparing SSM by 2D-SWE and LB [29, 32, 33]. Leung et al. [29] defined cut-off points able to discriminate between the different fibrosis stages (F1 vs F2 vs F3 vs F4; 19.4 vs 19.8 vs 20.6 vs 22 kPa, respectively) with a good diagnostic performance (AUROC 0.84; Sens 82%; Spec 81%).

However, up to now no meta-analyses are available to confirm and validate the diagnostic role of this technique for liver fibrosis assessment, and cut-off thresholds have not been well established. As illustrated in Table 8.2, SSM cirrhosis thresholds could vary as much as from 22 to 46 kPa or from 2.51 to 3.32 m/s. Nevertheless, available data indicate that SSM could be used as a surrogate of LSM or LB (especially when liver stiffness determination is not achieved or is unreliable) or as a complementary diagnostic approach to hepatic fibrosis stage.

8.4   Cirrhotic Portal Hypertension and Complications

In cirrhotic patients, portal hypertension (PH) is a mainly progressive condition leading to the development of ascites, gastroesophageal varices, variceal bleeding, hepatic encephalopathy, hepato-renal syndrome and hepatocellular carcinoma (HCC). These complications are the main determinants of the severe prognosis of decompensated cirrhosis and bear a close relationship with its mortality. Consequently, it is clinically relevant to evaluate the presence of PH and to monitor its aggravation over time, which is difficult to do on a general basis using the invasive HVPG technique. This has led proposing SSM as a safe and non-invasive diagnostic tool that could represent an alternative to HVPG measurements.

Table 8.2 Spleen stiffness measurement fibrosis/cirrhosis staging

Authors	Technique	Patients/controls	Etiology	Correlation with LB	Mean SSM Values	Endpoint	SS Cut-off	Sens.	Spec.	LR+	LR−	AUROC	Feasibility
Fraquelli et al. (2014) [19]	TE	132 CLD, 48 MD, 64 HC	Viral	0.550	25.7 kPa (HC) 55.6 kPa (MD) 37.1 kPa (CLD)	≥F2, significant fibrosis	36 kPa	76	80	3.9	0.3	0.750	75–83%
Hu et al. (2014) [27]	TE	6 ACLD, 54 CLD	HBV	0.833	13.82 kPa (S0)	F4, cirrhosis	46 kPa	89	78	4.5	0.1	0.840	100%
						S4 vs S0–S3	34.3 kPa	100	94.2	/	/	0.983	
						S3–S4 vs S0–S2	29.2 kPa	81.2	97.7	/	/	0.962	
						S2–S4 vs S0–S1	19.5 kPa	92	85.7	/	/	0.927	
						S1–S4 vs S0	18.5 kPa	69.8	100	/	/	0.902	
Bota et al. (2010) [30]	pSWE	57 ACLD, 10 CLD, 15 HC	Mixed	/	2.04 m/s (HC) 3.1 m/s (ACLD)	Prediction of cirrhosis	2.51 m/s	85.2	91.7	/	/	0.910	95%
Grgurevic et al. (2011) [28]	pSWE	18 CLD, 20 ACLD, 20 HC	HCV, HBV	0.352	2.27 m/s (HC) vs 2.58 (CLD) vs 3.29 m/s (ACLD)	Prediction of cirrhosis	2.73 m/s	90	77.8	/	/	0.822	100%
Chen et al. (2012) [97]	pSWE	163 CLD	HCV, HBV	0.721	2.7 m/s (F0–F3) 3.65 m/s (F4)	F1 vs F2–F4	2.74 m/s	75.2	79	3.58	−0.31	0.839	97%
						F1–F2 vs F3–F4	3.14 m/s	82.2	91.5	9.67	0.19	0.936	
						F1–F3 vs F4	3.32 m/s	80	88.4	6.90	0.23	0.932	

(continued)

Table 8.2 (continued)

Authors	Technique	Patients/controls	Etiology	Correlation with LB	Mean SSM Values	Endpoint	SS Cut-off	Sens.	Spec.	LR+	LR–	AUROC	Feasibility
Ye et al. (2012) [31]	pSWE	138 ACLD, 66 CLD, 60 HC	HBV	0.760	3.24 m/s (F4)	F0–F3 vs F4	2.72 m/s	88.4	93.2	/	/	0.960	100%
Leung et al. (2013) [29]	2D-SWE	226 ACLD, 171 HC	Mixed	0.670	17.3 kPa (HC) 13.3 kPa – 45.3 kPa (range in F1–F4)	≥F1 / ≥F2 / ≥F3 / F4	19.4 kPa / 19.8 kPa / 20.6 kPa / >22 kPa	66.3 / 75.8 / 79.8 / 82.4	85.9 / 84.8 / 82.8 / 80.9	/ / / /	/ / / /	0.810 / 0.820 / 0.830 / 0.840	/
Grgurevic, Puljiz, et al. (2015) [32]	2D-SWE	123 CLD	Viral	/	19.2 kPa (F0–F2) 22.8 kPa (F3–F4) 26.8 kPa (F5–F6)	≥F2 / >F5, cirrhosis	23 kPa / 24 kPa	59.4 / 66.7	93.8 / 86.7	/	/	0.838 / 0.821	53.7%
Pawlus, Inglot, et al. (2016) [98]	2D-SWE	80 CLD (<F2), 53 HC	HBV, HCV	/	SSM in HCV/HBV patients with F0–F1 (LSM < 7.1 kPa/6.5 kPa) is higher than SSM in HC	HC vs F0–F1	/			/	/		72%

2D-SWE 2-Dimensional Share Wave Elastography, *ACLD* Advanced Chronic Liver Disease, *AUROC* Area Under ROC Curve, *CLD* Chronic Liver Disease, *HBV* Hepatitis B Virus, *HC* Healthy Control, *HCV* Hepatitis C Virus, *LB* Liver Biopsy, *LR* Likelihood Ratio, *LSM* Liver Stiffness Measurement, *MD* Myeloproliferative Disorder, *pSWE* Point Share Wave Elastography, *SSM* Spleen Stiffness Measurement, *TE* Transient Elastography

In 2012, in a series of 100 consecutive HCV-related cirrhotic patients, we documented [13] a strong correlation between SSM and the whole range of HVPG values (r^2 = 0.85), suggesting that the increase in SSM is closely related to the progression of PH from early to late stages of cirrhosis. Moreover, SSM accurately predicted the presence of clinically significant portal hypertension (CSPH), denoting an HVPG $\geq$10 mmHg. In fact, SSM cut-offs of $\leq$40 and $\geq$52.8 kPa were able to rule-out and rule-in CSPH, respectively, values between 40 and 52.8 kPa representing a "grey zone" were neither the presence or absence of CSPH could be determined. These results were subsequently confirmed by others, using either TE [34–36] or different SWE methods [37–42]. Assessing SSM by pSWE in 78 patients with ACLD Attia et al. [37] documented that SSM could to identify an HVPG >10 mmHg (cut-off: 2.32 m/s) and an HVPG >12 mmHg (cut-off: 2.53 m/s) with a high diagnostic performance (AUC 0.97 and 0.95 respectively). Using 2D-SWE of liver and spleen in a large prospective multicentric study, Jansen et al. [42] recently identified an algorithm to rule-out and rule-in CSPH, with cut-offs of 21.7 for LS and 35.6 kPa for SS.

Mandorfer et al. [43] recently demonstrated a significant reduction in HVPG after direct-acting antiviral agents (DAAs) therapy achieving sustained virological response (SVR) rates in over 90% of the patients. The same group reported a close correlation between HVPG reduction and LSM variations [44]. In two additional studies [45, 46] assessing SSM after DAAs therapy showed a SSM reduction in 46% of the patients, but no statistically significant difference between SSM before and after treatment was found.

Regarding the use of SSM in monitoring the HVPG change in response therapy of PH, a recent preliminary report suggested that repeat measurements of SSM and of LSM could predict the HVPG response to non-selective beta blockers in the primary prophylaxis of esophageal variceal haemorrhage [47].

Table 8.3 summarizes the available studies assessing SSM as a non-invasive test to predict PH and CSPH. These results suggest that SSM can be an accurate non-invasive diagnostic tool for PH assessment that could replace HVPG measurements to detect the presence of CSPH.

8.4.1 Gastroesophageal Varices

Several studies have investigated the diagnostic/predictive role of SSM as a non-invasive tool in evaluating the presence and degree of esophageal varices (EV).

We showed [13] that SSM by TE was an accurate non-invasive test able to predict absence or presence of EV, with rule-out and rule-in cut-off of 41.3 and 55 kPa, respectively. Multiple studies have confirmed this result [12, 17, 19, 20, 34, 36, 48–54].

Many studies have been performed to evaluate the role of SSM by pSWE in EV detection [31, 37, 55–63]: in the largest one, a cohort of 340 patients with ACLD of mixed aetiology and 16 healthy controls, Takuma et al. [56] reported that cut-offs of

Table 8.3 Portal hypertension assessment by spleen stiffness measurement

Authors	Technique	Patients/controls	Etiology	SSM mean values (No CSPH vs CSPH)	Endpoint	SS Cut-off	Sens.	Spec.	LR+	LR−	AUROC	Feasibility	R^2
Colecchia et al. (2012) [13]	TE	141 ACLD	HCV	37 kPa vs 56 kPa	Rule-out CSPH	40 kPa	98.5	74.3	3.83	0.02	0.966	88.5%	0.85
					Rule-in CSPH	52.8 kPa	76.9	97.1	26.92	0.24			
					Rule-out SPH	41.3 kPa	98.1	674	3.01	0.03	0.959		
					Rule-in SPH	55 kPa	72.2	97.8	33.22	0.28			
Stefanescu et al. (2013) [34]	TE	37 ACLD	Mixed	33.1 kPa vs 65.8 kPa	CSPH	42.7 kPa	92.9	82.6	/	/	0.866	/	/
Zykus et al. (2015) [35]	TE	107 ACLD	Mixed	29.5 kPa vs 69.1 kPa	CSPH	47.6 kPa	77.3	79.2	/	/	0.846	99%	0.62
					SPH	50.7 kPa	78.1	77.1	/	/	0.869		
					SPH	2.53 m/s	94	89	8.45	0.1	0.950		
Elkrief et al. (2015) [36]	TE	79 ACLD	Mixed	56.3 kPa vs 73.5 kPa	CSPH by TE	56.3 kPa	73	67	/	/	0.640	42%	0.604
Rifai et al. (2011) [38]	pSWE	30 CLD with PH, 70 CLD without PH, 25 HC	Mixed	2.86 m/s vs 3.25 m/s	Prediction of PH	3.29 m/s	0.47	0.73	/	/	0.680	99%	/
Attia et al. (2015) [37]	pSWE	78 ACLD	Mixed	2.09 m/s vs 2.58 m/s	CSPH	2.32 m/s	96	89	3.63	0.05	0.968	100%	0.852
Takuma et al. (2016) [39]	pSWE	60 ACLD	Viral	/	Rule-out CSPH	3.1 m/s	97.1	57.7	2.29	0.05	0.943	96.8%	0.876
					Rule-out SPH	3.15 m/s	96.6	61.3	2.49	0.06	0.937		

Study												
Hirooka et al. (2011) [40]	2D-SWE	270 ACLD	Mixed	7.6	CSPH	8.24 m/s	/	/	/	0.978	97.8%	0.854
					SPH	9.99 m/s	/	/	/	0.948		
Procopet et al. (2015) [41]	2D-SWE	55 ACLD	Mixed	27.3 kPa vs 34.6 kPa	Rule-out CSPH	22.7 kPa	90	/	/	0.725	66%	0.514
					Rule-in CSPH	40 kPa	/	90	/			
Elkrief et al. (2015) [36]	2D-SWE	79 ACLD	Mixed	29.2 kPa vs 31.4 kPa	CSPH by 2D-SWE	34.7 kPa	40	100	/	0.630	44%	0.535
Jansen et al. (2016) [42]	2D-SWE	112 ACLD	Mixed	22.2 kPa vs 42.3 kPa	PH	24.6 kPa	/	/	/	0.900	91.2%	0.606
					CSPH	26.3 kPa	79.7	84.2	/	0.840		
					Rule-out CSPH	21.7 kPa	91.9	50	/	0.840		
					Rule-in CSPH	35.6 kPa	51.4	92	/	0.840		
					SPH	28.5 kPa	/	/	/	0.810		

2D-SWE 2-Dimensional Share Wave Elastography, ACLD Advanced Chronic Liver Disease, AUROC Area Under ROC Curve, CLD Chronic Liver Disease, CSPH Clinically Significant Portal Hypertension (HVPG ≥10 mmHg), HBV Hepatitis B Virus, HC Healthy Control, HCV Hepatitis C Virus, HVPG Hepatic Venous Pressure Gradient, LR Likelihood Ratio, LSM Liver Stiffness Measurement, PH Portal Hypertension (HVPG >5 mmHg), pSWE Point Share Wave Elastography, R Correlation Coefficient, SPH Severe Portal Hypertension (HVPG ≥12 mmHg), SSM Spleen Stiffness Measurement, TE Transient Elastography

3.18 m/s and 3.3 m/s were able to respectively detect EV and large EV with a good performance (AUROC >0.93).

To date, different studies have been conducted using 2D-SWE [25, 36, 40, 64, 65]; among them, Hirooka et al. [40] showed that SSM was able to predict EV with a AUROC of 0.91, and in a large study of 401 ACLD patients, Cassinotto et al. [25], documented that 25.6 kPa was an SSM cut-off able to predict large EV with high sensitivity and specificity.

The recent 2015 Baveno VI consensus workshop [66] highlighted the diagnostic role of non-invasive tests such as LSM in defining the presence of CSPH and EV. In particular, the so-called Baveno criteria were defined: patients with LSM <20 kPa (determined by TE) and a platelet count >150.000/mm^3 were considered to be very unlikely to have high-risk varices (<5%), and consequently in these patients, endoscopy could be safely avoided. The Baveno criteria can also be applied for longitudinal follow-up, prompting screening endoscopy if liver stiffness increases or platelet count decreases. In light of the substantial evidence regarding the role of SSM to predict the presence of varices with high risk of bleeding (F1 with red spots, F2–F3 varices), SSM could probably be proposed as a useful non-invasive test to exclude the presence of HRV.

Thus far, there are two meta-analyses [67, 68] on the role of SSM in predicting the presence of EV using all available ultrasound elastography methods. Ma et al. [67] assessed 16 published studies and found that SSM had a higher accuracy than LSM in predicting the presence of EV in ACLD patients. Even if the last world guidelines of non-invasive tests for the evaluation of liver disease did not suggest the use of SSM in clinical practice, according to the latest evidence, we believe that the assessment of SSM during the same LSM session could be a useful tool to predict the potential presence of EV.

The predictive role of SSM regarding variceal bleeding is still not well defined although two studies [52, 61] showed that SSM by TE (cut-off 42.6 kPa) or pSWE (cut-off 3.64 m/s) were able to predict variceal bleeding with a sensitivity of 89% and 79%, respectively. This should be further explored in prospective studies. Table 8.3 shows a summary of the above findings.

8.4.2   Clinical Decompensation and Mortality

The prognosis of compensated and decompensated liver cirrhosis is markedly different, thus it is of extreme importance to accurately identify those compensated patients at higher risk of decompensation [69]. The main predictor of decompensation is the presence of CSPH (a HVPG ≥10 mmHg) and its progression [70]; thus, several studies have proposed using SSM as a predictor of clinical decompensation in cirrhosis (Tables 8.4 and 8.5).

In a recent study by our group [14], SSM by TE and MELD were the only clinical variables independently associated with clinical decompensation; SSM values >54 kPa were related to risk of complications in the subsequent 2 years.

Table 8.4 Esophageal varices staging assess by spleen stiffness measurement

Authors	Technique	Patients/ controls	Etiology	Endpoint	Prevalence	SS Cut-off	Sens.	Spec.	LR+	LR−	AUROC	Feasibility
Stefanescu et al. (2011) [12]	TE	135 ACLD, 39 CLD, 17 HC	Alcohol, HCV	EV	84.9%	46.4 kPa	83.56	71.43	2.92	0.23	0.781	85.3%
Al-Dahshan (2012) [48]	TE	60 ACLD, 20 CLD, 10 HC	Mixed	EV	/	50.4 kPa	81.2	73.2	/	/	0.794	/
Colecchia et al. (2012) [13]	TE	141 ACLD	HCV	Rule-out EV	53%	41.3 kPa	98.1	66	2.88	0.03	0.941	88.5%
				Rule-in EV		55 kPa	71.7	95.7	16.85	0.30		
Liu et al. (2013) [49]	TE	259 ACLD	Mixed	EV	97.9%	44.5 kPa	88	68	/	/	0.804	/
Calvaruso et al. (2013) [17]	TE[a]	112 ACLD	HCV	EV	56%	50 kPa	65	61	1.70	0.50	0.701	85.7%
				LEV	27%	54 kPa	80	70	2	0.30	0.819	
Stefanescu et al. (2013) [34]	TE	118 ACLD	Mixed	LEV	40%	42.7 kPa	/	/	/	/	0.633	100%
Sharma et al. (2013) [50]	TE	200 ACLD	Mixed	EV	71%	40.8 kPa	94	76	3.90	0.08	0.898	87%
Goldschmidt et al. (2014) [20]	TE	Children, 62 CLD, 6 post-OLT, 31 HC	Mixed	EV	74%	75 kPa (with EV) vs 24 kPa (without EV)						96%
					47%	75 kPa (BEV history) vs 50.25 kPa (no history)						
Fraquelli et al. (2014) [19]	TE	132 ACLD, 48 MD, 64 HC	Viral	EV	10%	48 kPa	100	0.6	2.50	0.01	0.900	75–83%
Elkrief et al. (2015) [36]	TE	79 ACLD	Mixed	LEV	34%[b]	73.5 kPa	54	78	/	/	0.650	42%
Stefanescu et al. (2015) [99]	TE	136 ACLD	Mixed	HREV	53%	53 kPa	89	54	1.82	0.20	0.742	100%

(continued)

Table 8.4 (continued)

Authors	Technique	Patients/controls	Etiology	Endpoint	Prevalence	SS Cut-off	Sens.	Spec.	LR+	LR−	AUROC	Feasibility
Buechter et al. (2016) [52]	TE	143 ACLD	Mixed	Risk of BEV	75%	42.6 kPa	89	64	/	/	/	79%
Wong et al. (2016) [53]	TE	144 ACLD	HBV	Rule-out EV	21.5%	8.9 kPa	91.4	32.1	1.35	0.27	0.685	84.1%
				Rule-in EV		54.9 kPa	37.1	90.8	0.27	0.67		
Guo et al. (2016) [73]	TE	73 ACLD	/	LEV	/	40.3 kPa	/	/	/	/	0.788	/
Ye et al. (2012) [31]	pSWE	138 ACLD, 66 CLD, 60 HC	HBV	EV	65.7%	3.16	84.1	81	/	/	0.830	100%
				LEV	28.8%	3.39 m/s	78.9	78.3	/	/	0.830	
Bota et al. (2012) [55]	pSWE	140 ACLD	Mixed	LEV	43%	2.55 m/s	96.7	21.1	/	/	0.578	97.9%
Takuma et al. (2013) [56]	pSWE	340 ACLD, 16 HC	Mixed	EV	39%	3.18 m/s	98.5	60.1	2.47	0.03	0.933	95.5%
				LEV	26%	3.3 m/s[a]	98.9	62.9	2.66	0.02	0.930	
Rizzo et al. (2014) [57]	pSWE	54 ACLD, 27 CLD, 63 HC	HCV	EV	52%	3.1 m/s	96.4	88.5	8.36	0.04	0.959	/
Attia et al. (2015) [37]	pSWE	78 ACLD	Mixed	EV in CSFH	76%	2.55 m/s	95	90	9.06	0.05	0.899	100%
				EV in SPH		2.71 m/s	95	92	11.86	0.06	0.931	
Kim et al. (2015) [58]	pSWE	125 ACLD	Mixed	EV	62%	3.16 m/s	87	60.4	/	/	0.768	95%
				LEV	41.6%	3.4 m/s[a]	789	63	/	/	0.786	
Tomita et al. (2016) [59]	pSWE	33 ACLD	Biliary atresia	EV after OP[c]	31%	3.14 m/s	199	69.2	/	/	0.790	100%
Park et al. (2016) [60]	pSWE	366 ACLD	Mixed	EV	53%	29.9 kPa	85.1	79.1	/	/	0.859	60%

Study	Method	Population	Etiology	Target	%	Cutoff	Sens.	Spec.	LR		AUROC	
Takuma et al. (2016) [62]	pSWE	60 ACLD	Viral	Rule-out EV	40%	3.36 m/s	95.8	77.8	4.31	0.05	0.937	96.8%
				Rule-out LEV	26.7%	3.51 m/s	93.8	84.1	5.89	0.07	0.955	
Takuma et al. (2016) [39]	pSWE	446 ACLD		BEV	7.4%	3.64 m/s	78.8	/	/	/	0.857	/
Zhang et al. (2017) [100]	pSWE	42 ACLD, 28 HC	Biliary atresia	EV/GV after OP	55%	3.02 m/s	78.6	84.5	/	/	0.810	/
Hirooka et al. (2011) [40]	2D-SWE	270 ACLD	Mixed	EV	41.2%	8.24 / 9.99	98 / 26	93.8 / 99.4	/ /	/ /	0.908	97.8%
Grgurevic, Bokun, et al. (2015) [64]	2D-SWE	cACLD	Mixed	EV	36.4%	30.3 kPa	79.6	75.8	3.30	0.27	0.790	70.6%
Cassinotto, Charrie et al. (2015) [25]	2D-SWE	401 ACLD	Mixed	LEV	/	25.6 kPa	94	36	1.47	0.17	0.800	70.8%
Elkrief et al. (2015) [36]	2D-SWE	79 ACLD	Mixed	LEV	34%[b]	32.3 kPa	48	71	/	/	0.589	46%
Stefanescu et al. (2017) [65]	2D-SWE	73 cACLD	/	EV	60.3%	38 kPa	/	/	/	/	0.747	/

2D-SWE 2-Dimensional Share Wave Elastography, ACLD Advanced Chronic Liver Disease, AUROC Area Under ROC Curve, BEV Bleeding Esophageal Varices, cACLD compensated Advanced Chronic Liver Disease, CLD Chronic Liver Disease, EV Esophageal Varices, HBV Hepatitis B Virus, HC Healthy Control, HCV Hepatitis C Virus, HRV High Risk Varices, LEV Large Esophageal Varices, LR Likelihood Ratio, LSM Liver Stiffness Measurement, MD Myeloproliferative Disorder, OLT Orthotropic Liver Transplantation, OP Operation (Kasai's Procedure), pSWE Point Share Wave Elastography, SSM Spleen Stiffness Measurement, TE Transient Elastography

[a] SSM with modified software ranging from 1.5 kPa to 150 kPa

[b] The article claims no statistically difference between HRV e non, concluding that SSM cannot predict EV or HRV

[c] Although in the results, the author claims that there was no significant difference between EV e non EV

Table 8.5 Cirrhosis clinical decompensation and mortality assessment by spleen stiffness measurement

References	Method	Patients/controls	C-Index	OR/HR	Endpoint	SS Cut-off	Sens.	Spec.	LR+	LR−	AUROC	Feasibility
Radu et al. (2014) [71]	TE	52 ACLD	/	/	Decompensation Prediction Score (DPS)[a] for any event	73	/	/	/	/	0.700	/
Colecchia et al. (2014) [14]	TE	92 ACLD	0.87	OR = 1.11	Predictive equation for Any Event: **Upper Cut-Off**	0.76	/	/	11.58	/	/	90.3%
					Predictive equation for Any Event: **Lower Cut-Off**	0.22	/	/	/	0.06	/	/
					CD by SSM	54 kPa	97	63	/	0.05	/	/
Takuma, Morimoto et al. (2016) [61]	pSWE	393 ACLD (280 cALD)	0.856	HR = 14.5	CD	3.25 m/s	94.3	65.3	2.72	0.09	0.838	95.6%
Mori et al. (2013) [72]	pSWE	33 CLD, 14 HC	/	/	Prediction of ascites	3.34 m/s	73.3	77.8	3.30	2.92	0.800	100%
Grgurevic, Bokun, et al. (2015) [64]	2D-SWE	44 ACLD	/	HR = 3.99	Any event	31.7 kPa	P (event) > P (no event) Cumulative Risk: ↑1 kPa ->↑risk of CD by 9%;					/
Grgurevic, Puljiz, et al. (2015) [32]	2D-SWE	123 ACLD	/	/	CD	35 kPa	64.3	94.4	/	/	0.873	53.7%
Takuma, Morimoto, et al. (2016) [61]	pSWE	393 ACLD (280 cALD)	0.824 (univariate) 0.861 (multivariate)	/	**Mortality**	3.43 m/s	82.1	74.2	3.19	0.24	0.792	95.6%

2D-SWE 2-Dimensional Share Wave Elastography, *ACLD* Advanced Chronic Liver Disease, *AUROC* Area Under ROC Curve, *cACLD* compensated Advanced Chronic Liver Disease, *CD* Clinical Decompensation, *CLD* Chronic Liver Disease, *HC* Healthy Control, *LR* Likelihood Ratio, *LSM* Liver Stiffness Measurement, *OR/HR* Odd/Hazard ratio, *pSWE* Point Share Wave Elastography, *SSM* Spleen Stiffness Measurement, *TE* Transient Elastography

[a]$4.56 + (0.82*\textbf{mSSM}) + (0.496*\textbf{Bilirubin}) - (1.77*\textbf{Albumin})$

On the basis of these results, a predictive rule was proposed. Furthermore, the predictive accuracy of SSM, alone or combined with MELD, was at least not inferior to that of HVPG. After this observation other studies confirmed the role of SSM as a non-invasive alternative to HVPG to predict PH-related complications [32, 61, 64, 71, 72]. In fact, Takuma et al. [61] recently confirmed in a series of 393 ACLD patients that only SS by pSWE and MELD were significantly associated with development of clinical decompensation. In their study, patients with SSM <3.25 m/s had a 98.8% probability of remaining free of decompensation after a median follow-up of 44.6 months. Mori et al. [72] proposed a slightly higher cut-off, 3.34 m/s, to predict the development of ascites, while other study [64], using 2D-SWE, showed that an increase of 1 kPa in SSM was associated with a 9% increase in the risk of decompensation; in their model values of SSM above a cut-off of 31.7 kPa had an AUROC of 0.873 in predicting decompensated patients.

The MELD score and the Child-Pugh score are the tools most used in clinical practice in predicting mortality. However, these scores have drawbacks, leaving room for other non-invasive parameters to improve prognosis of ACLD. Takuma et al. [61] assessed the use of SSM by SWE in predicting mortality as a primary end point and reported that SSM had the best discriminative value among all other clinical variables, both in the univariate and in the multivariate analysis (AUROC 0.817). Each SSM unit (m/s) of increase by pSWE was associated with a 14.5-fold increase in the risk of death. The cut-off of 3.43 m/s had a 75.8% accuracy in predicting mortality after a median follow-up of 44.6 months.

Because of its prognostic value, SSM has been proposed for decompensated cirrhotic patients requiring transjugular intrahepatic portosystemic shunt (TIPS) with conflicting results [73–76]. Novelli et al. [74] showed that SSM decreased after TIPS placement only in 58% of patients; in addition there was no correlation between SSM and portal pressure measurement before and after TIPS placement. A more recent study by Gao et al. [73], using 2D-SWE, found that SSM values were significantly reduced after TIPS placement; in addition, they showed that SSM correlated with the post-TIPS portosystemic pressure gradient (PPG) and identified a SSM cut-off of 3.61 m/s able to detect TIPS dysfunction with good performance (AUROC 0.91), although with suboptimal specificity (Sens 92%, Spec 66%).

These data suggest that SSM could be a helpful adjunctive tool for physicians to better identify patients at higher risk of mortality and for a better stratification for specific treatments, and some studies suggest a good prognostic value in the context of liver transplantation, especially in patients with a MELD score ≥15 [20, 77]. In a small group of ACLD patients having liver transplantation, Chin et al. [77] reported that SSM decreased significantly from mean pre-LT values of 75 kPa to post-LT values of 35.8 kPa, suggesting that SSM mirrors PH changes after LT.

8.5   Non-Cirrhotic Portal Hypertension

PH is a condition related not only to cirrhosis of the liver, but occurs also in other conditions such as [78]:

• extrahepatic portal vein obstruction, mostly due to portal vein thrombosis and (Pre-Hepatic PH);
• Budd-Chiari syndrome, or hepatic vein thrombosis (Post-Hepatic PH);
• Portal-sinusoidal disease, known also as idiopathic non-cirrhotic portal hypertension/nodular regenerative hyperplasia/idiopathic portal fibrosis (Intra-Hepatic PH).

Portal hypertension without liver cirrhosis can also be found in hematological diseases like myelofibrosis, sinusoidal obstructive syndrome (SOS, previously known as Veno-Occlusive Disease, VOD) and some rare diseases (amyloidosis, arterio-portal venous fistulae).

When PH is clinically suspected, the first step is to evaluate its cause. Extra-hepatic causes of PH should be excluded by ultrasound, CT or MRI, whereas intra-hepatic causes in most cases require a liver biopsy and HVPG.

In the setting of hematological disease, in particular in myeloproliferative diseases, PH is a consequence of portal and/or hepatic vein thrombosis. Intrahepatic non-cirrhotic PH without portal or hepatic vein thrombosis is rarely described in these patients [79–81]. Two recent reports [82, 83] described the role of SSM in myelofibrosis, evaluated both by TE and p-SWE. In the first, Webb et al. [82] compared the spleen stiffness of patients with splenomegaly associated with myelofibrosis (without PH) to cirrhotic patients and to healthy volunteers, finding that SSM was increased but not able to distinguish patients with myelofibrosis from cirrhotic ones. Iurlo et al. [83] pointed out a potential use of SSM by TE in assessing the severity of primary myelofibrosis and, consequently, in monitoring the response to treatment.

A recent study [84] in patients with extra-hepatic portal vein obstruction (EHPVO), showed that while patients with EHPVO had normal or mild elevation of LSM (median 6.7 kPa), SSM was markedly elevated (median: 51.7 kPa) much higher than in control subjects. In addition, patients with a previous history of bleeding episodes had higher SSM than those without (60.4 kPa and 30.3 kPa respectively) suggesting that SSM could be of diagnostic and prognostic value in these patients.

There are currently no available data on SSM in patients with Budd-Chiari syndrome, even if it is very likely that both LSM and SSM could be increased due to venous congestion and PH [85]. As far as SOS/VOD we recently demonstrated that LSM suddenly increases a few days prior to the appearance of the typical clinical signs which allow suspecting the diagnosis (jaundice, weight gain, painful hepatomegaly, ascites) [86].

Considering idiopathic portal hypertension (IPH), a recent study [87] evaluated a possible diagnostic role of elastosonography based on the finding that LSM is only slightly increased in these patients, but is associated with marked increases in SSM

[88]. In order to help in the diagnosis, these authors proposed SSM/LSM (using pSWE) with a cut-off of 1.71 for differentiating patient with IPH from ACLD.

LSM and SSM could also be a useful tool to monitor patients with biliary atresia after Kasaii intervention [89, 90]; indeed, in one study [90] SSM correlated better with indirect signs of portal hypertension such as spleen diameter, portal vein diameter and development of collateral vessels than LSM. SSM was also studied for the prediction of outcomes in children receiving liver transplantation, mainly for biliary atresia (70%), which often results in venous complications leading to portal hypertension [91]; in these patients, SSM values decreased after curative intervention radiological procedures for portal or hepatic venous stenosis. In particular, the median spleen stiffness values were 2.70 and 4.00 m/s in patients without and with venous complications, with a cut-off value of 2.93 m/s having 100% sensitivity and 78.9% specificity.

In summary, SSM represents a promising tool to evaluate PH also in non-cirrhotic patients, to diagnose conditions other than liver cirrhosis that may lead to PH, and to follow up patients after liver transplantation and after radiology procedures focused on the splanchnic venous system.

Conclusion

Elastographic measurement of spleen stiffness is a new and useful tool for hepatologists, which can provide rapid and valuable information on liver fibrosis staging, presence and degree of portal hypertension, and predicting its complications. Spleen stiffness better represents the dynamic changes occurring in the advanced stages of liver cirrhosis than liver stiffness, and its diagnostic performance in detecting esophageal varices is higher. For the assessment of liver fibrosis SSM showed a good diagnostic accuracy. Up to now no meta-analysis is available to confirm these data; however SSM represents a useful tool when LSM is not reliable or its measurement is imperfect, and it is also a valuable adjunctive diagnostic instrument.

Regarding the detection of PH many single studies have showed an optimal diagnostic accuracy of SSM, particularly to rule out the presence of esophageal varices. To date two meta-analyses have been carried out, showing an adequate accuracy of SSM in detecting the presence of EV and HRV and that SSM was superior to LSM for predicting EV. Further studies are needed to confirm SSM as non-invasive tool for rule-out patients with HRV, with the purpose of sparing upper endoscopy and the rule on prediction of variceal bleeding. Encouraging data seem to show that SSM could have a role for monitoring the hemodynamic response to NSBB., Different studies have showed the role of SSM in predicting cirrhosis-related complication, TIPS function and PH resolution after LT, although further larger prospective studies are needed. Finally, SSM in non-cirrhotic portal hypertension will represent a promising further clinical application.

In conclusion, SSM, due to the wide diffusion of TE devices and of newest ultrasound elastography machines, will represent an useful and encouraging diagnostic and prognostic tool, thus allowing a rapid risk stratification of patients in order to better identify the best diagnostic and therapeutic strategy.

References

1. Groszmann RJ, Wongcharatrawee S. The hepatic venous pressure gradient: anything worth doing should be done right. Hepatology. 2004;39:280–2.
2. Carrión JA, Torres F, Crespo G, Miquel R, García-Valdecasas J-C, Navasa M, Forns X. Liver stiffness identifies two different patterns of fibrosis progression in patients with hepatitis C virus recurrence after liver transplantation. Hepatology. 2010;51:23–34.
3. Lemoine M, Katsahian S, Ziol M, Nahon P, Ganne-Carrie N, Kazemi F, Grando-Lemaire V, Trinchet J-C, Beaugrand M. Liver stiffness measurement as a predictive tool of clinically significant portal hypertension in patients with compensated hepatitis C virus or alcohol-related cirrhosis. Aliment Pharmacol Ther. 2008;28:1102–10.
4. Vizzutti F, Arena U, Romanelli RG, et al. Liver stiffness measurement predicts severe portal hypertension in patients with HCV-related cirrhosis. Hepatology. 2007;45:1290–7.
5. Bureau C, Metivier S, Peron JM, Selves J, Robic MA, Gourraud PA, Rouquet O, Dupuis E, Alric L, Vinel JP. Transient elastography accurately predicts presence of significant portal hypertension in patients with chronic liver disease. Aliment Pharmacol Ther. 2008;27:1261–8.
6. Bolognesi M, Merkel C, Sacerdoti D, Nava V, Gatta A. Role of spleen enlargement in cirrhosis with portal hypertension. Dig Liver Dis. 2002;34:144–50.
7. Mejias M, Garcia-Pras E, Gallego J, Mendez R, Bosch J, Fernandez M. Relevance of the mTOR signaling pathway in the pathophysiology of splenomegaly in rats with chronic portal hypertension. J Hepatol. 2010;52:529–39.
8. Giannini E, Botta F, Borro P, et al. Platelet count/spleen diameter ratio: proposal and validation of a non-invasive parameter to predict the presence of oesophageal varices in patients with liver cirrhosis. Gut. 2003;52:1200–5.
9. Giannini EG, Zaman A, Kreil A, et al. Platelet count/spleen diameter ratio for the noninvasive diagnosis of esophageal varices: results of a multicenter, prospective, validation study. Am J Gastroenterol. 2006;101:2511–9.
10. Kim BK, Han K-H, Park JY, Ahn SH, Kim JK, Paik YH, Lee KS, Chon CY, Kim DY. A liver stiffness measurement-based, noninvasive prediction model for high-risk esophageal varices in B-viral liver cirrhosis. Am J Gastroenterol. 2010;105:1382–90.
11. Berzigotti A, Seijo S, Arena U, Abraldes JG, Vizzutti F, Garcia Pagan JC, Pinzani M, Busch J. Elastography, spleen size, and platelet count identify portal hypertension in patients with compensated cirrhosis. Gastroenterology. 2013;144:102–111.e1.
12. Stefanescu H, Grigorescu M, Lupsor M, Procopet B, Maniu A, Badea R. Spleen stiffness measurement using Fibroscan for the noninvasive assessment of esophageal varices in liver cirrhosis patients. J Gastroenterol Hepatol. 2011;26:164–70.
13. Colecchia A, Montrone L, Scaioli E, et al. Measurement of spleen stiffness to evaluate portal hypertension and the presence of esophageal varices in patients with HCV-related cirrhosis. Gastroenterology. 2012;143:646–54.
14. Colecchia A, Colli A, Casazza G, et al. Spleen stiffness measurement can predict clinical complications in compensated HCV-related cirrhosis: a prospective study. J Hepatol. 2014;60:1158–64.
15. Piscaglia F, Salvatore V, Mulazzani L, et al. Differences in liver stiffness values obtained with new ultrasound elastography machines and Fibroscan: a comparative study. Dig Liver Dis. 2017. https://doi.org/10.1016/j.dld.2017.03.001.
16. Bonino F, Arena U, Brunetto MR, et al. Liver stiffness, a non-invasive marker of liver disease: a core study group report. Antivir Ther. 2010;15:69–78.
17. Calvaruso V, Bronte F, Conte E, Simone F, Craxi A, Di Marco V. Modified spleen stiffness measurement by transient elastography is associated with presence of large oesophageal varices in patients with compensated hepatitis C virus cirrhosis. J Viral Hepat. 2013;20:867–74.
18. Stefanescu H, Cales P, Fraquelli M, Ganne-Carrie N, Rosselli M, de Ledinghen V, Festi D. FRI-016 – performance of FibroScan® to detect large esophageal varices in chronic liver diseases is improved by a novel spleen-dedicated examination. J Hepatol. 2017. https://doi.org/10.1016/S0168-8278(17)31094-2.

19. Fraquelli M, Giunta M, Pozzi R, et al. Feasibility and reproducibility of spleen transient elastography and its role in combination with liver transient elastography for predicting the severity of chronic viral hepatitis. J Viral Hepat. 2014;21:90–8.
20. Goldschmidt I, Brauch C, Poynard T, Baumann U. Spleen stiffness measurement by transient elastography to diagnose portal hypertension in children. J Pediatr Gastroenterol Nutr. 2014;59:197–203.
21. Bota S, Herkner H, Sporea I, Salzl P, Sirli R, Neghina AM, Peck-Radosavljevic M. Meta-analysis: ARFI elastography versus transient elastography for the evaluation of liver fibrosis. Liver Int. 2013;33:1138–47.
22. Hudson JM, Milot L, Parry C, Williams R, Burns PN. Inter- and intra-operator reliability and repeatability of shear wave elastography in the liver: a study in healthy volunteers. Ultrasound Med Biol. 2013;39:950–5.
23. Cabassa P, Ravanelli M, Rossini A, Contessi G, Almajdalawi R, Maroldi R. Acoustic radiation force impulse quantification of spleen elasticity for assessing liver fibrosis. Abdom Imaging. 2015;40:738–44.
24. Ferraioli G, Tinelli C, Lissandrin R, Zicchetti M, Bernuzzi S, Salvaneschi L, Filice C. Ultrasound point shear wave elastography assessment of liver and spleen stiffness: effect of training on repeatability of measurements. Eur Radiol. 2014;24:1283–9.
25. Cassinotto C, Charrie A, Mouries A, et al. Liver and spleen elastography using supersonic shear imaging for the non-invasive diagnosis of cirrhosis severity and oesophageal varices. Dig Liver Dis. 2015;47:695–701.
26. Castera L, Forns X, Alberti A. Non-invasive evaluation of liver fibrosis using transient elastography. J Hepatol. 2008;48:835–47.
27. Hu X, Xu X, Zhang Q, Zhang H, Liu J, Qian L. Indirect prediction of liver fibrosis by quantitative measurement of spleen stiffness using the FibroScan system. J Ultrasound Med. 2014;33:73–81.
28. Grgurevic I, Cikara I, Horvat J, Lukic IK, Heinzl R, Banic M, Kujundzic M, Brkljacic B. Noninvasive assessment of liver fibrosis with acoustic radiation force impulse imaging: increased liver and splenic stiffness in patients with liver fibrosis and cirrhosis. Ultraschall Med. 2011;32:160–6.
29. Leung VY, Shen J, Wong VW, et al. Quantitative elastography of liver fibrosis and spleen stiffness in chronic hepatitis B carriers: comparison of shear-wave elastography and transient elastography with liver biopsy correlation. Radiology. 2013;269:910–8.
30. Bota S, Sporea I, Sirli R, Popescu A, Danila M, Sendroiu M, Focsa M. Spleen assessment by Acoustic Radiation Force Impulse Elastography (ARFI) for prediction of liver cirrhosis and portal hypertension. Med Ultrason. 2010;12:213–7.
31. Ye X-P, Ran H-T, Cheng J, Zhu Y-F, Zhang D-Z, Zhang P, Zheng Y-Y. Liver and spleen stiffness measured by acoustic radiation force impulse elastography for noninvasive assessment of liver fibrosis and esophageal varices in patients with chronic hepatitis B. J Ultrasound Med. 2012;31:1245–53.
32. Grgurevic I, Puljiz Z, Brnic D, Bokun T, Heinzl R, Lukic A, Luksic B, Kujundzic M, Brkljacic B. Liver and spleen stiffness and their ratio assessed by real-time two dimensional-shear wave elastography in patients with liver fibrosis and cirrhosis due to chronic viral hepatitis. Eur Radiol. 2015;25:3214–21.
33. Pawlus A, Inglot M, Chabowski M, Szymanska K, Inglot M, Patyk M, Slonina J, Caseiro-Alves F, Janczak D, Zaleska-Dorobisz U. Shear wave elastography (SWE) of the spleen in patients with hepatitis B and C but without significant liver fibrosis. Br J Radiol. 2016;89:20160423.
34. Stefanescu H, Procopet B, Platon-Lupsor M, Bureau C. Is there any place for spleen stiffness measurement in portal hypertension? Am J Gastroenterol. 2013;108:1660–1.
35. Zykus R, Jonaitis L, Petrenkiene V, Pranculis A, Kupcinskas L. Liver and spleen transient elastography predicts portal hypertension in patients with chronic liver disease: a prospective cohort study. BMC Gastroenterol. 2015;15:183.
36. Elkrief L, Rautou P-E, Ronot M, et al. Prospective comparison of spleen and liver stiffness by using shear-wave and transient elastography for detection of portal hypertension in cirrhosis. Radiology. 2015;275:589–98.

37. Attia D, Schoenemeier B, Rodt T, Negm AA, Lenzen H, TO L, Manns M, Gebel M, Potthoff A. Evaluation of liver and spleen stiffness with acoustic radiation force impulse quantification elastography for diagnosing clinically significant portal hypertension. Ultraschall Med. 2015;36:603–10.
38. Rifai K, Cornberg J, Bahr M, Mederacke I, Potthoff A, Wedemeyer H, Manns M, Gebel M. ARFI elastography of the spleen is inferior to liver elastography for the detection of portal hypertension. Ultraschall Med. 2011;32(Suppl 2):E24–30.
39. Takuma Y, Nouso K, Morimoto Y, Tomokuni J, Sahara A, Takabatake H, Matsueda K, Yamamoto H. Portal hypertension in patients with liver cirrhosis: diagnostic accuracy of spleen stiffness. Radiology. 2016;279:609–19.
40. Hirooka M, Ochi H, Koizumi Y, Kisaka Y, Abe M, Ikeda Y, Matsuura B, Hiasa Y, Onji M. Splenic elasticity measured with real-time tissue elastography is a marker of portal hypertension. Radiology. 2011;261:960–8.
41. Procopet B, Berzigotti A, Abraldes JG, Turon F, Hernandez-Gea V, Garcia-Pagan JC, Bosch J. Real-time shear-wave elastography: applicability, reliability and accuracy for clinically significant portal hypertension. J Hepatol. 2015;62:1068–75.
42. Jansen C, Bogs C, Verlinden W, et al. Algorithm to rule out clinically significant portal hypertension combining Shear-wave elastography of liver and spleen: a prospective multicentre study. Gut. 2016;65:1057–8.
43. Mandorfer M, Kozbial K, Schwabl P, et al. Sustained virologic response to interferon-free therapies ameliorates HCV-induced portal hypertension. J Hepatol. 2016;65:692–9.
44. Schwabl P, Mandorfer M, Steiner S, et al. Interferon-free regimens improve portal hypertension and histological necroinflammation in HIV/HCV patients with advanced liver disease. Aliment Pharmacol Ther. 2017;45:139–49.
45. Verlinden W, Francque S, Michielsen P, Vanwolleghem T. Successful antiviral treatment of chronic hepatitis C leads to a rapid decline of liver stiffness without an early effect on spleen stiffness. Hepatology. 2016;64:1809–10.
46. Knop V, Hoppe D, Welzel T, Vermehren J, Herrmann E, Vermehren A, Friedrich-Rust M, Sarrazin C, Zeuzem S, Welker M-W. Regression of fibrosis and portal hypertension in HCV-associated cirrhosis and sustained virologic response after interferon-free antiviral therapy. J Viral Hepat. 2016. https://doi.org/10.1111/jvh.12578.
47. Kim HY, Jung YJ, So YH, Woo H, Kim W. Noninvasive prediction of hemodynamic response to carvedilol therapy for primary prophylaxis in cirrhotic patients with esophageal varices: a prospective study. J Hepatol. 2017;66:S47.
48. Al-Dahshan M. Clinical application of transient elastography in prediction of portal hypertension related complication in patients with chronic liver diseases. J Egypt Soc Parasitol. 2012;42:79–88.
49. Liu F, Li T, Han T, Xiang H, Zhang H. Non-invasive assessment of portal hypertension in patients with liver cirrhosis using FibroScan transient elastography. Zhonghua Gan Zang Bing Za Zhi. 2013;21:840–4.
50. Sharma P, Kirnake V, Tyagi P, Bansal N, Singla V, Kumar A, Arora A. Spleen stiffness in patients with cirrhosis in predicting esophageal varices. Am J Gastroenterol. 2013;108:1101–7.
51. Stefanescu H, Radu C, Procopet B, Lupsor-Platon M, Habic A, Tantau M, Grigorescu M. Non-invasive menage a trois for the prediction of high-risk varices: stepwise algorithm using lok score, liver and spleen stiffness. Liver Int. 2015;35:317–25.
52. Buechter M, Kahraman A, Manka P, Gerken G, Jochum C, Canbay A, Dechene A. Spleen and liver stiffness is positively correlated with the risk of esophageal variceal bleeding. Digestion. 2016;94:138–44.
53. Wong GL-H, Kwok R, Chan HL-Y, Tang SP-K, Lee E, Lam TC-H, Lau TW-Y, Ma TM-K, Wong BC-K, Wong VW-S. Measuring spleen stiffness to predict varices in chronic hepatitis B cirrhotic patients with or without receiving non-selective beta-blockers. J Dig Dis. 2016;17:538–46.

54. Guo YL, Lu XL, Cheng Y, Shi HT, Xie DH, Li H, Dong L. Combination measurement of liver and spleen stiffness with portal vein width to evaluate risk of bleeding in esophageal and gastric varices patients. Zhonghua Gan Zang Bing Za Zhi. 2016;24:56–61.
55. Bota S, Sporea I, Sirli R, Focsa M, Popescu A, Danila M, Strain M. Can ARFI elastography predict the presence of significant esophageal varices in newly diagnosed cirrhotic patients? Ann Hepatol. 2012;11:519–25.
56. Takuma Y, Nouso K, Morimoto Y, et al. Measurement of spleen stiffness by acoustic radiation force impulse imaging identifies cirrhotic patients with esophageal varices. Gastroenterology. 2013;144:92–101.e2.
57. Rizzo L, Attanasio M, Pinzone MR, Berretta M, Malaguarnera M, Morra A, L'Abbate L, Balestreri L, Nunnari G, Cacopardo B. A new sampling method for spleen stiffness measurement based on quantitative acoustic radiation force impulse elastography for noninvasive assessment of esophageal varices in newly diagnosed HCV-related cirrhosis. Biomed Res Int. 2014;2014:365982.
58. Kim HY, Jin EH, Kim W, et al. The role of spleen stiffness in determining the severity and bleeding risk of esophageal varices in cirrhotic patients. Medicine (Baltimore). 2015;94:e1031.
59. Tomita H, Ohkuma K, Masugi Y, et al. Diagnosing native liver fibrosis and esophageal varices using liver and spleen stiffness measurements in biliary atresia: a pilot study. Pediatr Radiol. 2016;46:1409–17.
60. Park J, Kwon H, Cho J, Oh J, Lee S, Han S, Lee SW, Baek Y. Is the spleen stiffness value acquired using acoustic radiation force impulse (ARFI) technology predictive of the presence of esophageal varices in patients with cirrhosis of various etiologies? Med Ultrason. 2016;18:11–7.
61. Takuma Y, Morimoto Y, Takabatake H, Toshikuni N, Tomokuni J, Sahara A, Matsueda K, Yamamoto H. Measurement of spleen stiffness with acoustic radiation force impulse imaging predicts mortality and hepatic decompensation in patients with liver cirrhosis. Clin Gastroenterol Hepatol. 2016. https://doi.org/10.1016/j.cgh.2016.10.041.
62. Takuma Y, Nouso K, Morimoto Y, Tomokuni J, Sahara A, Takabatake H, Doi A, Matsueda K, Yamamoto H. Prediction of oesophageal variceal bleeding by measuring spleen stiffness in patients with liver cirrhosis. Gut. 2016;65:354–5.
63. Zhang GY, Tang Y, Niu NN, Wu HT. Clinical value of acoustic radiation force impulse technique to predict esophageal and gastric varices in patients with biliary atresia. Zhonghua Yi Xue Za Zhi. 2017;97:525–8.
64. Grgurevic I, Bokun T, Mustapic S, Trkulja V, Heinzl R, Banic M, Puljiz Z, Luksic B, Kujundzic M. Real-time two-dimensional shear wave ultrasound elastography of the liver is a reliable predictor of clinical outcomes and the presence of esophageal varices in patients with compensated liver cirrhosis. Croat Med J. 2015;56:470–81.
65. Stefanescu H, Allegretti G, Salvatore V, Piscaglia F. Bidimensional shear wave ultrasound elastography with supersonic imaging to predict presence of esophageal varices in cirrhosis. Liver Int. 2017. https://doi.org/10.1111/liv.13418.
66. de Franchis R, Baveno VI Faculty. Expanding consensus in portal hypertension: report of the Baveno VI Consensus Workshop: stratifying risk and individualizing care for portal hypertension. J Hepatol. 2015;63:743–52.
67. Ma X, Wang L, Wu H, Feng Y, Han X, Bu H, Zhu Q. Spleen stiffness is superior to liver stiffness for predicting esophageal varices in chronic liver disease: a meta-analysis. PLoS One. 2016;11:e0165786.
68. Singh S, Eaton JE, Murad MH, Tanaka H, Iijima H, Talwalkar JA. Accuracy of spleen stiffness measurement in detection of esophageal varices in patients with chronic liver disease: systematic review and meta-analysis. Clin Gastroenterol Hepatol. 2014;12:935–945.e4.
69. D'Amico G, Garcia-Tsao G, Pagliaro L. Natural history and prognostic indicators of survival in cirrhosis: a systematic review of 118 studies. J Hepatol. 2006;44:217–31.

70. Ripoll C, Groszmann R, Garcia-Tsao G, et al. Hepatic venous pressure gradient predicts clinical decompensation in patients with compensated cirrhosis. Gastroenterology. 2007;133:481–8.
71. Radu C, Stefanescu H, Procopet B, Lupsor Platon M, Tantau M, Grigorescu M. Is spleen stiffness a predictor of clinical decompensation in cirrhotic patients? J Gastrointestin Liver Dis. 2014;23:223–4.
72. Mori K, Arai H, Abe T, Takayama H, Toyoda M, Ueno T, Sato K. Spleen stiffness correlates with the presence of ascites but not esophageal varices in chronic hepatitis C patients. Biomed Res Int. 2013;2013:857862.
73. Gao J, Zheng X, Zheng Y-Y, Zuo G-Q, Ran H-T, Auh YH, Waldron L, Chan T, Wang Z-G. Shear wave elastography of the spleen for monitoring transjugular intrahepatic portosystemic shunt function: a pilot study. J Ultrasound Med. 2016;35:951–8.
74. Novelli PM, Cho K, Rubin JM. Sonographic assessment of spleen stiffness before and after transjugular intrahepatic portosystemic shunt placement with or without concurrent embolization of portal systemic collateral veins in patients with cirrhosis and portal hypertension: a feasibility study. J Ultrasound Med. 2015;34:443–9.
75. Ran H-T, Ye X-P, Zheng Y-Y, Zhang D-Z, Wang Z-G, Chen J, Madoff D, Gao J. Spleen stiffness and splenoportal venous flow: assessment before and after transjugular intrahepatic portosystemic shunt placement. J Ultrasound Med. 2013;32:221–8.
76. Gao J, Ran H-T, Ye X-P, Zheng Y-Y, Zhang D-Z, Wang Z-G. The stiffness of the liver and spleen on ARFI Imaging pre and post TIPS placement: a preliminary observation. Clin Imaging. 2012;36:135–41.
77. Chin JL, Chan G, Ryan JD, McCormick PA. Spleen stiffness can non-invasively assess resolution of portal hypertension after liver transplantation. Liver Int. 2015;35:518–23.
78. Garcia-Pagàn J, et al. EASL Clinical Practice Guidelines: vascular diseases of the liver. J Hepatol. 2016;64:179–202.
79. Alvarez-Larrán A, Abraldes JG, Cervantes F, Hernández-Guerra M, Vizzutti F, Miquel R, Gilabert R, Giusti M, Garcia-Pagan JC, Bosch J. Portal hypertension secondary to myelofibrosis: a study of three cases. Am J Gastroenterol. 2005;100:2355–8.
80. Angermayr B, Cejna M, Schoder M, Wrba F, Valent P, Gangl A, Peck-Radosavljevic M. Transjugular intrahepatic portosystemic shunt for treatment of portal hypertension due to extramedullary hematopoiesis in idiopathic myelofibrosis. Blood. 2002;99:4246–7.
81. Qi X, Jia J, Bai M, Fan D, Han G. Portal hypertension complicating myelofibrosis in a patient without portal or hepatic vein thrombosis. Ann Gastroenterol. 2014;27:188.
82. Webb M, Shibolet O, Halpern Z, Nagar M, Amariglio N, Levit S, Steinberg DM, Santo E, Salomon O. Assessment of liver and spleen stiffness in patients with myelofibrosis using FibroScan and shear wave elastography. Ultrasound Q. 2015;31:166–9.
83. Iurlo A, Cattaneo D, Giunta M, et al. Transient elastography spleen stiffness measurements in primary myelofibrosis patients: a pilot study in a single centre. Br J Haematol. 2015;170:890–2.
84. Sharma P, Mishra SR, Kumar M, Sharma BC, Sarin SK. Liver and spleen stiffness in patients with extrahepatic portal vein obstruction. Radiology. 2012;263:893–9.
85. Berzigotti A. Non-invasive evaluation of portal hypertension using ultrasound elastography. J Hepatol. 2017. https://doi.org/10.1016/j.jhep.2017.02.003.
86. Colecchia A, Marasco G, Ravaioli F, Kleinschmidt K, Masetti R, Prete A, Pession A, Festi D. Usefulness of liver stiffness measurement in predicting hepatic veno-occlusive disease development in patients who undergo HSCT. Bone Marrow Transplant. 2016;52(3):494–7.
87. Seijo S, Reverter E, Miquel R, Berzigotti A, Abraldes JG, Bosch J, García-Pagán JC. Role of hepatic vein catheterisation and transient elastography in the diagnosis of idiopathic portal hypertension. Dig Liver Dis. 2012;44:855–60.
88. Furuichi Y, Moriyasu F, Taira J, Sugimoto K, Sano T, Ichimura S, Miyata Y, Imai Y. Noninvasive diagnostic method for idiopathic portal hypertension based on measurements of liver and spleen stiffness by ARFI elastography. J Gastroenterol. 2013;48:1061–8.

89. Colecchia A, Di Biase AR, Scaioli E, et al. Non-invasive methods can predict oesophageal varices in patients with biliary atresia after a Kasai procedure. Dig Liver Dis. 2011;43:659–63.
90. Uchida H, Sakamoto S, Kobayashi M, et al. The degree of spleen stiffness measured on acoustic radiation force impulse elastography predicts the severity of portal hypertension in patients with biliary atresia after portoenterostomy. J Pediatr Surg. 2015;50:559–64.
91. Tomita H, Fuchimoto Y, Ohkuma K, et al. Spleen stiffness measurements by acoustic radiation force impulse imaging after living donor liver transplantation in children: a potential quantitative index for venous complications. Pediatr Radiol. 2015;45:658–66.
92. Lee M-J, Kim M-J, Han KH, Yoon CS. Age-related changes in liver, kidney, and spleen stiffness in healthy children measured with acoustic radiation force impulse imaging. Eur J Radiol. 2013;82:e290–4.
93. Karlas T, Lindner F, Troltzsch M, Keim V. Assessment of spleen stiffness using acoustic radiation force impulse imaging (ARFI): definition of examination standards and impact of breathing maneuvers. Ultraschall Med. 2014;35:38–43.
94. Canas T, Fontanilla T, Miralles M, Macia A, Malalana A, Roman E. Normal values of spleen stiffness in healthy children assessed by acoustic radiation force impulse imaging (ARFI): comparison between two ultrasound transducers. Pediatr Radiol. 2015;45:1316–22.
95. Balakrishnan M, Souza F, Munoz C, Augustin S, Loo N, Deng Y, Ciarleglio M, Garcia-Tsao G. Liver and spleen stiffness measurements by point shear wave elastography via acoustic radiation force impulse: intraobserver and interobserver variability and predictors of variability in a US population. J Ultrasound Med. 2016;35:2373–80.
96. Kassym L, Nounou MA, Zhumadilova Z, Dajani AI, Barkibayeva N, Myssayev A, Rakhypbekov T, Abuhammour AM. New combined parameter of liver and splenic stiffness as determined by elastography in healthy volunteers. Saudi J Gastroenterol. 2016;22:324–30.
97. Chen S-H, Li Y-F, Lai H-C, Kao J-T, Peng C-Y, Chuang P-H, Su W-P, Chiang I-P. Noninvasive assessment of liver fibrosis via spleen stiffness measurement using acoustic radiation force impulse sonoelastography in patients with chronic hepatitis B or C. J Viral Hepat. 2012;19:654–63.
98. Pawlus A, Inglot MS, Szymanska K, et al. Shear wave elastography of the spleen: evaluation of spleen stiffness in healthy volunteers. Abdom Radiol (NY). 2016;41:2169–74.
99. Stefanescu H, Procopet B, Platon Lupsor M. Modified spleen stiffness measurement: a step forward, but still not the solution to all problems in the noninvasive assessment of cirrhotic patients. J Viral Hepat. 2014;21:e54.
100. Han H, Yang J, Zhuge Y, Zhang M, Wu M. Point shear wave elastography to evaluate and monitor changing portal venous pressure in patients with decompensated cirrhosis. Ultrasound Med Biol. 2017. https://doi.org/10.1016/j.ultrasmedbio.2017.01.019.

Diagnostic Methods for Cirrhosis and Portal Hypertension: Imaging: Ultrasound and Doppler Ultrasonography

9

Soon Koo Baik and Moon Young Kim

Abbreviations

DI	Damping index
HV	Hepatic vein
HVPG	Hepatic venous pressure gradient
PH	Portal hypertension
PI	Pulsatility index
PV	Portal vein
RI	Resistive index
SV	Splenic vein
US	Ultrasonography

Because of its low cost, ease of use, and high patient compliance, ultrasonography (US) including Doppler US has been widely applied as an alternative diagnosis for hepatic fibrosis, cirrhosis and portal hypertension (PH) for several decades. Grayscale US and Doppler US have both their own advantages and limitations in clinical application. We overview the role of various US indices used in the diagnosis of cirrhosis and PH.

9.1 Grayscale US

Grayscale US (simple US) is a noninvasive, relatively simple, and inexpensive test that is used to study and follow-up patients with advanced chronic liver disease or cirrhosis. Various factors, including the liver size, bluntness of the liver edge,

S.K. Baik, M.D., Ph.D. (✉) • M.Y. Kim, M.D., Ph.D.
Department of Internal Medicine, Yonsei University, Wonju College of Medicine,
Wonju Severance Christian Hospital, Wonju, Republic of Korea
e-mail: baiksk@yonsei.ac.kr; drkimmy@yonsei.ac.kr

© Springer International Publishing AG, part of Springer Nature 2018
A. Berzigotti, J. Bosch (eds.), *Diagnostic Methods for Cirrhosis and Portal Hypertension*, https://doi.org/10.1007/978-3-319-72628-1_9

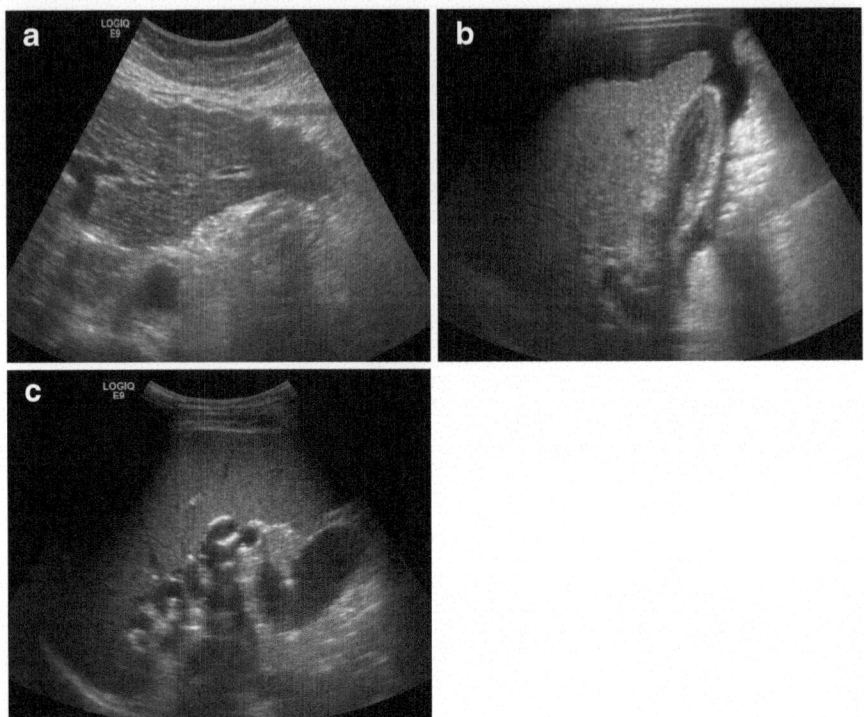

Fig. 9.1 Ultrasonography in liver cirrhosis shows irregular surface and blunted angle of the liver with coarse parenchymal echo pattern (**a**), right lobe atrophic change with ascites (**b**) and spleno-megaly with collaterals at the hilum (**c**)

coarseness of the liver parenchyma, nodularity of the liver surface, and spleen size have been suggested as useful parameters for US-based evaluation of advanced chronic liver disease (Fig. 9.1) [1–4]; among them, liver surface nodularity (prefer-ably assessed with linear high frequency probes) is the best single parameter associ-ated with the presence of cirrhosis [1–4]. In addition, US examination indicated that the thickness of the liver capsule, maximum oblique diameter of the right liver, diameter of the splenic vein (SV), and thickness of the spleen correlate with the staging of liver fibrosis. The use of multiple grey-scale US parameters (i.e., liver size, liver surface nodularity, spleen length, and SV respiratory variation) and one Doppler US variable (i.e., portal vein blood flow velocity, PVV) showed a diagnos-tic accuracy ranging from 73% for the diagnosis of significant fibrosis (METAVIR score of $\geq$F2) to 84% for severe fibrosis (METAVIR score of $\geq$F3) [5]. In another study, a combination of six US indices, namely liver surface and edge nodularity, parenchyma echogenicity, presence of right lobe atrophy, spleen size, SV diameter, and abnormality of hepatic waveform, also successfully diagnosed overt cirrhosis with 89.2% sensitivity and 69.4% specificity [6]. Another study introduced a US-based scoring system based on the surface pattern and appearance of the inter-nal echogenic bands, which indicate irregular liver texture, and demonstrated a significant correlation between the US-determined and histologically determined stages of fibrosis [7]. Moreover, abdominal US is invaluable in point of care detection of portal vein thrombosis, which should be ruled out in every single patient with PH irrespective of the presence of cirrhosis. The same holds true for the presence of hepatocellular carcinoma (HCC) and of direct signs of portal hypertension (ascites, portal-systemic collaterals). The presence of portal-systemic collaterals is a pathognomonic sign of portal hypertension, which should be always investigated and reported. The most frequently observed P-S collaterals include patency of paraumbilical vein (which indicates intra-hepatic portal hypertension=, epigastric collaterals through originating from the left gastric vein (coronaria stomacica), and collaterals in the left hypocondrium arising from spleno-renal circulation and short gastric veins. Despite its importance allowing diagnosing portal hypertension, the presence of porto-systemic collaterals does not allow differentiating between cirrhotic and non-cirrhotic causes of portal hypertension, and signs of cirrhosis vs. other potential etiologies should be therefore carefully assessed.

Although US can provide a qualitative assessment of diffuse liver disease, it is subjective, operator dependent, and not quantitative. Liver fibrosis and steatosis were reported to have similar appearances on US in studies performed in the '80s ("fatty fibrotic pattern") [8]; even if this may confound the actual diagnosis, advances in the ultrasound equipments allow nowadays a more accurate evaluation of the parenchyma characteristics. Regarding fibrosis in pre-cirrhotic stages, some studies have shown that the sensitivity and specificity of US are unacceptably low and that there is no correlation between US-estimated stages and the histologically determined stages by liver biopsy [9, 10]. However, the availability of ultrasound elastography techniques embedded in ultrasound devices has largely overcome this limitation (see specific chapters of this book).

9.2   Doppler US

Regional hepatic and systemic hemodynamic changes occur in patients with chronic liver disease and become important in patients with cirrhosis and portal hypertension [1]. Doppler US can assess hemodynamic changes in a non-invasive way; thus, many attempts using Doppler US have been made to investigate the hemodynamic alterations in cirrhosis and the response to medical treatment of portal hypertension (PH) [1, 2, 11–17]. Doppler US parameters that have been investigated include mean and maximum (time-averaged) portal vein (PV) velocity, blood flow volume of the portal vein (PVF), "congestion index" of the PV (which ratios the diameter and the blood flow velocity), effective portal liver perfusion, and resistance indices of arteries in the liver and spleen [1, 11–14]. A higher congestion index of the PV has been associated with a higher risk of bleeding from esophageal varices. Furthermore, pulsed wave Doppler can be used to determine the changes in waveforms of proper hepatic arteries, the PV, and the hepatic veins (HV). A reversal of portal blood flow in the main portal vein trunk usually indicates the presence of large portal-systemic collaterals upstream. Intrahepatic reversal of portal blood flow only in a segmental area should prompt the suspicion of intrahepatic shunts or artero-venous fistulae, which should be carefully ruled-out. The flow pattern in the right HV is triphasic in healthy individuals, and patients with a biphasic or mono-phasic flow pattern are at a higher risk of advanced fibrosis, cirrhosis and portal hypertension [1, 2, 11, 15, 17]. Some Doppler parameters have been proposed as candidate surrogates of the hepatic venous pressure gradient (HVPG) [11, 15]. However, on validation studies none has proved to be accurate enough, particularly to mirror changes of HVPG after pharmacological therapies. One of the possible reasons is that Doppler measurements can be influenced by many patient-related factors, such as respiration, food ingestion, vasoactive drugs, age, as well as by interobserver and interequipment variability. Furthermore, presence of portal-systemic collateral vessels, hepatic steatosis, and inflammation may all contribute to measurement variability [1, 15, 18]. Accuracy in the Doppler measurement are therefore key to provide reproducible and clinically meaningful data, and ultra-sound physician should follow the established international recommendations to perform and report Doppler in this field [19, 20].

9.3 Measurements of Doppler US Parameters

9.3.1 Blood Velocity and Flow

Doppler US makes it possible to examine the hemodynamics of abdominal vessels, including the measurement of blood flow velocity and flow volume in the hepatic and portal systems. This method is technically simple, and its clinical application for PH has been attempted. When measuring velocity, the angle between the Doppler beam and the long axis of the vessel should be less than $60°$ [1, 12, 14]. In line with these requirements, blood velocity and flow are easily measured for the PV and SV but are more difficult in the arterial vessels, even though the measurements are fea-sible at the superior mesenteric artery (Fig. 9.2). Portal venous flow (mL/min) is determined by the following formula: cross sectional area (cm^2) × mean velocity (cm/sec) × 60 [1, 12, 21]. The mean PV velocity is lower in cirrhotic patients than in healthy individuals due to increased intrahepatic vascular resistance (outflow resistance). Zironi et al. reported that the mean velocity values in the PV of cirrhotic patients and healthy individuals are 13.0 ± 3.2 cm/s vs. 19.6 ± 2.6 cm/s, respec-tively. A cutoff value of 15 cm/s showed a sensitivity and specificity of 88% and 96%, respectively, to diagnose cirrhosis [14]. PV velocity is lower in patients with more severe portal hypertension (i.e. large esophageal varices). However, clinical values of PV velocity may differ between patients with similar portal pressures because of the significant variability in portosystemic collateral patterns [1, 12, 13]. In addition, variability in PV velocity measurement is influenced by equipment-related factors as well as by intra- and inter-observer variance [18]. This can be reduced by proper training and standardization of measurement site. Splenic venous velocity and flow increase are associated with a dilated SV and an enlarged spleen in portal hypertensive patients. A splenic venous flow higher than portal venous

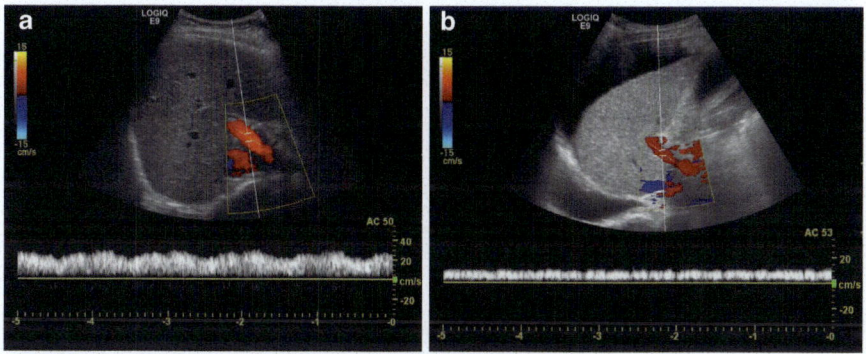

Fig. 9.2 Measurement of the portal venous velocity. Portal venous velocity in a patient with cirrhosis and portal hypertension (**a**) is lower than that in a healthy control (**b**)

flow may point out to the formation of portosystemic collaterals and gastroesophageal varices, and risk of variceal bleeding [16]. Overall, the results regarding the usefulness of Doppler US-determined SV and PV velocity for assessing the severity of PH in patients with cirrhosis are inconclusive [12–14, 16].

9.3.2 Resistive and Pulsatility Index

Regardless of the incidence angle, the resistances in the hepatic, splenic, and renal artery can be evaluated by measuring the resistive index (RI) and pulsatility index (PI) if the vessel is identified by color Doppler [1, 12, 22]. The RI [(peak systolic velocity − end diastolic velocity)/peak systolic velocity] and PI [(peak systolic velocity − end diastolic velocity)/mean velocity] can be estimated by measuring the peak systolic velocity, end diastolic velocity, and mean velocity (Fig. 9.3) [1, 12, 22]. With higher arterial resistance, peak systolic velocity increases and peak diastolic velocity decreases. Therefore, RI and PI increase with higher arterial resistance. PI is different from RI in that it uses the mean velocity as the denominator instead of peak velocity in its calculation eq. PI is superior to RI when arterial resistance is so high that end diastolic velocity is close to 0 (1). The splenic RI and hepatic PI increase in tandem with the increase in HVPG. Even though the kidney is an extrahepatic organ, measuring RI and PI in the kidney can be useful to diagnose PH and cirrhosis. Renal RI and PI are increased in patients with PH and cirrhosis, particularly in advanced stages because renal vasoconstriction is driven by a decrease in effective circulatory volume inducing an increase in sympathetic tone in cirrhosis (Fig. 9.4) [1, 12, 22]. Interestingly, renal RI predicts the onset of hepatorenal syndrome in patients with decompensated cirrhosis, and mirrors the improvement of kidney function in treated patients. However, like other Doppler indices, PI and RI also have limitations with regards to their clinical reproducibility (it is difficult to evaluate the RI and PI under the same conditions in different patients), and the accuracy of these parameters is matter of debate [1, 12].

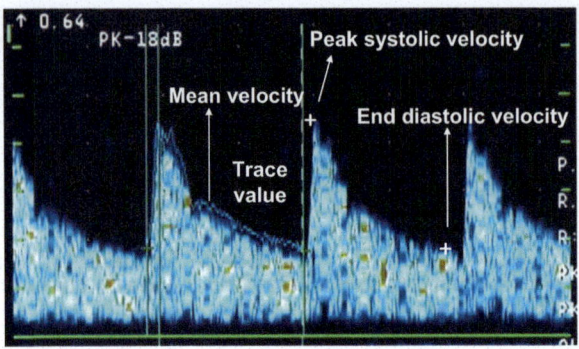

Fig. 9.3 Measurements of resistive index (RI) and pulsatility index (PI). RI = (peak systolic velocity − end diastolic velocity)/peak systolic velocity; PI = (peak systolic velocity − end diastolic velocity)/mean velocity

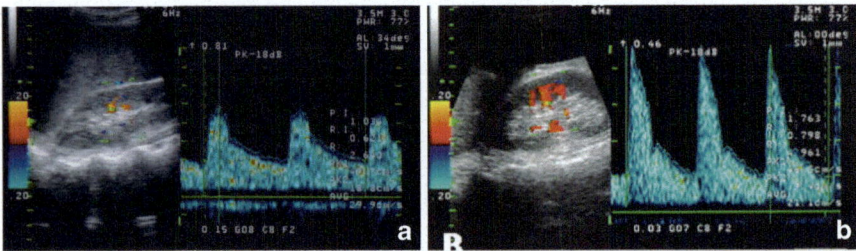

Fig. 9.4 Measurement of renal arterial pulsatility index (PI) and resistive index (RI). In a patient with Child-Pugh A, Doppler ultrasonography shows PI of 1.0 and RI of 0.6 in the renal artery, which are within the normal range (**a**). In a patient with Child-Pugh C, Doppler ultrasonography shows PI of 1.8 and RI of 0.8 in the renal artery, which are higher than the corresponding values for the patient with Child-Pugh A (**b**)

9.3.3 Hepatic Vein Waveform Analysis

The Doppler HV waveform in healthy individuals is triphasic (two negative waves and one positive) owing to variations in central venous pressure according to the cardiac cycle. In patients with cirrhosis, the presence of abnormal biphasic or monophasic HV waveforms has been confirmed by several studies (Fig. 9.5) [1, 2, 11, 15, 17]. The HV can be easily visualized along its longitudinal axis by color flow mapping in the supine position. In HV visualization, the flow appears blue in color flow mapping because it is away from the ultrasonic probe. In a study wherein Baik et al. prospectively examined the relationship between waveforms and the severity of PH as measured by HVPG, a correlation was found between abnormalities in HV waveforms and HVPG, i.e., with increasing HVPG, HV waveforms tended to flatten. Furthermore, a monophasic waveform was associated with severe PH (HVPG >15 mmHg) with relatively high sensitivity and specificity in that study population [11]. In addition, changes in HV waveforms following vasoactive agent

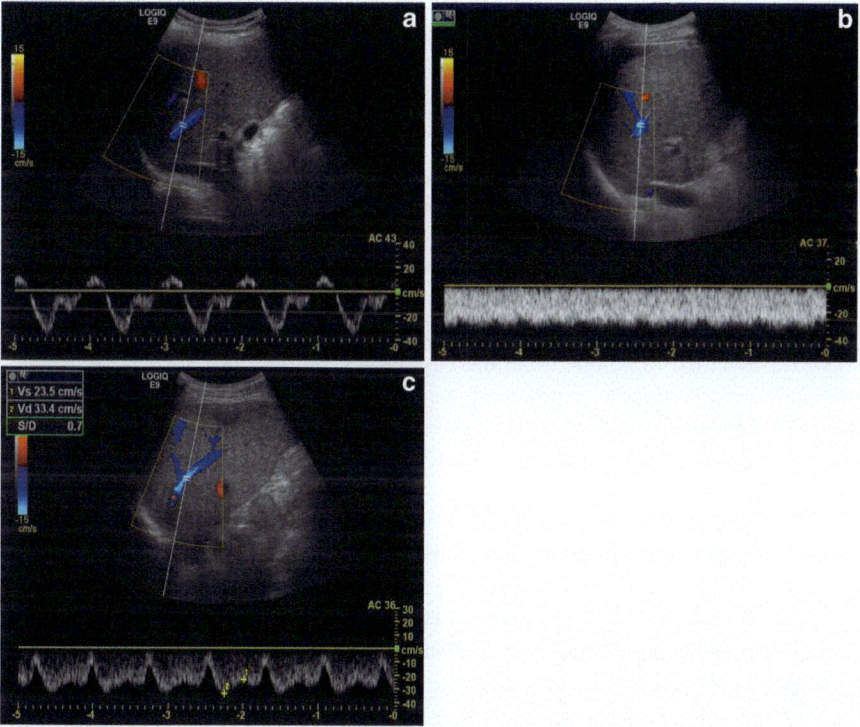

Fig. 9.5 Hepatic vein waveform on Doppler ultrasonography. Normal triphasic waveform comprises two forward flows and one reverse flow (**a**). In patients with liver cirrhosis and portal hypertension, an abnormal flat hepatic vein waveform (monophasic pattern) is observed (**b**). A monophasic pattern of hepatic vein waveform is associated with the presence of severe portal hypertension and advanced liver cirrhosis. (**c**) The measurement of damping index (0.7)

administration (which reduces the portal pressure) were also significantly correlated with changes in HVPG. Assessment of the damping index (DI) of the HV waveform allows for the quantification of the extent of its abnormality. Kim et al. prospectively evaluated the correlation between the extent of abnormal Doppler HV waveforms expressed as DI and HVPG and the response to propranolol in patients with cirrhosis. DI is calculated as minimum velocity/maximum velocity of the HV waveform. DI was significantly correlated with the grade of HVPG, i.e., with higher HVPG, increased DI was observed, and DI >0.6 was significantly more likely to indicate severe PH (sensitivity, 75.9% and specificity 81.8%) [15]. Regarding the evaluation of response to drugs, changes in DI following propranolol treatment also significantly correlated with changes in HVPG. Thus, these results suggest that when HVPG measurement is not feasible or available, the evaluation of the Doppler HV waveform may be a valuable supplementary tool to assess the therapeutic response to vasoactive drugs used to treat PH, although these findings require further validation and should be shown to be able to detect accurately decreases in HVPG of >10% and of >20% of baseline values, and of reaching a final HVPG

<12 mmHg. In a systematic review of 14 studies wherein the diagnostic performance of US for PH in patients with cirrhosis was evaluated [17], there was a statistically significant correlation between HVPG and HV, and the sensitivity and specificity of the HV waveform using HVPG as a reference are 75.9–77.8% were 81.8–100%, respectively.

The exact cause of these changes in the Doppler HV waveform remains unclear. The surrounding structural changes with increased rigidity of hepatic parenchyma and HV may be the main causes of this phenomenon. However, previous studies have shown that vasoactive agent-induced improvements in the waveforms, suggesting that hemodynamic effects linked to high portal pressure may also be a major factor of abnormal HV waveforms in PH [11, 15]. In other works, flattening of HV wave was deemed to be due to an increase in HV inflow from intrahepatic shunts implicated in PH, resulting in hemodynamic blunting of the effect of variations in central venous pressure during the cardiac cycle [1].

Conclusion

Grayscale and Doppler US are safe, inexpensive, and simple to use at the bedside or for outpatients; furthermore, they are important in examining morphological changes in the liver as well as hemodynamics of abdominal vessels of the hepatic and portal systems in patients with cirrhosis and PH. Therefore, US and Doppler US are useful tools for the diagnosis of cirrhosis and PH. Particularly, combining grey scale US and Doppler US parameters can improve the diagnostic accuracy of cirrhosis and PH.

References

1. Baik SK. Haemodynamic evaluation by Doppler ultrasonography in patients with portal hypertension: a review. Liver Int. 2010;30:1403–13.
2. Kim MY, Jeong WK, Baik SK. Invasive and non-invasive diagnosis of cirrhosis and portal hypertension. World J Gastroenterol. 2014;20(15):4300.
3. Colli A, Fraquelli M, Andreoletti M, et al. Severe liver fibrosis or cirrhosis: accuracy of US for detection – analysis of 300 cases. Radiology. 2003;227:89–94.
4. Shen L, Li JQ, Zeng MD, et al. Correlation between ultrasonographic and pathologic diagnosis of liver fibrosis due to chronic virus hepatitis. World J Gastroenterol. 2006;12:1292–5.
5. Aube C, Oberti F, Korali N, et al. Ultrasonographic diagnosis of hepatic fibrosis or cirrhosis. J Hepatol. 1999;30:472–8.
6. Moon KM, Kim G, Baik SK, et al. Ultrasonographic scoring system score versus liver stiffness measurement in prediction of cirrhosis. Clin Mol Hepatol. 2013;19:389–98.
7. Khan KN, Yamasaki M, Yamasaki K, et al. Proposed abdominal sonographic staging to predict severity of liver diseases – analysis with peritoneoscopy and histology. Dig Dis Sci. 2000;45:554–64.
8. Needleman L, Kurtz AB, Rifkin MD, et al. Sonography of diffuse benign liver disease: accuracy of pattern recognition and grading. AJR Am J Roentgenol. 1986;146(5):1011.
9. Chen CH, Lin ST, Yang CC, et al. The accuracy of sonography in predicting steatosis and fibrosis in chronic hepatitis C. Dig Dis Sci. 2008;53:1699–706.
10. Kutcher R, Smith GS, Sen F, et al. Comparison of sonograms and liver histologic findings in patients with chronic hepatitis C virus infection. J Ultrasound Med. 1998;17(5):321.

11. Baik SK, Kim JW, Kim HS, et al. Recent variceal bleeding: Doppler US hepatic vein wave-form in assessment of severity of portal hypertension and vasoactive drug response. Radiology. 2006;240:574–80.
12. Choi YJ, Baik SK, Park DH, et al. Comparison of Doppler ultrasonography and the hepatic venous pressure gradient in assessing portal hypertension in liver cirrhosis. J Gastroenterol Hepatol. 2003;18:424–9.
13. Merkel C, Sacerdoti D, Bolognesi M, et al. Doppler sonography and hepatic vein catheteriza-tion in portal hypertension: assessment of agreement in evaluating severity and response to treatment. J Hepatol. 1998;28:622–30.
14. Zironi G, Gaiani S, Fenyves D, et al. Value of measurement of mean portal flow velocity by Doppler flowmetry in the diagnosis of portal hypertension. J Hepatol. 1992;16:298–303.
15. Kim MY, Baik SK, Park DH, et al. Damping index of Doppler hepatic vein waveform to assess the severity of portal hypertension and response to propranolol in liver cirrhosis: a prospective nonrandomized study. Liver Int. 2007;27:1103–10.
16. Nelson RC, Sherbourne GM, Spencer HB, et al. Splenic venous flow exceeding portal venous flow at Doppler sonography – relationship to portosystemic varices. Am J Roentgenol. 1993;161:563–7.
17. Kim G, Cho YZ, Baik SK, et al. The accuracy of ultrasonography for the evaluation of portal hypertension in patients with cirrhosis: a systematic review. Korean J Radiol. 2015;16:314–24.
18. Jee MG, Baik SK, Park DH, et al. Interequipment variability of Doppler ultrasonographic indices in patients with liver cirrhosis. Korean J Hepatol. 2006;12:539–45.
19. Berzigotti A, Piscaglia F. Ultrasound in portal hypertension—part 1. Ultraschall Med. 2011;32:548–68. quiz 569–571
20. Berzigotti A, Piscaglia F, Education E, et al. Ultrasound in portal hypertension—part 2—and EFSUMB recommendations for the performance and reporting of ultrasound examinations in portal hypertension. Ultraschall Med. 2012;33:8–32. quiz 30–31
21. Baik SK, Park DH, Kim MY, et al. Captopril reduces portal pressure effectively in portal hypertensive patients with low portal venous velocity. J Gastroenterol. 2003;38:1150–4.
22. Baik SK, Jee MG, Jeong PH, et al. Relationship of hemodynamic indices and prognosis in patients with liver cirrhosis. Korean J Intern Med. 2004;19:165–70.

Contrast-Enhanced Ultrasonography for the Diagnosis of Portal Hypertension

10

Hitoshi Maruyama and Naoya Kato

10.1 Introduction

Portal hypertension is the major pathogenesis of cirrhosis and non-cirrhotic portal hypertension [1, 2]. The increase in portal venous pressure determines the severity of portal hypertension, which is associated with various manifestations such as development of gastroesophageal varices, portal hypertensive gastropathy, ascites, and hepatic encephalopathy [3]. Because portal pressure is also a significant prognostic factor for patients with portal hypertension, it is recognized as a key parameter in their medical care.

Hepatic venous pressure gradient (HVPG) is a surrogate marker for portal venous pressure, and is obtained by invasive procedures using hepatic venous catheterization. Recently, the increasing need of measuring the HVPG due to its many valuable applications has encouraged to introduce non-invasive markers that may replace invasive procedures to reduce the burden on patients [4, 5].

Ultrasound (US) is a minimally invasive technique that enables simple and real-time observations of the hemodynamics and anatomical structures under physiological conditions [6]. It may be the most frequently used imaging tool in the practical management of patients with chronic liver disease. Given the introduction of microbubble contrast agents, along with the development of digital technologies, contrast-enhanced US (CEUS) has become a popular imaging modality for the detailed assessment of liver diseases [7–9]. This chapter describes the concept, benefits, and limitations of CEUS for the non-invasive assessment of portal hypertension.

H. Maruyama, M.D., Ph.D. (✉) • N. Kato, M.D., Ph.D.
Department of Gastroenterology, Chiba University Graduate School of Medicine, Chiba, Japan
e-mail: maru-cib@umin.ac.jp

10.2   Contrast Agents

Contrast agents for US are microbubble-based materials with various properties depending on the kinds of gas and other chemical substances [10]. The latter, such as proteins, lipids, or polymers, are used as a shell to enhance stabilization. Because the diameter of microbubbles is smaller than that of red blood cells, when administered intravenously, they move freely in the bloodstream.

Levovist is the first-generation contrast agent characterized by galactose-based, air-filled microbubbles with palmitic acid (Schering AG, Berlin, Germany) [10]. The newer generations consist of less diffusible gas cores with very flexible and soft envelopes to improve stability and persistence [10].

There are three types of second-generation microbubble agents available for the abdomen [11]: *SonoVue* (sulfur hexafluoride; Bracco, Milan, Italy), *Sonazoid* (perfluorobutane; GE Healthcare UK Ltd., Pollards Wood, UK), and *Definity* (perflutren lipid microsphere; Lantheus Medical Imaging, Billerica, MA, USA). SonoVue and Definity are so-called blood pool contrast agents that travel in the vascular space without accumulating property, whereas Sonazoid is captured in the reticuloendothelial systems such as the Kupffer cells.

There are possible side effects when using microbubble contrast agents, and severe hypersensitivity events related to CEUS may occur [10]. However, the incidence is much lower than that with iodinated contrast materials and is comparable to that of the contrast materials for magnetic resonance imaging (MRI) [10, 11]. It should be emphasized that microbubble contrast agents are safe, nonetheless the CEUS examinations should be performed in the appropriate facilities for emergency management and the operators should be trained in resuscitation. There is limited data on the usage of microbubble contrast agents in pregnancy, during breast feeding or in pediatrics.

10.3   Phases of Contrast Effect

Contrast-enhanced appearance in the liver changes over time because of the nature of dual vascular supply by the arteries and portal veins. The phases in CEUS are defined in a time-related manner: the arterial phase from 10–20 s to 30–45 s (Fig. 10.1a), the portal venous phase from 30–45 s to 120 s (Figs. 10.1b and 10.2), and the late phase after 120 s to the time of microbubble disappearance [11]. Sonazoid-induced enhancement after 10 min or later is called the "post-vascular phase" created by the accumulated microbubbles (Fig. 10.3). Needless to say, the time definition is sensitive to individual differences.

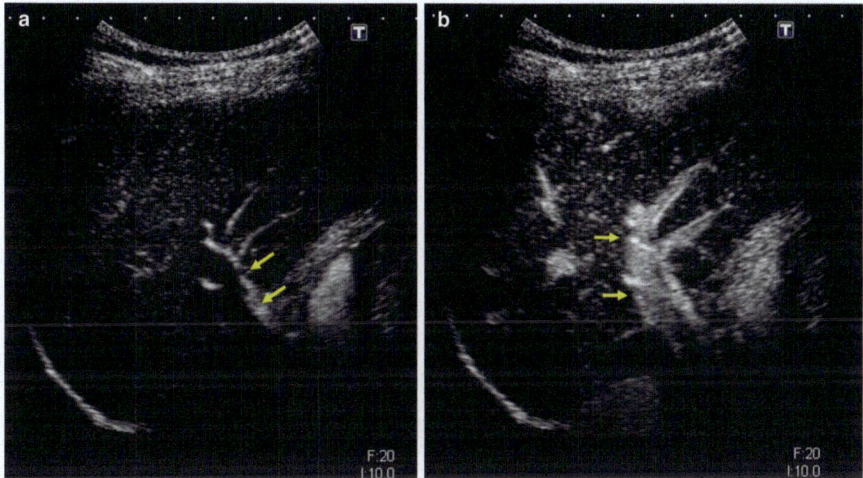

Fig. 10.1 Contrast-enhanced sonograms of the liver (Sonazoid; non-B non-C cirrhosis, 52-year-old female). (**a**) Arterial phase. The image shows the enhancement in the right hepatic artery (arrows). (**b**) Portal venous phase. The image shows the enhancement in the right portal vein (arrows)

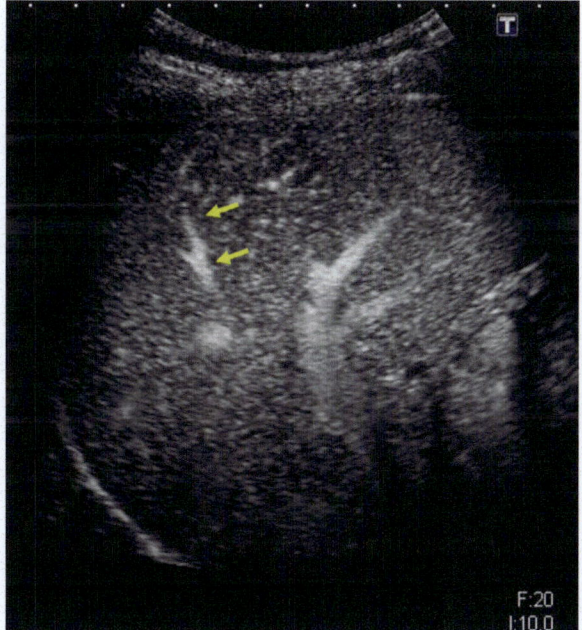

Fig. 10.2 Arrival of the contrast effect in the hepatic vein (Sonazoid; non-B non-C cirrhosis, 52-year-old female). The image shows the contrast enhancement in the right hepatic vein (arrows)

Fig. 10.3 Contrast-enhanced sonogram of the liver at the post-vascular phase (Sonazoid; 15 min after the injection, non-B non-C cirrhosis, 52-year-old female). The right lobe liver parenchyma is homogeneously enhanced with the disappearance of enhancement in the intrahepatic portal vein (arrow) and hepatic vein (arrowheads)

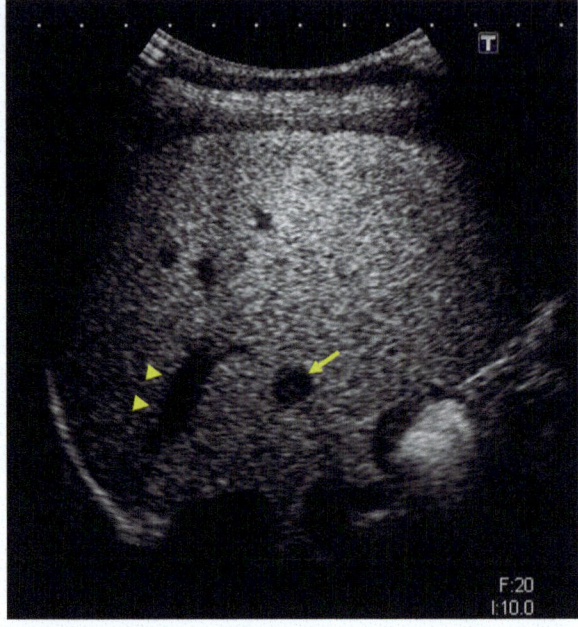

10.4 US for Dynamic Microbubbles

10.4.1 Images and Parameters

The detailed observation of earlier-phase contrast enhancement by circulating micro-bubbles allows an assessment of hepatic hemodynamics, which is closely correlated with the pathophysiology of portal hypertension. A difference in the time of appearance and/or in the intensity change is used as a marker for dynamic microbubble studies [9]. Measurement of the time difference between different vessels is a representative parameter for this purpose, reported as the transit time. Albrecht et al. initially reported this parameter, which depends on the severity of liver disease [12].

10.4.2 Severity of Portal Hypertension

The degree of portal pressure appears to affect the in vivo behavior of dynamic microbubbles. An intensity-based study by Berzigotti et al. showed a correlation between regional hepatic perfusion using SonoVue and HVPG (R = 0.279, $P = 0.041$) and hyperdynamic syndrome markers [13]. Qu et al. reported that the portal vein/hepatic artery time-intensity curve ratio (Qp/Qa), portal vein/hepatic artery strength ratio (Ip/Ia), and portal vein/hepatic artery wash-in perfusion slope ratio (βp/βa) had close correlations with portal pressure [14]. An animal study published later examined the diagnostic abilities using the same parameters: the area under the receiver operating characteristic curve (AUROC) was 0.866 by Qp/Qa for elevated portal pressure (≥18 cm H_2O) with a sensitivity of 76% and a specificity of 86%, and 0.895 by Ip/Ia with a sensitivity of 85% and a specificity of 87% [15].

With regard to the diagnostic performance, a study with a large patient population showed that the AUROC of the hepatic vein arrival time (HVAT) using SonoVue was 0.973 for HVPG >10 mmHg in compensated cirrhosis with a sensitivity of 92.7%, a specificity of 86.7%, a positive predictive value of 90.5%, a negative predictive value of 89.7%, a positive likelihood ratio of 6.95, and a negative likelihood ratio 0.08 under a cut-off value of 14 s [16] (Table 10.1). Another study also reported the usefulness of HVAT, that is, the diagnostic ability of HVAT (SonoVue) for HVPG >12 mmHg had a sensitivity of 88.9%, a specificity of 58.1% to 62.8%, and an AUROC of 0.72 under a cut-off of 19 s [17]. However, an intrahepatic transit time under 6 s offered better diagnostic ability, showing a sensitivity of 85.3% to 91.2%, a specificity of 77.8% to 88.9%, and an AUROC of 0.94 (all, $P < 0.05$) [17].

There is a new dimension in the research field of vascular and hemodynamics. Amat-Roldan et al. demonstrated that the clustering coefficient of the hepatic vascular connectome created by computer-based graph analysis using contrast sonograms (SonoVue) was lower in patients with HVPG ≥10 mmHg than in those with HVPG <10 mmHg ($P = 0.006$) [20]. Further, the model derived by the distribution

Table 10.1 Comparison of diagnostic abilities in contrast-enhanced ultrasound parameters for grading portal hypertension

Author	Contrast agent	N	Parameter (Cut-off value)	Grade of PH	Se/Sp/PPV/NPV/Ac/PLR/NLR	AUROC
Kim [16]	SonoVue	71	HVAT (14 s)	CSPH	93/87/91/90/−/6.95/0.08	0.973
Jeong [17]	SonoVue	53	HVAT (19 s)	SPH	56/89/95/35/63/−/−, R1[a]	0.72
					(50/89/94/32/58/−/−, R2[a])	0.71
			ITT (6 s)	SPH	91/89/97/73/91/−/−, R1[a]	0.94
					(85/78/94/58/84/−/−, R2[a])	0.90
Eisenbrey [18]	Sonazoid	45	SHAPE	CSPH	89/88/−/−/−/−/−	0.90
				SPH	100/81/−/−/−/−/−	0.94
Shimada [19]	Sonazoid	91	SA-SV[b] (13.5 s)	CSPH	71/68/69/70/−/−/−	0.76
			SA-SV[b] (14.5 s)	SPH	60/80/75/67/−/−/−	0.76

PH portal hypertension, *Se* sensitivity, *Sp* specificity, *PPV* positive predictive value, *NPV* negative predictive value, *Ac* accuracy, *PLR* positive likelihood ratio, *NLR* negative likelihood ratio, *AUROC* area under the receiver operating characteristic curve, *HVAT* hepatic vein arrival time, *CSPH* clinically significant portal hypertension (HVPG ≥10 mmHg), *ITT* intrahepatic transit time, *SPH* severe portal hypertension (HVPG ≥12 mmHg), *SHAPE* subharmonic aided pressure estimation
[a]R1, reader 1, R2, reader 2
[b]The interval time from the contrast onset in the splenic artery to the time to reach the maximum intensity level in the splenic vein

of the clustering coefficient (10 bins) of hepatic vascular connectome was highly correlated with the value of HVPG (r = 0.97; P < 0.0001). However the study used a short number of patients and has not yet been externally validated. Another approach is the subharmonic-aided pressure estimation (SHAPE) [21]. An animal study clearly disclosed a significant correlation between subharmonic signal amplitude changes and portal venous pressure. A clinical study performed by the same group reported that the SHAPE gradient between the portal vein and the hepatic veins showed good overall agreement with HVPG (r = 0.82) [18]. Furthermore, the SHAPE had 89% sensitivity and 88% specificity in detecting patients with HVPG ≥10 mmHg and 100% sensitivity and 81% specificity in detecting patients with HVPG ≥12 mmHg.

A recent study examined the splenic circulation using Sonazoid instead of the hepatic hemodynamics [19]. It found that the microbubble transit time from the splenic artery to the splenic vein reflects the severity of portal hypertension, probably due to the modification of the splenic hemodynamics caused by the increased portal pressure. The study showed an AUROC of 0.76 for detecting HVPG ≥10 mmHg and an AUROC of 0.76 for detecting HVPG ≥12 mmHg, indicating a moderate applicability of this technique for detecting the severity of portal hypertension.

10.5   US for Static Microbubbles

10.5.1 Images and Parameters

Sonazoid is the only second-generation contrast agent with the intrahepatic accumulating property used for the abdominal field. The post-vascular phase (10 min or later) is the time for the observation of accumulated microbubbles. Generally, scanning and observation may be much easier in the post-vascular phase than in the arterial/portal phase due to the motionlessness of the target. However, when interpreting the image, care should be taken about the source of enhancement because the duration of the availability of the circulating microbubbles depends on individual factors [22], and the image may not be necessarily originated from signals by accumulated microbubbles alone.

Transmission with higher power (high mechanical index) easily destroys microbubbles; therefore, it is applicable to estimate the amount of accumulated intrahepatic microbubbles by the subtraction of intensity between before and after microbubble disruption by high power transmission [23]. With the use of this technique, the assessment of the post-vascular phase image can be used for grading hepatic fibrosis in diffuse liver disease. A prospective study performed in 203 subjects reported that signal intensity analysis with Sonazoid showed AUROCs of 0.88 for ≥F2, 0.95 for ≥F3, and 0.97 for cirrhosis, being superior to those obtained with FIB4 (age [years] × aspartate aminotransferase [U/L]/[platelet (10^9/L) × alanine aminotransferase$^{1/2}$ (U/L)]; 0.85 for ≥F2, P = 0.15; 0.89 for ≥F3, P = 0.057; 0.90 for cirrhosis, P = 0.017) [24]. These interesting findings should be further validated and compared with other non-invasive methods, including MRI or ultrasound based hepatic elastography measurements. The potential role of the assessment of the accumulated microbubbles in predicting the actual portal pressure has not been determined.

10.6   Complications of Portal Hypertension

Portal vein thrombosis is a common cause of portal hypertension (pre-hepatic portal vein obstruction). In addition, it is also a relatively common and severe complication of patients with portal hypertension [1–3]. There are two aspects in the application of CEUS for portal vein thrombosis; one is the differentiation from tumoral "thrombosis" (venous invasion and occlusion of the portal vein or its branches, most commonly due to hepatocellular carcinoma) [25], and the other is the prediction of the effectiveness of anticoagulation [26, 27].

Imaging of the gastrointestinal tract is another target of CEUS. A recent study conducted a quantitative analysis of the contrast enhancement with Sonazoid in the stomach wall, which was effective to detect portal hypertensive gastropathy [28]. The other study focused on the intestinal hemodynamics in cirrhosis and showed that a prolonged transit time of microbubbles from the superior mesenteric artery to the superior mesenteric vein was a characteristic appearance in cirrhosis [29]. CEUS findings are also effective to assess the function of a transjugular intrahepatic portosystemic shunt [30].

A recent unique study examined the microbubble delivery time from the hepatic artery to maximum enhancement of the liver parenchyma on the sonogram, defined as the "hepatic filling rate" [31]; a prolonged hepatic filling rate was related to a poor prognosis and a higher occurrence of hepatocellular carcinoma (HCC) in cirrhosis. It may be caused by the presence of severely diminished liver function revealed by the impaired hepatic circulation comprehensively assessed with the analysis of microbubble movement.

10.7   Differential Diagnosis between Cirrhosis and Idiopathic Portal Hypertension

Idiopathic portal hypertension (IPH) represents non-cirrhotic portal hypertension, presenting typically with gastroesophageal varices, ascites, splenomegaly and portal vein thrombosis [32]. In addition, IPH offers characteristic features of a lower incidence of developing into HCC and a better survival rate than cirrhosis. Because of the necessity of different management, these two diseases should be strictly differentiated. However, imaging is not necessarily effective for differentiation due to their similarities: atrophy and deformity of the liver, splenomegaly, gastroesophageal varices and ascites.

There are three studies that reported the utility of CEUS with Sonazoid to differentiate between cirrhosis and IPH. The first study focused on the unique structure of the intrahepatic portal vein characteristic of IPH, showing the efficacy of three-dimensional CEUS with a similar diagnostic ability to direct portography [33]. The second study found that a delayed arterial phase peri-portal hepatic enhancement strongly suggests a diagnosis of IPH [34]. The third study examined the degree of contrast effect by intrahepatic accumulated microbubbles at the post-vascular phase and reported a significantly higher microbubble accumulation in IPH livers than in those with cirrhosis [23]. These data strongly suggest that the use of CEUS with Sonazoid has unique properties useful to identify IPH.

10.8   Limitations

CEUS offers various benefits in the assessment of portal hemodynamics with a possible prediction of the severity and the outcomes of patients with portal hypertension and for making a differential diagnosis. However, there are still several limitations. A major problem is inherent to US examinations, the dependency on the operator's experience and skill, and the difficulty in the assessment in obese subjects. Even after using a contrast agent, these problems might remain in some cases. Second, the optimal parameter and imaging method to determine the severity of portal hypertension has not been determined. This may be partly due to an insufficient understanding of the in vivo behavior of microbubbles that may vary according to the type of materials. Third, the number of studies is still not enough to get firm conclusions, specially considering that only a few studies have compared the diagnostic capacity of CEUS and other non-invasive markers, including serum markers, elastography, and MRI. Additional studies with large patient populations using multiple contrast agents and head to head comparisons with other non-invasive techniques are required to solve these problems.

Conclusion
Evidence has proved the significant effect of CEUS in the management of patients with portal hypertension. Further studies may enhance the value of this technique as a non-invasive tool that is an alternative to invasive procedures such as catheterization and biopsy.

References

1. Tsochatzis EA, Bosch J, Burroughs AK. Liver cirrhosis. Lancet. 2014;383:1749–61.
2. Sanyal AJ, Bosch J, Blei A, Arroyo V. Portal hypertension and its complications. Gastroenterology. 2008;134:1715–28.
3. Maruyama H, Sanyal AJ. 14, Portal hypertension: non-surgical and surgical management. In: Schiff's diseases of the liver. 11th ed. Oxford, UK: Wiley-Blackwell; 2012. p. 326–60.
4. Thabut D, Moreau R, Lebrec D. Noninvasive assessment of portal hypertension in patients with cirrhosis. Hepatology. 2011;53:683–94.

 5. de Franchis R. Expanding consensus in portal hypertension: Report of the Baveno VI Consensus Workshop: Stratifying risk and individualizing care for portal hypertension. J Hepatol. 2015;63:743–52.
 6. Baik SK. Haemodynamic evaluation by Doppler ultrasonography in patients with portal hypertension: a review. Liver Int. 2010;30:1403–13.
 7. Lencioni R, Piscaglia F, Bolondi L. Contrast-enhanced ultrasound in the diagnosis of hepatocellular carcinoma. J Hepatol. 2008;48:848–57.
 8. Maruyama H, Sekimoto T, Yokosuka O. Role of contrast-enhanced ultrasonography with Sonazoid for hepatocellular carcinoma: evidence from a 10-year experience. J Gastroenterol. 2016;51:421–33.
 9. Maruyama H, Shiha G, Yokosuka O, et al. Non-invasive assessment of portal hypertension and liver fibrosis using contrast-enhanced ultrasonography. Hepatol Int. 2016;10:267–76.
10. Bouakaz A, de Jong N. WFUMB safety symposium on Echo-contrast agents: nature and types of ultrasound contrast agents. Ultrasound Med Biol. 2007;33:187–96.
11. Claudon M, Dietrich CF, Choi BI, et al. Guidelines and good clinical practice recommendations for contrast enhanced ultrasound (CEUS) in the liver – update 2012: a WFUMB-EFSUMB initiative in cooperation with representatives of AFSUMB, AIUM, ASUM, FLAUS and ICUS. Ultrasound Med Biol. 2013;39:187–210.
12. Albrecht T, Blomley MJ, Cosgrove DO, et al. Non-invasive diagnosis of hepatic cirrhosis by transit-time analysis of an ultrasound contrast agent. Lancet. 1999;353:1579–83.
13. Berzigotti A, Nicolau C, Bellot P, et al. Evaluation of regional hepatic perfusion (RHP) by contrast-enhanced ultrasound in patients with cirrhosis. J Hepatol. 2011;55:307–14.
14. Qu EZ, Zhang YC, Li ZY, Liu Y, Wang JR. Contrast-enhanced sonography for quantitative assessment of portal hypertension in patients with liver cirrhosis. J Ultrasound Med. 2014;33:1971–7.
15. Zhai L, Qiu LY, Zu Y, et al. Contrast-enhanced ultrasound for quantitative assessment of portal pressure in canine liver fibrosis. World J Gastroenterol. 2015;21:4509–16.
16. Kim MY, Suk KT, Baik SK, et al. Hepatic vein arrival time as assessed by contrast-enhanced ultrasonography is useful for the assessment of portal hypertension in compensated cirrhosis. Hepatology. 2012;56:1053–62.
17. Jeong WK, Kim TY, Sohn JH, Kim Y, Kim J. Severe portal hypertension in cirrhosis: evaluation of perfusion parameters with contrast-enhanced ultrasonography. PLoS One. 2015;10:e0121601.
18. Eisenbrey JR, Dave JK, Halldorsdottir VG, et al. Chronic liver disease: noninvasive subharmonic aided pressure estimation of hepatic venous pressure gradient. Radiology. 2013;268:581–8.
19. Shimada T, Maruyama H, Kondo T, Sekimoto T, Takahashi M, Yokosuka O. Impact of splenic circulation: non-invasive microbubble-based assessment of portal hemodynamics. Eur Radiol. 2015;25:812–20.
20. Amat-Roldan I, Berzigotti A, Gilabert R, Bosch J. Assessment of hepatic vascular network connectivity with automated graph analysis of dynamic contrast-enhanced US to evaluate portal hypertension in patients with cirrhosis: a pilot study. Radiology. 2015;277:268–76.
21. Dave JK, Halldorsdottir VG, Eisenbrey JR, et al. Investigating the efficacy of subharmonic aided pressure estimation for portal vein pressures and portal hypertension monitoring. Ultrasound Med Biol. 2012;38:1784–98.
22. Maruyama H, Matsutani S, Okugawa H, et al. Microbubble disappearance-time is the appropriate timing for liver-specific imaging after injection of Levovist. Ultrasound Med Biol. 2006;32:1809–15.
23. Maruyama H, Ishibashi H, Takahashi M, et al. Effect of signal intensity from the accumulated microbubbles in the liver for differentiation of idiopathic portal hypertension from liver cirrhosis. Radiology. 2009;252:587–94.
24. Ishibashi H, Maruyama H, Takahashi M, et al. Demonstration of intrahepatic accumulated microbubble on ultrasound represents the grade of hepatic fibrosis. Eur Radiol. 2012;22:1083–90.

25. Rossi S, Ghittoni G, Ravetta V, et al. Contrast-enhanced ultrasonography and spiral computed tomography in the detection and characterization of portal vein thrombosis complicating hepatocellular carcinoma. Eur Radiol. 2008;18:1749–56.
26. Maruyama H, Ishibashi H, Takahashi M, Shimada T, Kamesaki H, Yokosuka O. Prediction of the therapeutic effects of anticoagulation for recent portal vein thrombosis: a novel approach with contrast-enhanced ultrasound. Abdom Imaging. 2012;37:431–8.
27. Maruyama H, Takahashi M, Shimada T, Yokosuka O. Emergency anticoagulation treatment for cirrhosis patients with portal vein thrombosis and acute variceal bleeding. Scand J Gastroenterol. 2012;47:686–91.
28. Kiyono S, Maruyama H, Kobayashi K, et al. Non-invasive diagnosis of portal hypertensive gastropathy: quantitative analysis of microbubble-induced stomach wall enhancement. Ultrasound Med Biol. 2016;42:1792–9.
29. Sekimoto T, Maruyama H, Kondo T, Shimada T, Kiyono S, Yokosuka O. Potential stagnation in the splanchnic hemodynamics demonstrated by the dynamic microbubble in chronic liver disease. J Gastroenterol Hepatol. 2015;30:1001–8.
30. Micol C, Marsot J, Boublay N, et al. Contrast-enhanced ultrasound: a new method for TIPS follow-up. Abdom Imaging. 2012;37:252–60.
31. Sekimoto T, Maruyama H, Kiyono S, et al. Hepatic filling rate by a microbubble agent: a novel predictor of long-term outcomes in patients with cirrhosis. Ultrasound Med Biol. 2014;40:2082–8.
32. Maruyama H, Kondo T, Sekimoto T, Yokosuka O. Differential clinical impact of ascites in cirrhosis and idiopathic portal hypertension. Medicine. 2015;94:e1056.
33. Maruyama H, Okugawa H, Kobayashi S, et al. Non-invasive portography: a microbubble-induced three-dimensional sonogram for discriminating idiopathic portal hypertension from cirrhosis. Br J Radiol. 2012;85:587–95.
34. Maruyama H, Shimada T, Ishibashi H, Takahashi M, Kamesaki H, Yokosuka O. Delayed periportal enhancement: a characteristic finding on contrast ultrasound in idiopathic portal hypertension. Hepatol Int. 2012;6:511–9.

Subharmonic Aided Pressure Estimation (SHAPE)

11

Ipshita Gupta, John R. Eisenbrey, and Flemming Forsberg

11.1 Introduction and Background

11.1.1 Portal Hypertension and HVPG

Portal hypertension (PH) results from obstruction of the portal blood flow. Cirrhosis of the liver is the most common cause of PH in western countries, followed by portal vein thrombosis [1]. An increase of over 5 mmHg in the pressure gradient between the portal vein and the inferior vena cava (IVC) or the hepatic vein is defined as portal hypertension [2]. Portal pressure in cirrhosis is estimated clinically by the hepatic venous pressure gradient (HVPG), the difference between the wedged and free hepatic venous pressures [3]. This technique is invasive and requires insertion of a balloon catheter via a transjugular approach into the hepatic vasculature [4]. PH becomes clinically significant when the HVPG is above 10 mmHg and there is higher probability of presence of varices, while an HVPG of 12 mmHg or more increases the risk of variceal bleeding [5–7].

Noninvasive techniques such as ultrasound, magnetic resonance imaging (MRI) and computed tomography (CT) have very poor sensitivity for portal pressure estimation and are therefore, not accurate enough to be used routinely for diagnosing PH [4]. Currently ultrasound is used for observing abdominal portosystemic collaterals in clinically significant portal hypertensive (CSPH) patients, however only 20–54% of cirrhotic patients show collaterals on imaging [4]. A noninvasive technique to monitor liver stiffness as an indirect indicator of HVPG showed a correlation with HVPG, but this is not close enough to substitute HVPG measurements [8]. The use of grayscale and Doppler ultrasound to study PH has limitations [9–11], including operator dependency,

I. Gupta • J.R. Eisenbrey (✉) • F. Forsberg
Thomas Jefferson University, Philadelphia, PA, USA
e-mail: John.Eisenbrey@jefferson.edu

© Springer International Publishing AG, part of Springer Nature 2018   159
A. Berzigotti, J. Bosch (eds.), *Diagnostic Methods for Cirrhosis and Portal Hypertension*, https://doi.org/10.1007/978-3-319-72628-1_11

timing of meals and difference in equipment. Currently non-invasive blood-based markers are also insufficient for evaluating PH [12]. Thus, an alternative accurate, noninvasive ultrasound based procedure would be a major development in the diagnosis of portal hypertension making the diagnosis safer, quicker and relatively cheaper.

11.1.2 Ultrasound Contrast Agents (UCAs) and Imaging

UCAs are gas filled microbubbles having a lipid, protein or polymer shell that oscillate nonlinearly within ultrasound waves emitted at higher incident acoustic pressures (>200 kPa). These UCAs have diameters less than 8 μm and can traverse the entire vasculature including capillaries [13]. The gas within these microbubbles has high compressibility and thus, generate a much higher echogenicity than the surrounding tissues. Hence, the microbubbles enhance the backscattered ultrasound signal (about 10–30 dB enhancement). This aids in contrast enhanced imaging of the blood vessels carrying these UCAs and in differentiating the vessels from the surrounding tissues [14]. The UCA's nonlinear oscillations occur over a wide range of frequencies from subharmonics ($f_0/2$) to second harmonics ($2f_0$) and ultraharmonics ($3f_0/2$) of the insonation frequency (f_0) as well as its multiples (Fig. 11.1). These signals can be used to create contrast specific imaging modes, such as subharmonic imaging (SHI), harmonic imaging (HI) and superharmonic imaging, respectively [16]. Harmonic imaging where ultrasound is transmitted at f_0 and received at $2f_0$ is the most common commercial contrast imaging mode, but HI suffers from restricted bandwidth since the tissue produces significant harmonic energy and leads to reduced blood to tissue contrast. SHI is an imaging mode that transmits at double the resonance frequency and receives at half the transmit frequency i.e., $f_0/2$ [16, 17]. Since the surrounding tissue does not generate a subharmonic response at the low power levels used, SHI has an excellent contrast-to-tissue ratio i.e., the ratio of the mean bubble and tissue signal amplitudes. Contrast to tissue ratio values as high as 20 dB have been reported *in vitro* by Daechin et al. [18].

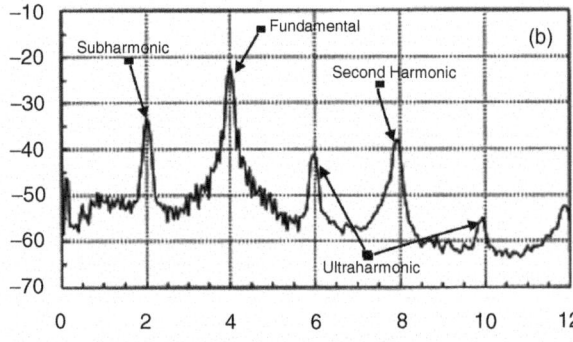

Fig. 11.1 Frequency spectrum of nonlinearly oscillating microbubbles [15]

11.1.3 The Concept of SHAPE

Our group has proposed the use of ultrasound contrast agents as pressure sensors (i.e., Subharmonic Aided Pressure Estimation, SHAPE) for noninvasive, quantitative pressure estimation in portal hypertension [16, 19]. The non-linear response of microbubbles depends strongly on the incident acoustic pressure, and undergoes three stages: occurrence, growth and saturation (Fig. 11.2, left) [19, 20]. In the

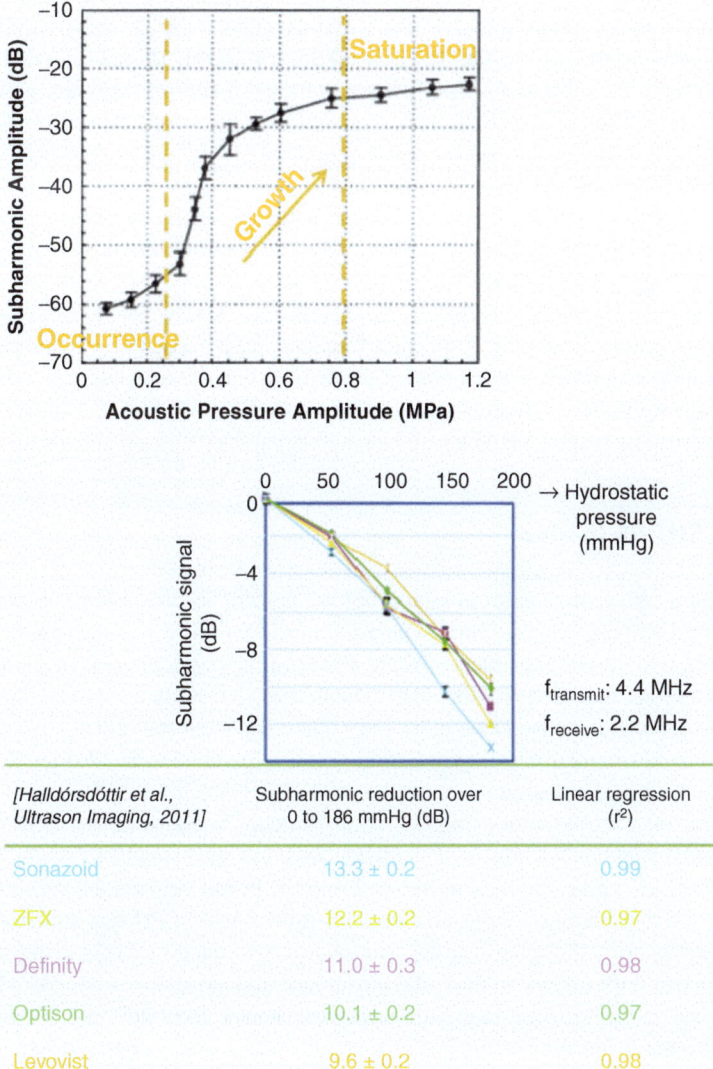

[Halldórsdóttir et al., Ultrason Imaging, 2011]	Subharmonic reduction over 0 to 186 mmHg (dB)	Linear regression (r²)
Sonazoid	13.3 ± 0.2	0.99
ZFX	12.2 ± 0.2	0.97
Definity	11.0 ± 0.3	0.98
Optison	10.1 ± 0.2	0.97
Levovist	9.6 ± 0.2	0.98

Fig. 11.2 (Left) Characteristic s-curve obtained from subharmonic emissions of the microbubbles with increasing input acoustic pressures. Three distinct phases are seen, Occurrence, Growth and Saturation [19]. (Right) Results from a previous study comparing six different contrast agents, shows inverse linear relationship between subharmonic amplitude and ambient pressure, with the best results seen for Sonazoid in blue [16, 19, 20]

growth stage the subharmonic component increases rapidly with acoustic power. In this stage subharmonic microbubble signals (i.e., SHAPE) have the highest sensitivity to pressure changes and an inverse linear relation with the ambient pressure [16, 19]. Using an *in vitro* system, based on single element transducers, changes in the first, second, and subharmonic amplitudes of six different ultrasound contrast agents with a square input pulse wave were measured at hydrostatic pressures from 0–186 mmHg (i.e., the range of human blood pressures), and frequencies of 2.5–6.6 MHz [20]. As the pressure was increased, the first and second harmonic amplitudes reduced by approximately 2 dB for all contrast agents, but the subharmonic amplitudes decreased by 10–14 dB and excellent correlations were achieved with the ambient pressure variations (r = −0.98, p < 0.001) (Fig. 11.2, right) [20]. This matching of subharmonic amplitude variations to ambient pressure variations represents the basis of SHAPE. Sonazoid proved to be the most sensitive for SHAPE with the highest gradient in subharmonic amplitude as the pressure was increased and a correlation coefficient of 0.99 (Fig. 11.2, right), hence has been selected for our study. Sonazoid contains a perfluorobutane gas encapsulated in a membrane of hydrogenated egg phosphatidyl serine, have a volume median diameter of 2.6 ± 0.1 μm and contain about $1.2 * 10^9$ microbubbles per ml [21]. Sonazoid microbubbles are commercially available, have a proven safety profile [22] and are approved for clinical use [23]. A transmit frequency of 2.5 MHz was the most sensitive operating frequency. These results demonstrate that the dependence of the subharmonic amplitude on hydrostatic pressure can be employed for non-invasive pressure estimation (i.e., SHAPE).

11.2   SHAPE In Vivo

Following *in vitro* studies, an *in vivo* proof of concept for using SHAPE was performed by Forsberg et al. in 2005 where the aortic pressure was measured in two dogs using two single transducers giving a maximum standard error of 5.4 mmHg relative to actual recorded pressure [16]. The first *in vivo* study of SHAPE for portal hypertension was done by Dave et al. [24]. They analyzed the efficacy of SHAPE with Sonazoid microbubbles in predicting portal hypertension in 14 dogs. In eight dogs, a slow-flow (increased resistance) model of PH was induced by embolization of the liver microcirculation using Gelfoam (Ethicon, Somerville, NJ, USA) injection. Approximately 2–3 sheets of Gelfoam were cut into small pieces and mixed with 4–5 mL of saline and then introduced into the portal vein via the surgical inlet [24]. For the remaining six dogs, an increased-flow model of PH was induced surgically by connecting the splenic or the femoral artery to the portal vein using a three-way stopcock with extension tube, thereby creating an arterial-venous (AV) fistula. An external saline infusion bag with a pressure sensor and cuff were additionally used to increase the flow volume. For both of these models of PH induction, the portal vein pressures were continuously monitored via a Millar pressure catheter.

At a transmit frequency of 2.5 MHz (i.e., receiving at 1.25 MHz) and after optimizing the input acoustic power in the growth phase, the changes in subharmonic signal amplitude correlated with changes in portal vein pressures; correlation coefficients ranged from −0.82 to −0.94 and from −0.70 to −0.73 for the two PH models considered separately or together, respectively [24]. These *in vivo* studies proved that SHAPE is an effective technique for measuring pressures noninvasively.

11.3   SHAPE in Humans—Pilot Study

A pilot study was conducted to compare *in vivo* quantitative SHAPE to HVPG measurements to determine the presence of portal hypertension in patients undergoing a transjugular liver biopsy [25]. The hypothesis of this study was that portal vein pressures can be monitored and quantified noninvasively in humans using SHAPE.

Patients get random liver biopsies for hepatic dysfunction; most commonly in individuals with cirrhosis from hepatitis or alcohol abuse. Additionally, the biopsy allows the treating physician to get an estimate of the severity of the inflammatory change within the liver (i.e., grading) as well as determine the stage of fibrosis (i.e., staging) [26]. In patients considered to be at high risk for complications from percutaneous biopsy, a biopsy performed from a transjugular approach is now standard clinical practice [10]. The HVPG is measured in all patients undergoing a transjugular liver biopsy.

A total of 45 patients underwent the SHAPE study. The patients enrolled in this project were adults over the age of 21 scheduled for a transjugular liver biopsy and written informed consent was obtained from everyone. Forty-five patients completed this study, 27 (60%) were men and 18 (40%) were women. Thirty-nine patients (87%) were white and the remaining six (13%) were African-American. Twelve patients (27%) had previously undergone liver transplantation. Disease etiology was hepatitis C in 21 patients (47%), nonalcoholic steatohepatitis in 13 patients (29%), hepatitis B in three patients (7%), cryptogenic cirrhosis in three patients (7%), amyloidosis in one patient (2%), alcoholic hepatitis in one patient (2%), venous outflow obstruction with possible autoimmune hepatitis in one patient (2%), adenocarcinoma from primary breast cancer in one patient (2%), and primary sclerosing cholangitis in one patient (2%). Subharmonic signals from the portal vein were successfully obtained in all 45 patients, while signals from the hepatic vein were obtained in 42 patients because of scanning difficulties in three obese individuals (BMIs of 37, 40, and 51 kg/m^2). Data from an additional nine patients were removed because of inadequate signal within the hepatic vein.

An ultrasound scanner (Logiq 9; GE Healthcare, Milwaukee, WI) with a 4C curvilinear probe was modified to acquire radiofrequency data within a selected region of interest (ROI) during scanning. Within 2 h post biopsy, the SHAPE scan was performed. To select the correct acoustic window, an experienced sonographer identified the portal vein and the hepatic vein in the same plane and approximately similar depths. The depth and diameters of the portal and hepatic veins were determined by the sonographer and saved as a reference image (Fig. 11.3). Sonazoid was infused IV (0.72 mL microbubbles per kilogram of body weight per hour, and saline at 120 mL/h). Once the sonographer confirmed the patency of the portal and

Fig. 11.3 Example
acoustic window selection
showing regions of interest
in the hepatic and portal
veins (circled)

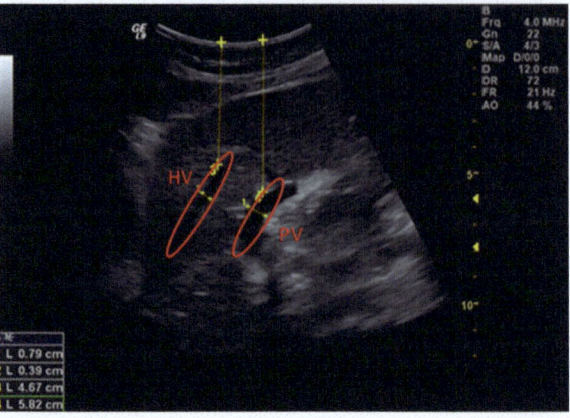

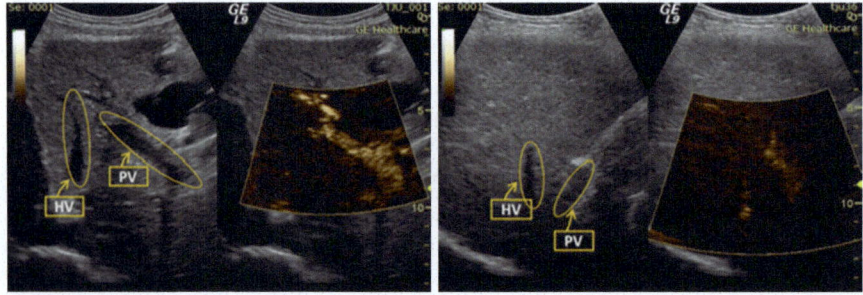

Fig. 11.4 Example of two typical SHAPE acquisitions for a normal and a portal hypertensive
patient. In each case, Dual Imaging on B mode with the selected areas of interest for portal vein
(PV) and hepatic vein (HV) are shown on the left and SHI on the right frame. (Left) A patient with
normal HVPG values, having a bright SHI signal from the PV and not much SHI signal from the
HV. (Right) A patient with a HVPG of 12, having considerable SHI signal in both PV and HV

hepatic veins and the presence of microbubbles, the automated optimization code
to select the optimum acoustic power [27] was run. This code is built into the modified Logiq 9 scanner and runs automatically in Matlab (The MathWorks, Inc.,
Natick, MA, USA).

This scanner provides dual mode imaging i.e., both the regular B Mode image
and the contrast mode SHI image are displayed at the same time as shown in
Fig. 11.4. This provided for easier navigation and identification of the vascular
structures of interest; namely, the portal and the hepatic vein. The B mode was set
to operate at 4.0 MHz and the SHAPE mode was set to transmit four-cycle pulses at
2.5 MHz and to receive subharmonic signals at 1.25 MHz.

Subharmonic data from the microbubbles (i.e., SHAPE) was acquired at the optimal acoustic power setting in 5 s segments during the infusion of the Sonazoid
suspension from both the portal and hepatic veins. All measurements were repeated
three times. The average frame rate was 8 fps. The average radiofrequency signal
over all the frames in the 0.5 MHz bandwidth around 1.25 MHz gave the mean

subharmonic signal in each vessel. The SHAPE gradient was calculated as the difference in the mean subharmonic signal between the portal vein and the hepatic vein. The SHAPE gradient was compared to the catheter based pressure measurements of the HVPG. The SHAPE pressure gradient was also compared to the MELD score that assesses the severity of chronic liver disease [26, 28]. Figure 11.4 show two typical images from SHAPE acquisitions for a normal and a portal hypertensive patient.

Portal hypertension patients presented a larger signal in the hepatic vein, compared to normal pressure patients, suggesting that SHAPE evaluation of the hepatic vein could be a useful sign to suspect portal hypertension.

The SHAPE gradient and HVPG values for the entire data set showed a linear correlation of 0.82 (and 0.97 for patients with a HVPG >12 mmHg) [25].

The results from this study indicate that SHAPE can be a viable tool for noninvasively measuring the portal pressure gradient. If these results can be validated in a larger patient population, it would represent a major breakthrough [25]. In identifying patients with HVPG >10 mmHg, SHAPE had a sensitivity of 89% and specificity of 88%, which changed to a 100% and 81%, respectively, for subjects with HVPG >12 mmHg. Patients at increased risk for variceal hemorrhage (HVPG >12 mmHg) had significantly higher subharmonic gradients than patients with lower HVPGs (1.93 dB ± 0.61 [standard deviation] vs −1.47 dB ± 0.29, p = 0.001). These results strongly suggest that SHAPE could be a useful tool for screening patients for clinically significant portal hypertension (CSPH) and for risk of variceal bleeding.

Moderate to poor correlations were observed between the SHAPE gradient and the patients' MELD score (r = 0.38) and fibrosis score (r = 0.13). The correlations between HVPG and MELD score (r = 0.24) and HVPG and fibrosis score (r = 0.19) were also poor. Our results are not unexpected and show that liver function and portal pressure gradient are not strictly correlated and should be measured independently.

Many alternative ultrasound techniques have been tried and tested for non invasive estimation of portal hypertension however, none are robust enough. As examples, Choi et al. checked whether Doppler ultrasonography correlate with HVPG [11]. They also attempted to distinguish responders from non responders to the treatment for cirrhosis. None of the ultrasound parameters (PV velocity, splenic venous velocity, resistive index of hepatic, splenic and renal arteries) correlated with HVPG [11]. Mariyuma et al. used ultrasound with Sonazoid to distinguish idiopathic PH (IPH) from cirrhosis. They studied 101 patients, 8 with IPH, 57 with cirrhosis and 36 controls. They found no significant difference in the hepatic and portal enhancement onset time between the IPH and cirrhotic group [29]. Zhang et al. tested for the correlation between hepatic vein–hepatic artery transit time of a ultrasound contrast agents and portal pressure and reported a good correlation between these two parameters (r = −0.90); however, the study looked at portal pressure and not HVPG [30].

A recent study by Kumar et al. looked retrospectively at the correlation between transient elastography (TE) and HVPG in 326 patients [8]. The results showed a moderate correlation between the two (r = 0.36) [8]. Jansen et al. investigated the use of spleen and liver sheer wave elastography (LSWE and SSWE) to predict clinically significant PH. They showed a correlation of r = 0.62 between LSWE and HVPG and r = 0.60 between SSWE and HVPG [31].

11.4 Current State of a Multi-Center Trial

Based on the encouraging results from the pilot study, a large scale, multi-center blinded clinical trial has been started. The Institutional Review Boards at Thomas Jefferson University (TJU) and the Hospital of the University of Pennsylvania (HUP) approved this study. A total of 103 patients have been enrolled to date in this ongoing clinical study. The infusion rate of Sonazoid has been doubled to avoid losing data due to lack of signal from HV. The infusion rate used is 0.024 µL/kg/min. We have also optimized the input ultrasound pulse shape for optimal performance of SHAPE and are now using a Gaussian windowed binomial filtered square wave as opposed to a square wave used in the pilot study [32]. The linear relationship between the SHAPE gradient and HVPG till now shows good correlation (r = 0.76). There was a significant difference in SHAPE gradient when patients were separated into two groups according to the HVPG being below than or equal/greater than 10 mmHg (-1.58 ± 3.50 vs -4.86 ± 2.63 dB; p < 0.001). The study aims at enrolling 300 patients. Apart from the correlation between SHAPE gradient and HVPG, other parameters such as the BMI, MELD and fibrosis score of the patients will be compared with the SHAPE and HVPG values.

Conclusion

There is a good overall correlation between SHAPE and HVPG values which indicates that SHAPE is a useful tool for noninvasive estimation of portal hypertension. SHAPE was also useful in identifying patients with a HVPG ≥ 10 mmHg and those at a higher risk of variceal bleeding i.e., having a HVPG ≥ 12 mmHg.

While our results are promising, there were several limitations to this study. The research software on the Logiq 9 scanner is still in the development phase. Hence it is fragile and prone to crashes. Also, as described above, selecting the optimal acoustic power in the growth phase is crucial for best SHAPE performance. However, the existing optimization algorithm is user dependent and vulnerable to breathing artefacts. This can lead to noisy s-curves and multiple points of inflection leading to inaccurate selection of acoustic power. Although rare, sometimes the hepatic vein cannot be catheterized and therefore HVPG cannot be measured. Lastly, the U.S. Food and Drug Administration (FDA) has yet to approve Sonazoid for clinical use. In our study, we chose to use this UCA because our previous *in vitro* work showed its subharmonic amplitude to be the most sensitive to hydrostatic pressures of all commercially available agents [20]. However, SHAPE has also been shown to be feasible when performed with other FDA approved UCAs [20, 33], and the usage of such agents could potentially result in more rapid clinical translation of SHAPE.

In conclusion, SHAPE measurements appear to correlate well with transjugular HVPG measurements. The technique allows identification of patients with clinically significant PH and those at elevated risk of variceal bleeding.

References

1. Navarro V, Rossi S, Herrine S. Hepatic cirrhosis. Pharmacology and therapeutics: principles to practice. Saunders-Elsevier, Philadelphia, PA, USA. 2008. p. 505–26.
2. Sanyal AJ, Bosch J, Blei A, Arroyo V. Portal hypertension and its complications. Gastroenterology. 2008;134(6):1715–28.
3. Bosch J, Garcia-Pagan JC, Berzigotti A, Abraldes JG. Measurement of portal pressure and its role in the management of chronic liver disease. Semin Liver Dis. 2006;26(4):348–62.
4. Iwakiri Y. Pathophysiology of portal hypertension. Clin Liver Dis. 2014;18(2):281–91.
5. Garcia-Tsao G, Groszmann RJ, Fisher RL, et al. Portal pressure, presence of gastroesophageal varices and variceal bleeding. Hepatology. 1985;5(3):419–24.
6. Groszmann RJ, Garcia-Tsao G, Bosch J, et al. Beta-blockers to prevent gastroesophageal varices in patients with cirrhosis. N Engl J Med. 2005;353(21):2254–61.
7. Kalambokis G, Manousou P, Vibhakorn S, et al. Transjugular liver biopsy – indications, adequacy, quality of specimens, and complications – a systematic review. J Hepatol. 2007;47(2):284–94.
8. Kumar A, Khan NM, Anikhindi SA, et al. Correlation of transient elastography with hepatic venous pressure gradient in patients with cirrhotic portal hypertension: a study of 326 patients from india. World J Gastroenterol. 2017;23(4):687–96.
9. Cokkinos DD, Dourakis SP. Ultrasonographic assessment of cirrhosis and portal hypertension. Curr Med Imaging Rev. 2009;5(1):62–70.
10. Lafortune M, Marleau D, Breton G, et al. Portal venous system measurements in portal-hypertension. Radiology. 1984;151(1):27–30.
11. Choi YJ, Baik SK, Park DH, et al. Comparison of Doppler ultrasonography and the hepatic venous pressure gradient in assessing portal hypertension in liver cirrhosis. J Gastroenterol Hepatol. 2003;18(4):424–9.
12. Kim MY, Jeong WK, Baik SK. Invasive and non-invasive diagnosis of cirrhosis and portal hypertension. World J Gastroenterol. 2014;20(15):4300–15.
13. Goldberg BB, Liu JB, Forsberg F. Ultrasound contrast agents – a review. Ultrasound Med Biol. 1994;20(4):319–33.
14. Stride EP, Coussios CC. Cavitation and contrast: the use of bubbles in ultrasound imaging and therapy. Proc Inst Mech Eng H. 2010;224(H2):171–91.
15. Forsberg F, Shi WT, Goldberg BB. Subharmonic imaging of contrast agents. Ultrasonics. 2000;38(1–8):93–8.
16. Forsberg F, Liu JB, Shi WT, et al. In vivo pressure estimation using subharmonic contrast microbubble signals: proof of concept. IEEE Trans Ultrason Ferroelectr Freq Control. 2005;52(4):581–3.
17. Shankar PM, Krishna PD, Newhouse VL. Subharmonic backscattering from ultrasound contrast agents. J Acoust Soc Am. 1999;106(4):2104–10.
18. Daeichin V, Bosch JG, Needles A, et al. Subharmonic, non-linear fundamental and ultraharmonic imaging of microbubble contrast at high frequencies. Ultrasound Med Biol. 2015;41(2):486–97.
19. Shi WT, Forsberg F, Raichlen JS, Needleman L, Goldberg BB. Pressure dependence of subharmonic signals from contrast microbubbles. Ultrasound Med Biol. 1999;25(2):275–83.
20. Halldorsdottir VG, Dave JK, Leodore LM, et al. Subharmonic contrast microbubble signals for noninvasive pressure estimation under static and dynamic flow conditions. Ultrason Imaging. 2011;33(3):153–64.

21. Sontum PC. Physicochemical characteristics of sonazoid (tm), a new contrast agent for ultrasound imaging. Ultrasound Med Biol. 2008;34(5):824–33.
22. Landmark KE, Johansen PW, Johnson JA, et al. Pharmacokinetics of perfluorobutane following intravenous bolus injection and continuous infusion of sonazoid (tm) in healthy volunteers and in patients with reduced pulmonary diffusing capacity. Ultrasound Med Biol. 2008;34(3):494–501.
23. Bouakaz A, De Jong N. Wfumb safety symposium on echo-contrast agents: nature and types of ultrasound contrast agents. Ultrasound Med Biol. 2007;33(2):187–96.
24. Dave JK, Halldorsdottir VG, Eisenbrey JR, et al. Investigating the efficacy of subharmonic aided pressure estimation for portal vein pressures and portal hypertension monitoring. Ultrasound Med Biol. 2012;38(10):1784–98.
25. Eisenbrey JR, Dave JK, Halldorsdottir VG, et al. Chronic liver disease: noninvasive subharmonic aided pressure estimation of hepatic venous pressure gradient. Radiology. 2013;268(2):581–8.
26. Malinchoc M, Kamath PS, Gordon FD, et al. A model to predict poor survival in patients undergoing transjugular intrahepatic portosystemic shunts. Hepatology. 2000;31(4):864–71.
27. Dave JK, Halldorsdottir VG, Eisenbrey JR, et al. On the implementation of an automated acoustic output optimization algorithm for subharmonic aided pressure estimation. Ultrasonics. 2013;53(4):880–8.
28. Kamath PS, Wiesner RH, Malinchoc M, et al. A model to predict survival in patients with end-stage liver disease. Hepatology. 2001;33(2):464–70.
29. Maruyama H, Shimada T, Ishibashi H, et al. Delayed periportal enhancement: a characteristic finding on contrast ultrasound in idiopathic portal hypertension. Hepatol Int. 2012;6(2):511–9.
30. Zhang CX, Hu J, Hu KW, et al. Noninvasive analysis of portal pressure by contrast-enhanced sonography in patients with cirrhosis. J Ultrasound Med. 2011;30(2):205–11.
31. Jansen C, Bogs C, Verlinden W, et al. Shear-wave elastography of the liver and spleen identifies clinically significant portal hypertension: a prospective multicentre study. Liver Int. 2017;37(3):396–405.
32. Gupta I, Eisenbrey J, Stanczak M, et al. Effect of pulse shaping on subharmonic aided pressure estimation in vitro and in vivo. J Ultrasound Med. 2017;36(1):3–11.
33. Halldorsdottir VG, Dave JK, Eisenbrey JR, et al. Subharmonic aided pressure estimation for monitoring interstitial fluid pressure in tumours – in vitro and in vivo proof of concept. Ultrasonics. 2014;54(7):1938–44.

Endoscopic Ultrasound and Portal Hypertension

12

Oriol Sendino and Angels Ginès

12.1 Introduction

Since the 1980s, endoscopic ultrasonography (EUS) has been useful in the evaluation of portal hypertension, either for diagnostic aspects or for the evaluation of therapy and risk of bleeding. More recently, it has been described as a method for guiding interventions such as variceal injection or coiling, portal vein catheterization, and in animal models even for creating an intrahepatic portosystemic shunt (Table 12.1).

12.2 EUS Visualization of Vascular Abnormalities in Portal Hypertension

EUS is a reliable tool for assessment of vascular abnormalities within and outside the gastrointestinal wall in patients with portal hypertension, and adds information to the standard endoscopic examination (described in a separate chapter in this book).

Table 12.1 Summary of utility of EUS in portal hypertension

Diagnosis of portal hypertension and prediction of cirrhosis
Diagnosis of gastroesophageal varices
Visualization of collateral veins
Prediction of bleeding and evaluation of the endoscopic treatment response
Therapy of gastroesophageal and ectopic varices (sclerotherapy, cyanocrylate injection, coiling)

O. Sendino, M.D., Ph.D. • A. Ginès, M.D., Ph.D., M.M.Sc. (✉)
Endoscopy Unit, Hospital Clínic, IDIBAPS, CIBERehd, Barcelona, Spain
e-mail: sendino@clinic.cat; magines@clinic.cat

© Springer International Publishing AG, part of Springer Nature 2018
A. Berzigotti, J. Bosch (eds.), *Diagnostic Methods for Cirrhosis and Portal Hypertension*, https://doi.org/10.1007/978-3-319-72628-1_12

Fig. 12.1 Perforating vein
(yellow arrow). Vein path
is perfectly seen going
from outside the
muscularis propria to
inside the wall

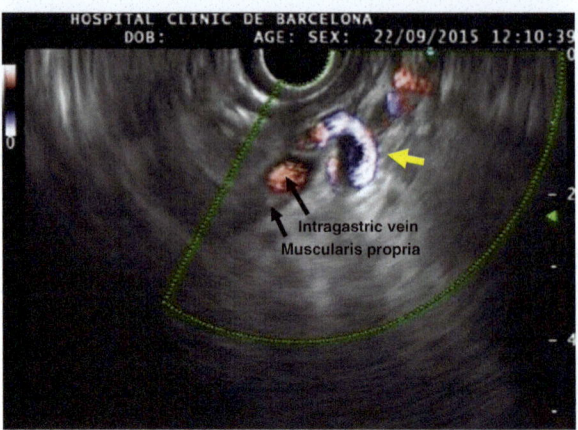

The venous anatomy of the lower esophagus and upper stomach has been described into four layers: intraepithelial channels, superficial venous plexus, deep venous plexus and adventitial veins [1, 2]. The deep venous plexus is composed by the periesophageal collateral veins, adjacent to the muscularis propria and the para-esophageal collateral veins, external to the muscularis propria. The same applies to perigastric and paragastric collaterals veins. Perforating veins are seen as serpiginous echofree tubular structures, usually of smaller diameter than varices, located in the submucosa and connecting periesophagogastric collateral veins with luminal gastroesophageal varices (Fig. 12.1). On EUS, esophageal varices (EV) are visualized as rounded anechoic structures just beneath the mucosal and submucosal layers. Gastric varices (GV) are seen on EUS as anechoic serpiginous structures within the gastric wall, mainly in the fundus or at the cardia, below the esophagogastric junction [3].

Portal vein (PV) and splenic vein (SV) can be easily traced from the hepatic and splenic hilum to the porto-spleno-mesenteric confluence by EUS examination. The length of the PV is approximately 6–8 cm with a mean diameter of 1.09 cm. The SV drains the lower esophagus (esophageal veins), stomach (short gastric and left gastro-epiploic veins), pancreas (pancreas veins) and first portion of the duodenum. The SV diameter is less than 0.45 cm. The azygos vein (AV) which plays an important role in porto-systemic collateral circulation draining the gastroesophageal varices to the superior vena cava, is also visualized on EUS images at the central mediastinum as a round and anechoic structure between the esophageal wall, the aorta and the spine. In patients with portal hypertension all these veins are significantly dilated. The thoracic duct may be identified by EUS in the posterior mediastinum, adjacent to the azygos vein in the majority of patients with portal hypertension [4]. Some studies demonstrated that EUS is a useful tool to detect gastrorenal shunts or portosystemic shunts [5, 6].

Superficial gastric layers may display some abnormalities typical of portal hypertension. Portal hypertensive gastropathy appears as numerous rounded echo-free structures within the submucosa of the stomach. Besides hypertensive gastropathy, gastric mucosa and submucosal layers are often thickened in patients with portal hypertension, most likely because of relative outflow obstruction of venous and lymphatic flow [7].

Although EUS is not a routine procedure in clinical practice in patients with portal hypertension, it allows for a noninvasive evaluation of the hemodynamic changes linked to this condition. Kassem and colleagues [8] demonstrated that EUS and Doppler EUS are useful to detect the hemodynamic changes in the azygos vein after variceal obliteration by endoscopic injection sclerotherapy (EIS). These investigators studied 40 patients with portal hypertension and bleeding varices who had injection sclerotherapy. The study assessed AV diameter, maximal velocity and blood flow volume index as measured by Doppler EUS before and 1 week after variceal obliteration, and found a significant increase in AV diameter and blood flow volume index. This technique has been validated with reference to the standard invasive techniques to test hemodynamic changes in cirrhotic patients with portal hypertension after administration of pharmacologic agents such as somatostatin or octreotide [9]. In this study, color Doppler EUS was used to assess rapid changes in AV blood flow after administration of placebo, somatostatin or octreotide in a random and blinded manner and the study confirmed the transient effects of these drugs on AV blood flow and gastric mucosal perfusion. In another study, 18 patients with portal hypertension were randomly selected to receive a bolus injection of terlipressin, somatostatin or saline [10]. AV blood flow was measured by color Doppler EUS before and 5 and 10 min after the administration of the vasoactive agents or placebo. This study also concluded that Doppler EUS is a useful technique for monitoring the effects of vasoactive agents. In a study by Faigel et al. [11], paraesophageal varices were detected in 97% of cirrhotic patients (n = 66) and 3% of control patients (n = 32) (P < 0.001) and were a more sensitive predictor of cirrhosis than varices at endoscopy (74%, P < 0.0001). In another study, 16 children, median age 13 months (range, 7–88 months), being assessed for intestinal transplant underwent simultaneous upper endoscopy and EUS to evaluate for portal hypertension and therefore if combined liver-intestine transplantation was needed. In 56.2% of patients the results of upper endoscopy and EUS were concordant for the detection of gastroesophageal varices. In seven patients, gastroesophageal varices were only identified by EUS and liver biopsy was avoided in four of these cases [12].

12.3 Detection and Grading of Gastroesophageal Varices

EUS was found to be inferior to conventional endoscopy in detecting and grading EV but superior to detect GV. Caletti and colleagues [13] compared vascular findings in 40 patients with portal hypertension with those in 48 control subjects. EUS did not display EV or GV, periesophageal collaterals or portal hypertensive gastropathy in control subjects, whereas the AV, SV and PV were seen in both patients and controls. In this study, EUS was significantly inferior to upper endoscopy in detecting and grading EV, but superior in displaying GV. Detection of periesophageal veins increased with the diameter of the varices (57%, 89%, and 100% in grades 1, 2, and 3, respectively), as well as the diameter of the AV. In another study, EUS findings were compared with upper endoscopy in 58 patients with portal hypertension and controls [14]. Esophageal, gastric, periesophageal and perigastric varices, perforating veins, dilation of portal, splenic, upper mesenteric, azygos veins and the thoracic duct were seen in a high percentage of patients, but none of these changes was observed in controls. In this study, the assessment of GV was superior with EUS than with upper endoscopy. Upper endoscopy, however, was more sensitive than EUS in detecting and grading EV. Esophageal wall compression by the balloon of the echoendoscope or the close proximity of the tip of the echoendoscope to the esophageal wall, which is not within the focal zone of the transducer, may explain these observations. Similar observations have been made by other investigators [15]. The visualization of the EV may improve by using high-frequency miniprobes, as demonstrated in several studies [16, 17]. In a study by Choudhuri et al. [18], only 45% of small varices was seen while all the patients with large varices were correctly diagnosed. However, GV were detected significantly more often by EUS (66%) compared with endoscopy (17; 34%, P < 0.005). Lee et al. [19] compared 52 cirrhotic and 166 dyspeptic patients to assess gastroesophageal varices and extraluminal venous abnormalities sonographically. EUS identified EV endoscopically in 53.8% with good correlation with upper endoscopy (r = 0.855, P < 0.001); furthermore, it detected GV in 30.8%, compared with 17.3% detected by upper endoscopy. Extraluminal venous abnormalities were detected in 92% of patients with cirrhosis.

Owing to the location in the deep submucosal layer of the stomach, GV may be difficult to detect or differentiate from prominent gastric folds or submucosal lesions on endoscopy. As mentioned above, several studies have demonstrated that EUS is superior to upper endoscopy in identifying GV [13, 14, 19 22]. Doustiere et al. [15] found that the use of EUS increases the detection of fundal varices sixfold. Even when detected by endoscopy, the visualized portion may be only the tip of the iceberg. A recent study indicated that the GV diameter, which was independent from the variceal form, Child-Pugh Classification and the presence of hepatocellular carcinoma was closely related to the GV flow volume [13].

Similarly, in the rectum, EUS is able to identify colorectal varices and congestive rectopathy in patients with portal hypertension [23]. EUS may also be useful for the evaluation of intramural vessels of uncommon locations, such as duodenal varices [24, 25].

12.4   Prediction of Bleeding, Recurrence and Evaluation of the Treatment Response

One study [20] collected 30 consecutive patients with EV at high risk of bleeding. Simultaneous conventional endoscopy and EUS were performed before endoscopic therapy. The study showed that EUS revealed cardial submucosal varices in all patients, while conventional endoscopy showed varices in 70% of patients. Furthermore, patients with recurrent EV were more likely to have severe-grade perforating veins prior to treatment (71.4%) compared to patients without recurrence (12.5%), and patients with severe as opposed to mild-grade perforating veins before treatment had a significantly higher recurrence rate (90.9% vs. 21.0%). Collateral deep veins were associated with recurrence of varices seen on high frequency (20 MHz) ultrasound catheter probe while the presence of veins at the gastroesophageal junction did not correlate with recurrence. Another study [26] used EUS to examine 38 patients who had undergone endoscopic injection sclerotherapy (EIS). EUS found a significantly higher incidence of severe-type periesophageal collateral veins and significantly larger and more perforating veins in patients with endoscopic recurrences of EV compared to patients without recurrence. Sato et al. [27] used Color Doppler (CD-EUS) EUS to study 306 patients in which EV had been treated with EIS. These patients underwent CD-EUS before EIS and 3–5 months after EIS. The results showed that the predictors of early recurrence of EV within 1 year included more perforating veins and the inflowing type of perforating veins before EIS, and more cardiac intramural veins and perforating veins and the inflowing type of perforating veins after EIS. Lo and colleagues [21] showed that EUS is a reliable technique to assess paraesophageal veins after sclerotherapy or ligation. These investigators studied two groups of patients with esophageal variceal bleeding treated with endoscopic ligation (EL) (n = 44) or sclerotherapy (n = 35). The prevalence of paraesophageal veins was 86% in the ligation group and 51% in the sclerotherapy group. Esophageal varices recurred in 70% and 43% in the ligation and injection group, respectively and, moreover, patients in both groups with more severe paraesophageal varices had a significantly higher rate of variceal recurrence. The rate of recurrent bleeding was also significantly higher in patients with paraesophageal varices. A possible explanation for the results could be that ligation only affects the varices in the mucosal and submucosal layers, leaving the perforating veins untouched. Based on these studies, it has been suggested that a closer follow-up and retreatment may be needed in patients with prominent paraesophageal veins.

With EUS, it is possible to evaluate successful EIS by demonstrating a reduction in the number and size of paraesophageal collateral vessels and the disappearance of perforating veins [28]. In a study [29] aimed at investigating whether follow-up EUS in conjunction with endoscopy after variceal ligation would be helpful in predicting the recurrence of bleeding from varices, Leung and colleagues showed that patients with large paraesophageal varices are those at highest risk of variceal recurrence and rebleeding after EL. These investigators studied 40 patients, who had ligation after an episode of variceal bleeding, with EUS and gastroscopy 4 weeks after obliteration of varices and every 6 months for up to 1 year. The proportion of patients developing recurrent submucosal esophageal varices as well as recurrent bleeding was significantly higher in the group of patients presenting with large paraesophageal varices. Leung and colleagues concluded that EUS can accurately identify a subset of patients with large paraesophageal varices who are at high risk of rebleeding, and they proposed careful endoscopic monitoring in these patients.

EUS also enabled visualization of the left gastric vein. Hino and colleagues [30] examined the hemodynamics and morphology of the left gastric vein (which is the main vessel feeding esophageal varices) by CD-EUS to identify factors that contributed to recurrence of varices and bleeding after endoscopic treatment. The investigators found that a low hepatofugal flow velocity in the left gastric vein trunk was the only factor associated with the efficacy of the endoscopic therapy. Moreover, the incidence of the anterior branch dominant type of the left gastric vein was significantly less in the responders to therapy. Kuramochi et al. [31] included 68 patients treated for moderate or large EV who underwent CD-EUS after EL and EIS. Patients with a high hepatofugal flow velocity in the LGV (>12 cm/s) or an anterior branch dominant pattern, were classified into a high-risk group. Half of the patients showed a recurrence of EV within half a year, whereas it took nearly 2 years for half of the patients in the other group to exhibit a recurrence. The hazard ratio of these features for early recurrence was 3.0.

Lee et al. [32] demonstrated that performing EUS to monitor GV obliteration after glue injection and performing repeated cyanocrylate injections when incompletely obliterated, reduced the risk of bleeding with a possible reduction in mortality when compared with "on-demand" injections alone. Similarly, Iwase et al. [33] showed that residual patency of treated varices correlated with rebleeding risk after glue injection. Varix obliteration can be confirmed by the absence of blood flow on CD-EUS.

12.5 EUS-Guided Therapy of Esophageal Varices

EUS enables the visualization of perforating veins and collaterals for targeted sclerotherapy. Lahoti et al. [34] first reported the use of EUS-guided sclerotherapy to achieve variceal obliteration. The injection of sclerosant was directed at the perforating vessels until flow was no longer seen. All five treated patients achieved variceal obliteration after an average of 2.2 sessions. No recurrent bleeding was reported after a mean follow-up period of 15 months. De Paulo et al. [35] reported a randomized controlled trial of 50 patients comparing EIS and EUS-guided sclerotherapy of esophageal collateral veins. They found similar rebleeding rates after similar numbers of sessions to achieve obliteration, but rebleeding was found to be significantly associated with the presence of collateral vessels. Currently EUS-guided sclerotherapy of EV could be an optional therapy for patients with bleeding refractory to band ligation and conventional sclerotherapy.

12.6 EUS-Guided Therapy of Gastric Varices

EUS has conceptual advantages to guide the injection of glue into GV. EUS-guided glue injection is attractive as it enables sonographic visualization of glue delivery into the varix lumen avoiding a paravariceal injection. Furthermore, it allows for visualization of deeper varices as well as the feeding vein system. Another advantage of EUS-guided treatment is that varix lumen can be accurately targeted for glue injection even in the presence of retained food or blood that may obstruct the endoscopic view.

In a case series of five patients [36], EUS-guided injection of a 1:1 mixture of N-butyl-2-cyanoacrylate and lipiodol was performed in perforating veins feeding GV. It was found that this technique was beneficial in eradicating the GV in all patients without complications after a mean of 1.6 sessions, and moreover, there was no recurrence of bleeding during 10 months of follow-up. However, the identification of the feeder vessel with EUS can sometimes be difficult and time-consuming and has been considered a limitation of this technique for some authors.

To avoid complications related to the use of glue, mostly systemic embolization, Levy et al. [37] reported the first case of EUS guided coil injection for acute ectopic gastric variceal bleeding. They advanced a total of three embolization microcoils through a 22-gauge EUS-FNA needle for variceal obliteration. Rebleeding occurred, but was successfully treated with two additional coils placed into untreated varices.

A multicenter study [38] retrospectively compared EUS-guided coil injection to EUS-guided glue injection of feeding gastric varices. Thirty consecutive patients received either cyanocrylate injection (19 patients) or coils (11 patients) and they were followed up to 6 months. The results showed similar obliteration rates (94% vs 90% respectively), but fewer endoscopy sessions were required in the coil group (82% obliteration in a single session compared to 53%). Of note, the intended therapy was for coil injection in all, but technical difficulties hindering the use of coils were encountered in 19 of 30 patients, resulting in only 11 treated with coils. The rates of adverse events were significantly higher in the cyanocrylate vs. the coil group (58% vs. 9%), although nine of the 11 adverse events in the cyanocrylate group were asymptomatic pulmonary glue embolisms found on routine postprocedure tomography which means that glue embolization is likely more common than appreciated, but that it rarely causes symptoms.

Bhat et al. [39] evaluated the long-term outcomes of EUS-guided injection of coils and glue for therapy of GV in a retrospective study. The authors enrolled 152 patients with GV. Seven (5%) had active hemorrhage, 105 (69%) had recent bleeding, and 40 (26%) were treated for primary prophylaxis. Treatment was technically successful in 151 patients (>99%). Mean number of coils was 1.4 and mean volume of cyanocrylate was 2 mL. Mean Follow-up was 436 days. Among 100 patients with follow-up EUS examinations, complete obliteration of GV was confirmed in 93 (93%). Post-treatment bleeding from obliterated GV occurred in 3 of 93 patients (3%). Twenty-five patients who had clinical and/or upper endoscopy follow-up had three post-treatment bleeding episodes after a median follow-up of 324 days. Among the 40 patients treated for primary prophylaxis, 28 underwent follow-up EUS and 27 (96%) had confirmed obliteration. Clinical signs of pulmonary embolization were seen in one patient (1%). Another four patients (3%) presented with minor delayed upper gastrointestinal bleeding from coil and glue extrusion.

Comparative studies are needed to determine the benefit of combined cyanocrylate and coil treatment of GV (Fig. 12.2) over cyanocrylate alone, as well as the advantages of EUS-guidance over endoscopy-guidance.

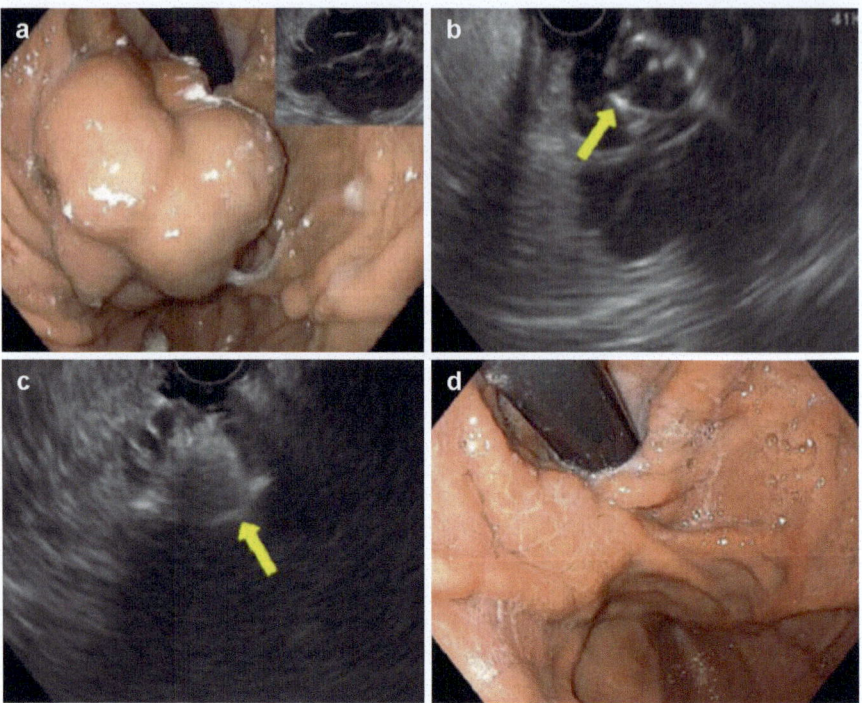

Fig. 12.2 EUS-guided treatment of gastric fundal varices with combined injection of coils and cyanocrylate glue. (**a**) Evident gastric varices on gastroscopy and EUS. (**b**) EUS vue of the coil inside the varix (arrow). (**c**) EUS vue of the obliterated varix after glue injection (arrow). (**d**) Erradicated varices after treatment

12.7   EUS-Guided Therapy of Ectopic Varices

EUS-guided therapy has been described in case reports for variceal bleeding at other anatomical sites. So et al. [40] described the use of an EUS-guided coil to treat massive duodenal variceal bleeding. The use of CYA glue in this scenario has also been described. Rectal varices are common but have a smaller risk of bleeding than their gastroduodenal counterparts. The uses of both, EUS-guided CYA injection and combination therapy with EUS-guided coil/CYA for rectal varices, have been described [41, 42]. EUS has also been used to direct glue into parastomal varices [43]. While there is currently insufficient evidence to recommend EUS-guided treatment as first line in these cases, it has emerged as a viable option for rescue therapy.

12.8   EUS-Guided Portal Vein Interventions

The ability of EUS to access the PV potentially enables a broad spectrum of diagnostic, staging, and therapeutic interventions (Table 12.2).

Table 12.2 EUS-guided portal vein interventions	PV pressure measurement (human studies)
	Intrahepatic portosystemic shunt (animal studies)
	Sampling of PV thrombosis (human studies)
	Sampling of circulating tumor cells in PV (human studies)
	Selective PV embolization (animal studies)

12.8.1 EUS-Guided Portal Vein Pressure Measurement

EUS may permit PV access, contrast injection and monitoring the PV pressure. Lai and colleagues [44] catheterized the extrahepatic PV in 14 pigs with portal hypertension and seven controls. A 22-gauge (22 G) needle was advanced under EUS guidance and pressure measurements were successfully obtained in 18 of 21 (86%) swine. A good correlation with those obtained by transhepatic catheterization was observed, but one of these pigs developed severe intraperitoneal bleeding. Small caliber of the needle and difficulty in maintaining a stable needle position were the reported challenges. Giday et al. [45] performed EUS-guided transhepatic PV catheterization in three pigs with a modified ERCP catheter, which allowed them to perform portal angiography and obtain continuous portal pressure readings over 1 h. Results showed minimal variability within each animals and no complications were observed. Successful and reproducible EUS-guided portal pressure measurements by using a digital pressure wire (Pressure Wire Aeris; St. Jude Medical, St. Paul, Minn) advanced through a 22 G needle were reported in five Yorkshire pigs [46]. EUS-guided measurement of the portal pressure gradient was reported by using a 25 G needle and a small battery-operated manometer; the left PV, right hepatic vein, and intrahepatic inferior vena cava were accessed in three Yorkshire pigs to obtain these measurements [47].

Recently one report [48] published the first human report demonstrating the feasibility and safety of PV and hepatic vein pressure measurements by EUS allowing diagnosis of arteriovenous malformations in a patient with Noonan syndrome. Following this report, a human pilot study [49] was performed in 28 patients with a history of liver disease or suspected cirrhosis. They underwent EUS-guided portal pressure gradient measurement by using a 25 G needle and a new compact manometer (Cook Medical, Bloomington, Ind). Measurements were recorded in the intrahepatic PV near its bifurcation and in the hepatic vein or directly from the intrahepatic inferior vena cava when hepatic vein access was not possible. A good correlation between the measured portal pressure gradients and clinical parameters of portal hypertension was observed and no adverse events were noted.

Direct measurement of PV pressure with EUS guidance represents a novel approach; however, a disadvantage is represented by the lack of simultaneous measurement of the systemic venous pressure, (hence, no hepatic pressure gradient calculation). Well-designed, comparative trials to determine the accuracy and safety of this technique compared with transjugular hepatic venous pressure measurements are essential.

12.8.2 EUS-Guided Intraportal Portosystemic Shunt

Decompression of the portal system by placement of a transjugular intrahepatic portosystemic shunt (TIPS) is frequently used for the treatment of portal hypertension and its complications. TIPS is a widely used technique, predominantly performed by interventional radiologists, and limited to tertiary-referral centers. Buscaglia et al. first described EUS-guided creation of an intrahepatic portosystemic shunt (IPS) in a total of ten pigs [50]. Under direct EUS observation, the left hepatic vein and the left PV were sequentially punctured with a 19 G needle. A guidewire was advanced through the needle into the PV. A self-expandable tubular metal stent was advanced over the guidewire and deployed with its distal end inside the PV and the proximal end inside the HV. Four pigs required a second stent. No adverse events were reported. Two groups [51, 52] have reported use of a fully covered lumen-apposing metal stent to create an IPS in a live swine model by using a similar technique. In one of these studies, three of five animals were noted to have partial in-stent thrombosis at necropsy 2 weeks after the procedure. These early investigations suggest that EUS-guided creation of an IPS is feasible and may offer an alternative approach, but further refinement of devices and techniques is needed.

12.8.3 EUS-Guided FNA of PV Thrombosis for Staging of Hepatocellular Carcinoma

Distinguish a portal vein tumoral thrombus secondary to invasion of hepatocellular carcinoma from a bland thrombus can be sometimes challenging. Successful trans-duodenal EUS-FNA of malignant PV thrombi by using 25 G needles has been reported without adverse events [53–56]. Some case reports have described the diagnosis of hepatocellular carcinoma by EUS-FNA of malignant PV thrombi in patients with no hepatic mass visualized on cross-sectional imaging [53, 54].

12.8.4 EUS-Guided PV Embolization

Selective embolization of the right or left branch of the PV to produce a compensatory hypertrophy of the contralateral hepatic lobe before resection for hepatic malignancy has been described. Preliminary results from an animal model [57] suggest EUS-guided microcoil embolization of the right PV can produce intended hypertrophy of the left hepatic lobe. Matthes et al. [58] reported a successful embolization of the PV using a polymer (Enteryx) in a pig.

12.8.5 EUS-Guided Portal Injection Chemotherapy

EUS-guided PV injection of chemotherapy (EPIC) by using drug-eluting micro-beads or nanoparticles was successfully demonstrated in 24 anesthetized pigs [59].

Significantly higher hepatic drug levels and significantly lower systemic drug levels were observed. Although further evaluation of this technique is warranted, this study demonstrated that EPIC is feasible in a nonsurvival animal model and could be a therapeutic option for patients with diffuse liver metastases or even primary liver malignancies.

12.8.6 EUS-Guided PV Sampling of Circulating Tumor Cells in Pancreaticobiliary Cancers

A single-center prospective study [60] reported the safety and feasibility of EUS-guided sampling of intrahepatic PV to detect circulating tumor cells using a 19 G needle in 18 patients with metastatic and nonmetastatic pancreatic and biliary cancers to evaluate for CTCs. Although not demonstrated in hepatocellular carcinoma, it could be a diagnostic tool in the future for these patients.

12.9 Summary

EUS is a readily available, minimally-invasive technique to explore vascular changes in patients with portal hypertension, but currently it does not have an established role in clinical practice. Several studies have demonstrated that EUS is superior to upper endoscopy in identifying gastric varices and for the evaluation of collateral vessels, which is useful to predict the risk of bleeding and the response to therapy.

Vascular access and therapy are emerging applications for EUS-based interventions. EUS may be of help in guiding endoscopic therapy of varices, such as EUS-guided sclerotherapy of esophageal collateral vessels and EUS-guided glue injection or coiling of gastric varices. However data are still very limited. Prospective and controlled trials are needed to show clinical effectiveness and safety in humans as well as the advantages of EUS-guidance over endoscopy-guidance.

EUS-guided PV access and therapeutic interventions represent an exciting new technical advance in interventional EUS. Several technical applications have been shown to be feasible in animal models and in small, preliminary human studies. The development of new tools designed for EUS-guided vascular therapy is essential. Moreover, well-designed studies will be needed to establish the efficacy and safety profile of these interventions in comparison to any current competing techniques and will be crucial in determining their eventual clinical use.

References

1. Kitano S, Terblanche J, Kahn D, et al. Venous anatomy of the lower oesophagus in portal hypertension: practical implications. Br J Surg. 1986;73:525–31.
2. Hashizume M, Kitano S, Sugimachi K, et al. Threedimensional view of the vascular structure of the lower esophagus in clinical portal hypertension. Hepatology. 1988;8:1482–7.

3. Irisawa A, Obara K, Sato Y, et al. EUS analysis of collateral veins inside and outside the esophageal wall in portal hypertension. Gastrointest Endosc. 1999;50:374–80.
4. Parasher VK, Meroni E, Malesci A, et al. Observation of thoracic duct morphology in portal hypertension by endoscopic ultrasound. Gastrointest Endosc. 1998;48:588–92.
5. Wiersema MJ, Chak A, Kopecky KK, et al. Duplex Doppler endosonography in the diagnosis of splenic vein, portal vein, and portosystemic shunt thrombosis. Gastrointest Endosc. 1995;42:19–26.
6. Kakutani H, Hino S, Ikeda K, et al. Use of the curved linear-array echo endoscope to identify gastrorenal shunts in patients with gastric fundal varices. Endoscopy. 2004;36:710–4.
7. Avunduk C, Hampf F. Endoscopic ultrasound in the diagnosis of watermelon stomach. J Clin Gastroenterol. 1996;22:104–6.
8. Kassem AM, Salama ZA, Zakaria MS, et al. Endoscopic ultrasonography study of the azygos vein before and after endoscopic obliteration of esophagogastric varices by injection sclerotherapy. Endoscopy. 2000;32:630–4.
9. Nishida H, Giostra E, Spahr L, et al. Validation of color Doppler EUS for azygos blood flow measurement in patients with cirrhosis: application to the acute hemodynamic effects of somatostatin, octreotide, or placebo. Gastrointest Endosc. 2001;54:24–30.
10. Lee YT, Sung JJY, Yung MY, et al. Use of color Doppler EUS in assessing azygos blood flow for patients with portal hypertension. Gastrointest Endosc. 1999;50:47–52.
11. Faigel DO, Rosen HR, Sasaki A, et al. EUS in cirrhotic patients with and without prior variceal hemorrhage in comparison with noncirrhotic control subjects. Gastrointest Endosc. 2000;52:455–62.
12. McKiernan PJ, Sharif K, Gupte GL. The role of endoscopic ultrasound for evaluating portal hypertension in children being assessed for intestinal transplantation. Transplantation. 2008;86:1470–3.
13. Caletti G, Brocchi E, Baraldini M, et al. Assessment of portal hypertension by endoscopic ultrasonography. Gastrointest Endosc. 1990;36:S21–7.
14. Burtin P, Calès P, Oberti F, et al. Endoscopic ultrasonographic signs of portal hypertension in cirrhosis. Gastrointest Endosc. 1996;44:257–61.
15. Boustiere C, Dumas O, Jouffre C, et al. Gastric endoscopic ultrasonography: a new approach to the diagnosis of portal hypertension in cirrhotic patients. Hepatology. 1991;14:85,
16. Liu JD, Miller LS, Feld RI, et al. Gastric and esophageal varices: 20-MHz transnasal endoluminal US. Radiology. 1993;187:363–6.
17. Suzuki T, Matsutani S, Umebara K, et al. EUS changes predictive for recurrence of esophageal varices in patients treated by combined endoscopic ligation and sclerotherapy. Gastrointest Endosc. 2000;52:611–7.
18. Choudhuri G, Dhiman RK, Agarwal DK. Endosonographic evaluation of the venous anatomy around the gastro-esophageal junction in patients with portal hypertension. Hepato-Gastroenterology. 1996;43:1250–5.
19. Lee YT, Chan FK, Ching JY, et al. Diagnosis of gastroesophageal varices and portal collateral venous abnormalities by endosonography in cirrhotic patients. Endoscopy. 2002;34:391–8.
20. Konishi Y, Nakamura T, Kida H, et al. Catheter US probe EUS evaluation of gastric cardia and perigastric vascular structures to predict esophageal variceal recurrence. Gastrointest Endosc. 2002;55:197–203.
21. Lo GH, Lai KH, Cheng JS, et al. Prevalence of paraesophageal varices and gastric varices in patients achieving variceal obliteration by banding ligation and by injection sclerotherapy. Gastrointest Endosc. 1999;49:428–36.
22. Pontes JM, Leitao MC, Portela FA, et al. Endoscopic ultrasonography in the treatment of esophageal varices by endoscopic sclerotherapy and band ligation: do we need it. Eur J Gastroenterol Hepatol. 1995;7:41–6.
23. Goenka MK, Kochhar R, Nagi B, et al. Rectosigmoid varices and other mucosal changes in patients with portal hypertension. Am J Gastroenterol. 1991;86:1185–9.
24. Wu CS, Chen CM, Chang KY. Endoscopic injection sclerotherapy of bleeding duodenal varices. J Gastroenterol Hepatol. 1995;19:481–3.

25. Palazzo L, Hochain P, Helmer C, et al. Biliary varices on endoscopic ultrasonography: clinical presentation and outcome. Endoscopy. 2000;32:520–4.
26. Irisawa A, Saito A, Obara K, et al. Endoscopic recurrence of esophageal varices is associated with the specific EUS abnormalities: severe periesophageal collateral veins and large perforating veins. Gastrointest Endosc. 2001;53:77–84.
27. Sato T, Yamazaki K, Toyota J, et al. Endoscopic ultrasonographic evaluation of hemodynamics related to variceal relapse in esophageal variceal patients. Hepatol Res. 2009;39:126–33.
28. Dhiman RK, Choudhuri G, Saraswat VA, et al. Role of paraesophageal collateral and perforating veins on outcome of endoscopic sclerotherapy for esophageal varices: an endosonographic study. Gut. 1996;38:759–64.
29. Leung VK, Sung JJ, Ahuja AT, et al. Large paraesophageal varices on endosonography predict recurrence of esophageal varices rebleeding. Gastroenterology. 1997;112(6):1811.
30. Hino S, Kakutani H, Ikeda K, et al. Hemodynamic analysis of esophageal varices using color Doppler endoscopic ultrasonography to predict recurrence after endoscopic treatment. Endoscopy. 2001;33:869–72.
31. Kuramochi A, Imazu H, Kakutani H, et al. Color Doppler endoscopic ultrasonography in identifying groups at high-risk of recurrence of esophageal varices after endoscopic treatment. J Gastroenterol. 2007;42:219–24.
32. Lee YT, Chan FK, Ng EK, et al. EUS-guided injection of cyanoacrylate for bleeding gastric varices. Gastrointest Endosc. 2000;52:168–74.
33. Iwase H, Suga S, Morise K. Color Doppler endoscopic ultrasonography for the evaluation of gastric varices and endoscopic obliteration with cyanoacrylate glue. Gastrointest Endosc. 1995;41:150–4.
34. Lahoti S, Catalano M, Alcocer E, et al. Obliteration of esophageal varices using EUS-guided sclerotherapy with color Doppler. Gastrointest Endosc. 2000;51(3):331.
35. De Paulo GA, Ardengh JC, Nakao FS, et al. Treatment of esophageal varices: a randomized controlled trial comparing endoscopic sclerotherapy and EUSguided sclerotherapy of esophageal collateral veins. Gastrointest Endosc. 2006;63:396–402.
36. Romero-Castro R, Pellicer-Bautista FJ, Jiménez-Saenz M, et al. EUS-guided injection of cyanoacrylate in perforating feeding veins in gastric varices: results in 5 cases. Gastrointest Endosc. 2007;66:402–7.
37. Levy M, Wong Kee Song L, Kendrick M. EUS-guided coil embolization for refractory ectopic variceal bleeding. Gastrointest Endosc. 2008;67:572–4.
38. Romero-Castro R, Ellrichmann M, Ortiz-Moyano C, et al. EUS-guided coil versus cyanoacrylate therapy for the treatment of gastric varices: a multicenter study (with videos). Gastrointest Endosc. 2013;78:711–21.
39. Bhat YM, Weilert F, Fredrick RT, et al. EUS-guided treatment of gastric fundal varices with combined injection of coils and cyanoacrylate glue: a large U.S. experience over 6 years (with video). Gastrointest Endosc. 2016;83(6):1164–72.
40. So H, Park do H, Jung K, Ko HK. Successful endoscopic ultrasound-guided coil embolization for severe duodenal bleeding. Am J Gastroenterol. 2016;111:925.
41. Sharma M, Somasundaram A. Massive lower GI bleed from an endoscopically inevident rectal varices: diagnosis and management by EUS (with videos). Gastrointest Endosc. 2010;72:1106–8.
42. Weilert F, Shah JN, Marson FP, et al. EUS-guided coil and glue for bleeding rectal varix. Gastrointest Endosc. 2012;76:915–6.
43. Tsynman DN, DeCross AJ, Maliakkal B, et al. Novel use of EUS to successfully treat bleeding parastomal varices with N-butyl-2-cyanoacrylate. Gastrointest Endosc. 2014;79:1007–8. discussion 1008
44. Lai L, Poneros J, Santilli J. EUS-guided portal vein catheterization and pressure measurement in an animal model: a pilot study of feasibility. Gastrointest Endosc. 2004;59:280–3.
45. Giday S, Clarke J, Buscaglia J, et al. EUS-guided portal vein catheterization: a promising novel approach for portal angiography and portal vein pressure measurements. Gastrointest Endosc. 2008;67:338–42.

46. Schulman AR, Thompson CC, Ryou M. EUS-guided portal pressure measurement using a digital pressure wire with real-time remote display: a novel, minimally invasive technique for direct measurement in an animal model. Gastrointest Endosc. 2016;83:817–20.
47. Huang JY, Samarasena JB, Tsujino T, et al. EUS-guided portal pressure gradient measurement with a novel 25-gauge needle device versus standard transjugular approach: a comparison animal study. Gastrointest Endosc. 2016;84:358–62.
48. Fujii-Lau LL, Leise MD, Kamath PS, et al. Endoscopic ultrasonography-guided portal-systemic pressure gradient measurement. Endoscopy 2014;46(S01):E654–E656.
49. Huang JY, Samarasena JB, Tsujino T, et al. EUS-guided portal pressure gradient measurement with a simple novel device: a human pilot study. Gastrointest Endosc. Epub 2016 Sep 29
50. Buscaglia JM, Dray X, Shin EJ, et al. A new alternative for a transjugular intrahepatic portosystemic shunt: EUS-guided creation of an intrahepatic portosystemic shunt (with video). Gastrointest Endosc. 2009;69:941–7.
51. Schulman AR, Ryou M, Aihara H, et al. EUS-guided intrahepatic portosystemic shunt with direct portal pressure measurements: a novel alternative to transjugular intrahepatic portosystemic shunting. Gastrointest Endosc. 2017;85:243–7.
52. Binmoeller KF, Shah JN. EUS-guided transgastric intrahepatic portosystemic shunt using the axios stent [abstract]. Gastrointest Endosc. 2011;73:AB167.
53. Lai R, Stephens V, Bardales R. Diagnosis and staging of hepatocellular carcinoma by EUS-FNA of a portal vein thrombus. Gastrointest Endosc. 2004;59:574–7.
54. Michael H, Lenza C, Gupta M, et al. Endoscopic ultrasound-guided fineneedle aspiration of a portal vein thrombus to aid in the diagnosis and staging of hepatocellular carcinoma. Gastroenterol Hepatol. 2011;7:124–9.
55. Storch I, Gomez C, Contreras F, et al. Hepatocellular carcinoma (HCC) with portal vein invasion, masquerading as pancreatic mass, diagnosed by endoscopic ultrasound-guided fine needle aspiration (EUS-FNA). Dig Dis Sci. 2007;52:789–91.
56. Kayar Y, Turkdogan KA, Baysal B, Unver N, et al. EUS-guided FNA of a portal vein thrombus in hepatocellular carcinoma. Pan Afr Med J. 2015;21:86.
57. Vazquez-Sequeiros E, Olcina JRF. Endoscopic ultrasound guided vascular access and therapy: a promising indication. World J Gastrointest Endosc. 2010;2:198–202.
58. Matthes K, Sahani D, Holalkere NS, et al. Feasibility of endoscopic ultrasound guided portal vein embolization with Enteryx. Acta Gastroenterol Belg. 2005;68:412–5.
59. Faigel D, Lake D, Landreth T, et al. Endoscopic ultrasonography-guided portal injection chemotherapy for hepatic metastases. Endosc Ultrasound. 2014;3(Supp 1):S1.
60. Catenacci DVT, Chapman CG, Xu P, et al. Acquisition of portal venous circulating tumor cells from patients with pancreaticobiliary cancers by endoscopic ultrasound. Gastroenterology. 2015;149:1794–803.e4.

Computed Tomography

13

Maxime Ronot, Romain Pommier, Paul Calame,
Yvonne Purcell, and Valérie Vilgrain

Abbreviations

CT	Computed tomography
DE-CT	Dual-energy computed tomography
fEES	Fractional extravascular extracellular space
HCC	Hepatocellular carcinoma
HH	Hepatic hydrothorax
HPS	Hepatopulmonary syndrome
HVPG	Hepatic venous pressure gradient
LSN	Liver surface nodularity
MRI	Magnetic resonance imaging
PCT	Perfusion tomography perfusion
PHT	Portal hypertension
TIPS	Transjugular intrahepatic portosystemic shunt

M. Ronot, M.D., Ph.D. (✉) • V. Vilgrain, M.D., Ph.D.
Department of Radiology, Hôpitaux Universitaires Paris Nord Val de Seine, Beaujon,
Clichy, Hauts-de-Seine, France

University Paris Diderot, Sorbonne Paris Cité, Paris, France

INSERM U1149, Centre de Recherche Biomédicale Bichat-Beaujon, CRB3, Paris, France
e-mail: maxime.ronot@aphp.fr

R. Pommier, M.D. • P. Calame, M.D.
Department of Radiology, Hôpitaux Universitaires Paris Nord Val de Seine, Beaujon,
Clichy, Hauts-de-Seine, France

University Paris Diderot, Sorbonne Paris Cité, Paris, France

Y. Purcell
Department of Radiology, Hôpitaux Universitaires Paris Nord Val de Seine, Beaujon,
Clichy, Hauts-de-Seine, France

© Springer International Publishing AG, part of Springer Nature 2018
A. Berzigotti, J. Bosch (eds.), *Diagnostic Methods for Cirrhosis and Portal
Hypertension*, https://doi.org/10.1007/978-3-319-72628-1_13

13.1 Introduction

Cirrhosis is a heterogeneous and dynamic condition, associated with the progressive deposition of hepatic fibrosis that leads to increased vascular resistance at the level of the hepatic sinusoids, and to portal hypertension. Cirrhosis accounts for 90% of the causes of portal hypertension (PHT) in adults [1]. Increased portal pressure is the main factor determining the clinical course of cirrhosis [2]. An accurate estimation of the severity of fibrosis and PHT is essential to evaluate the disease state and prognosis, and is often the first step towards the optimization of treatment. Liver biopsy and invasive measurement of hepatic venous pressure gradient (HVPG) are the gold standard techniques for the estimation of hepatic fibrosis and PHT, respectively. However, both are invasive and, as such, cannot be used repeatedly in clinical practice [3]. As a consequence, the need for non-invasive diagnosis tests for cirrhosis and PHT is major.

Computed Tomography (CT) is a fast, standardized, and cheap cross-sectional imaging technique based on 3D X-ray technology that provides an anatomical exploration of organs. In the field of hepatology it is routinely used for the exploration of patients with chronic liver disease and portal hypertension, but also for the characterization of focal liver lesions.

This chapter aims to review the role of CT in the diagnosis, grading, and prognosis of hepatic fibrosis and portal hypertension. After technical considerations about CT, its role in the depiction of hepatic and splenic morphological and functional changes in cirrhosis (part I), and screening for porto-systemic collaterals and organomegaly in portal hypertension (part II) will be detailed and discussed. The third part is dedicated to the non-invasive assessment of the severity of disease, the prediction of related events, and screening for complications. Finally, this chapter will close on future technical perspectives regarding the assessment of cirrhosis and portal hypertension. Extrahepatic portal vein thrombosis, and idiopathic portal hypertension will be discussed in other chapters.

13.2 Technical Considerations

13.2.1 CT Protocol and Contrast Injection

Classically, contrast-enhanced computed tomography (CECT) is used to assess chronic liver disease and portal hypertension, with three or four phases: unenhanced phase, arterial phase (start delay, 30–35 s after the beginning of contrast injection), portal venous phase (start delay, 70–80 s) and, delayed phase when considered necessary (start delay, 180 s). The use of non-ionic contrast material injected at a rate of 2–3 mL/s using an automatic injector system through an 18–20 gauge cannula placed in an antecubital vein is the most common technique for contrast medium injection. The unenhanced phase allows an analysis of the spontaneous attenuation of the parenchyma and liquids, as well as the depiction of calcifications or iron overload. Analysis of the arterial network (branches of the celiac trunk and of the superior mesenteric artery), and detection of hypervascular hepatic lesions are performed on arterial phase images. The enhancement of parenchyma (hepatic, splenic, mucosal, etc.), the further characterization of hepatic lesions, together with portal and systemic venous mapping are carried out on the portal phase images. A delayed phase is mostly performed for the characterization of focal liver lesions. Dual-energy CT can be used in patients with chronic liver disease as it can quantify hepatic iron and fat content as well as quantification of tissue perfusion by providing iodine maps. However, this technique is mostly used in patients with high suspicion of hepatocellular carcinoma. The drawbacks of CT are well known and include exposure to ionizing radiation, the risk of allergic reactions and iodine contrast material-related nephrotoxicity.

13.2.2 CT Post-Treatment

Routine CT protocol is normally sufficient for the evaluation of liver parenchyma and contours, and stigmata of portal hypertension such as esophageal varices. As an example, Park et al. [4] reported no influence of section thickness (i.e. 1, 3, or 5 mm) for the detection and grading of esophageal varices in cirrhotic patients. When defining larger varices as vessels larger or equal to 3 mm, sensitivity, specificity, and predictive values were comparable among the three image datasets. On the other hand, Yu et al. [5] demonstrated an increase in specificity of CT for the risk stratification of esophageal varices from the 1- to 3-mm multiplanar reformat or surface-shaded display compared with the standard 5-mm images. Yet, to date, most CT scans include 1- or 3-mm sections, with multiplanar reconstruction (MPR), and maximum intensity projection (MIP) for the analysis of vessels.

13.2.3 Esophagus Distension

Classically, on CT images the esophageal lumen appears collapsed. This may hamper the detection of submucosal anomalies that may be associated with PHT. Some consider that esophageal distension may improve the quality of three-dimension (3D) CT reconstructions. Ingestion of effervescent powder mixed with water both prior to intravenous contrast agent administration, and immediately after the acquisition of arterial phase images, has been proposed to obtain effective distention of the esophageal lumen [6], and therefore to increase the accuracy of CT for the diagnosis of esophageal varices [7]. The use of air injected through a mechanical inflator into a catheter placed in the upper esophagus was also evaluated by Kim et al. and compared with endoscopic findings. Authors reported a high sensitivity and specificity of CT (93% and 97%, respectively) in detecting varices with high risk of bleeding [8]. Yet, and despite these results, the vast majority of CT scans are acquired without esophagueal distension in routine practice.

13.3   Part I: Hepatic and Splenic Morphological and Functional Changes in Cirrhosis

Cirrhosis and portal hypertension lead to progressive morphological changes of the liver and spleen. In cirrhosis, the progressive deposition and accumulation of fibrosis, together with nodular regeneration, cause diffuse disorganization of hepatic morphology, with a progressive redistribution of portal venous flow into the different parts of the liver. Liver trophicity is regionally altered, leading to progressive atrophy of segments, while other segments partially compensate by hypertrophying. CT or MR imaging are insensitive to early changes and many patients with cirrhosis and portal hypertension may appear normal. Later, parenchymal heterogeneity and surface nodularity are observed [9], with progressive liver atrophy.

13.3.1 Morphological Changes of the Liver

Liver dystrophy corresponds with modifications of normal hepatic morphology and segment volumes (Fig. 13.1) [10]. The two most characteristic morphologic features of liver cirrhosis are atrophy of segment 4 and hypertrophy of the caudate lobe [9]. Although atrophy of segment 4 (defined as a segment 4 diameter of less than 30 mm) has been compared with controls on ultrasound, this finding is also easy to detect on CT [11]. The caudate lobe may show wide morphological changes in normal adults and therefore has been subject to several studies. The first study has shown that a ratio of transverse caudate lobe width to right lobe width greater than or equal to 0.65 constitutes a positive indicator for the diagnosis of cirrhosis with an accuracy of 94% [12]. More recently, a modified caudate lobe width to right lobe width ratio (mC/RLr), using the right portal vein instead of the main portal vein to set the lateral boundary, has been reported to be more accurate. By using a mC/RLr greater than 0.90, the accuracy for the diagnosis of cirrhosis was 74.2% on MRI [13]. Indeed, hypertrophy of the caudate lobe is not specific to cirrhosis and has also been reported in patients with Budd–Chiari syndrome and/or cavernous transformation of the portal vein. Other CT morphological changes are hypertrophy of the left lobe of the liver and atrophy affecting the right posterior segments (6 and 7). Other changes such as the enlargement of hilar periportal space >10 mm [14, 15] or a narrowing of the right hepatic vein <5 mm [16], a right posterior hepatic notch sign [17, 18], an expanded gallbladder fossa [19] and generalized widening of the interlobar fissures are also considered typical findings of cirrhosis. However, these morphologic features (Table 13.1) suffer from moderate sensitivity, moderate interobserver agreement due to the subjective nature of these signs, and are not always present at earlier stages of fibrosis [20]. Therefore, caution should be taken before excluding liver fibrosis in a patient with normal liver morphology. Indeed, 15–20% of patients with advanced fibrosis/cirrhosis and elevated stiffness on MR elastography showed normal morphologic features on conventional MR imaging [21, 22]. Regional changes in hepatic volume correlate well with the degree of fibrosis.

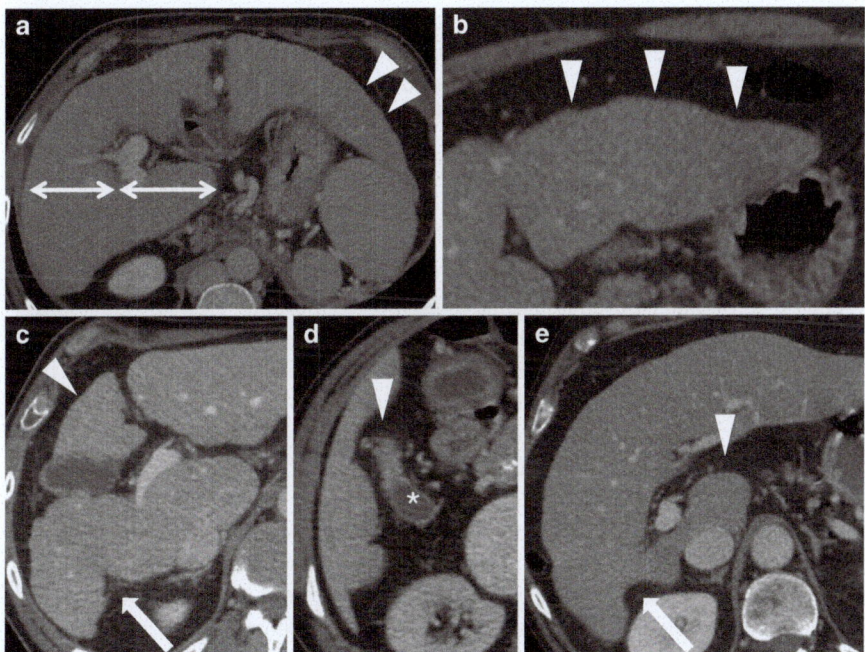

Fig. 13.1 Cirrhosis features on CT. Portal venous phase CT scan on different cirrhotic patients shows (**a**). An atrophy-hypertrophy complex associating an atrophy of the right lobe and an enlarged caudate lobe and left liver lobe. The caudate lobe width to right lobe width ratio, using the right portal vein, is higher than 0.9; (**b**) A hepatic surface nodularity with lobulated margins (white arrowheads) of the hypertrophic left lobe; (**c**) An atrophy of the segment 4 (white arrowhead) and a right posterior hepatic notch sign (white arrow); (**d**) An enlarged gallbladder (asterisk) fossa (white arrowhead); (**e**) An enlarged porta hepatis (white arrowhead)

Table 13.1 Cirrhosis features on CT scan

Statistical characteristics	Se (%)	Sp (%)	Acc (%)	PPV (%)
Surface nodularity [20]	91.8	84.3	88	–
Caudate to right lobe ratio > 0.90 [13]	71.7	77.4	74.2	–
Atrophy of segment 4 [11]	74.2	100	–	100
Right hepatic posterior notch [17, 18]	72	98	82	99
Expanded gallbladder fossa [19]	68	98	80	98
Expanded hilar periportal space [14, 15]	93	92	92	91
Narrow right hepatic vein [16]	59	99	–	–

Se sensitivity, *Sp* specificity, *Acc* accuracy, *PPV* positive predictive value

13.3.2 Liver Heterogeneity: Nodules, Fibrosis

Nodular regeneration and nodule formation is part of the pathological definition of cirrhosis as chronic injury of the liver. Regenerative nodules are micronodular (diameter between 3 and 9 mm) or macronodular (diameter greater than 9 mm).

Regenerative nodules are iso-attenuating to surrounding liver parenchyma on pre-contrast CT images and therefore difficult to detect [23]. Unenhanced CT can detect regenerative nodules when surrounded by hypoattenuating fibrotic bands or when they appear hyperattenuating, due to the accumulation of iron (siderotic nodules). On contrast-enhanced images, they are also isoattenuating to the liver [24]. Indeed, regenerative nodules receive predominantly portal venous flow and do not usually demonstrate marked enhancement on the arterial phase. In the liver periphery, nodules are responsible for the lobulated surface margin. This nodularity of the liver surface is the single most accurate feature of cirrhosis [25]. More recently, a computer-based quantitative method to measure liver surface nodularity from routine CT images with 5.0-mm section thickness has been developed. Liver surface nodularity, as a noninvasive biomarker to differentiate cirrhotic from non-cirrhotic livers, was shown to be significantly more accurate (area under the receiver operating characteristic curve [AUC] 0.929) than splenic volume (AUC, 0.835) or left lateral segment to total liver volume ratio measurements (AUC, 0.753) [26].

Fibrosis, as a scaring process in chronic liver diseases, presents classically with two different patterns: patchy fibrosis, and focal and confluent mass-like fibrosis. Patchy fibrosis, described as a lacelike pattern, consists of thin or thick bands that surround regenerative nodules, best depicted on non-enhanced CT, is usually not well seen on the portal venous phase [27] but is more evident on delayed phase images, as fibrosis enhances over time. Focal confluent fibrosis is observed in end-stage liver disease and is usually a wedge-shaped lesion located in the subcapsular portion of segments 4, 5 or 8, with associated capsular retraction. Focal confluent fibrosis rarely shows enhancement on arterial phase images and may be mistaken for hepatocellular carcinoma. However, persistent contrast enhancement on the delayed phase is typically observed and is due to the retention of contrast by the fibrotic tissue. This feature, along with the characteristic capsular retraction and typical location and shape, help distinguish confluent fibrosis from hepatocellular carcinoma [9].

13.3.3 Focal and Diffuse Perfusion Changes

Focal perfusion anomalies are increasingly being observed in cirrhotic patients because of the increasing use of multiphasic thin-sliced CT [28, 29]. Perfusion anomalies are likely due to intrahepatic shunts between peripheral hepatic arterial branches and small portal veins. Such transient hepatic attenuation differences are only seen on the arterial phase and could mimic hypervascular hepatic tumors. Perfusion anomalies can also result from occlusion of a portal venous branch with compensatory increased arterial flow causing arterial phase hyperenhancement [30]. These pseudolesions can usually be distinguished from tumors by their peripheral location, wedge shape, lack of mass effect, and isoattenuation with the liver on all other phases [9, 31]. Lack of growth and disappearance on subsequent imaging are other keys to diagnosing these vascular anomalies.

Diffuse perfusion alterations are also observed in cirrhosis. The liver has a dual blood supply and receives approximately 25% of its blood from the hepatic artery and the remaining 75% from the portal vein. There is no hepatic capillary network *per se*. It is replaced by fenestrated sinusoids. These two afferent vascular systems communicate through trans-sinusoidal and transvasal communications as well as the peribiliary plexuses. One of the fundamental adaptive mechanisms involved in vascular abnormalities of the liver is the presence of an arterioportal balance called the 'hepatic buffer response' characterized by a compensatory increase in arterial blood supply when portal supply decreases, although the reverse does not occur [32].

Dilatation of hepatic and extra-hepatic arteries on CT can be easily seen in cirrhotic patients, more particularly the splenic artery and right inferior phrenic artery. Attributed to the increase in splenic blood flow associated with PHT [33], splenic artery aneurysms (SAA) are more frequent in adults with cirrhosis, with a reported incidence between 7% and 17% [33–37]. Most SAA are small, solitary and located in the distal part of the splenic artery, and well visualized on CT, especially on the arterial phase. Kaya et al. found that enlargement of the splenic vein was a significant positive predictive factor (hazard ratio 1.23) for the development of SAA [37]. Esen et al. also showed a linear relationship between phrenic artery diameter and the severity of liver disease [38].

The development and progression of liver fibrosis to cirrhosis is associated with micro-architectural vascular changes and modified perfusion: sinusoids gradually convert into continuous non-fenestrated capillaries with an organized basal membrane containing laminin, an increase in vascular resistance and a decrease in portal perfusion, partly compensated by an increase in arterial perfusion (buffer response) and later by an overall decrease in global perfusion. The first studies evaluating chronic liver diseases with perfusion CT were published in the 1990s. Miles et al. and Bloomey et al. described the buffer response [39, 40], and Van Beers et al. reported an increase in the arterial fraction and mean transit time in a group of patients with cirrhosis compared to a control group using a compartmental model [41]. They also confirmed the decrease in total liver blood flow in patients with cirrhosis compared to controls. The increase in mean transit time was attributed to the reduced mobility of low molecular weight tracer molecules in the space of Disse in fibrotic livers, since mobility was preserved and the distribution of volumes was unchanged. We showed that perfusion CT could identify the early stages of fibrosis [42]. More perfusion CT advances are detailed in Part IV.

13.3.4 Liver and Spleen Volumes

Total liver volume is a very poor predictor of underlying fibrosis. On the other hand, splenomegaly correlates with cirrhosis and the severity of liver disease [43] but this feature has a sensitivity of 60–65% in patients with cirrhosis [44]. Of course, splenomegaly is also strongly associated with PHT (see part III). Yet, it is not only caused by parenchymal congestion, but also to tissue hyperplasia and fibrosis.

Splenomegaly is accompanied by a parallel increase in splenic blood flow, which probably participates in the pathogenesis of PHT [45]. Classically, splenomegaly has been reported more frequently in patients with post-hepatitis cirrhosis than in patients with alcoholic cirrhosis [44, 46]. According to Pickhardt et al., hepato-splenic volume assessment is comparable to liver elastography for fibrosis staging and can easily be performed retrospectively [47].

The most accurate method is the volumetric evaluation of the spleen and an upper limit of normal of 314.5 cm³ has been proposed by Prassopoulos et al. [48]. However, volumetric measurement is time-consuming and not useful in routine clinical practice. This is why Bezerra et al. developed a single measurement of splenic length (splenomegaly defined as greater than 9.76 cm) that proved comparable with a multiple-measurement method [49]. The assessment of spleen volume by CT is also important to guide specific treatments to control portal hypertension and its complications (thrombocytopenia) such as splenic embolization or splenectomy [50].

13.3.5 Etiological Approaches with CT Scan

Different causes of chronic liver disease may show distinctive features on CT, with different distorted hepatic morphologies. For instance, alcoholic cirrhosis induces a significant enlargement of the total liver volume at early stages [51], while the total liver volume significantly decreases with progression of cirrhosis with atrophy/hypertrophy as previously described. In compensated cirrhosis, hypertrophy of the caudate lobe has been shown to be more pronounced in patients with alcoholic or metabolic diseases than in virus-related cirrhosis. Hypertrophy of the left lobe of the liver, and atrophy of segment 4 and the right lobe of the liver, progress less rapidly in patients with non-alcoholic steato-hepatitis than in those with virus-related and alcoholic cirrhosis [52].

Of course, CT can also depict steatosis in the former patients. Indeed, steatosis causes reduced liver attenuation compared with the spleen on unenhanced imaging, classically less than 40 Hounsfield Units (HU), with relatively hyperattenuating intrahepatic vessels on the portal venous phase after injection. Non-fatty liver is normally 6–12 HU greater in density than the spleen. If the attenuation of the liver is at least 10 HU less than that of the spleen, the diagnosis of fatty liver is made [53]. In contrast, iron overload is associated with a marked homogeneous increase in liver attenuation on unenhanced CT (typically between 72 and 130 HU) [54]. As a consequence, portal and hepatic veins appear hypoattenuating relative to the liver. CT has low sensitivity (63%) but high specificity (96%) for the diagnosis of iron overload [55]. Dual-energy CT has recently been proposed to quantify iron deposition [56].

Primary sclerosing cholangitis induces end-stage cirrhosis and pseudotumoral enlargement of the caudate lobe is observed in virtually all patients, along with atrophy of the peripheral hepatic segments resulting in a lobulated liver contour. Concomitant multiple irregular strictures of the intra- and extrahepatic bile ducts are also observed [57]. Finally, primary biliary cirrhosis typically produces early signs of portal hypertension while the liver is enlarged, along with prominent "lacelike fibrosis," regenerative nodules, and lymphadenopathy. Late-stage primary biliary cirrhosis is indistinguishable from other etiologies. Patchy fibrosis is seen in about one-third of patients with primary biliary cirrhosis, regardless of stage [58].

13.4   Part II: Screening for Porto-Systemic Collaterals and Organomegaly in Portal Hypertension

The portal vein, formed by the confluence of the splenic and superior mesenteric veins, carries blood from the mesenteric and splenic circulation to the liver. Cirrhotic liver is highly resistant to portal inflow and the systemic response that increases the splanchnic flow worsens the situation, creating a vicious cycle that may result in the development of PHT. Decompression of the portal pressure is achieved by formation of porto-systemic collaterals bypassing the liver [59], increased spleen volume and, in the case of decompensation, ascites. CT is accurate in mapping porto-systemic collaterals (Fig. 13.2). This venous network appears as a dilated portal

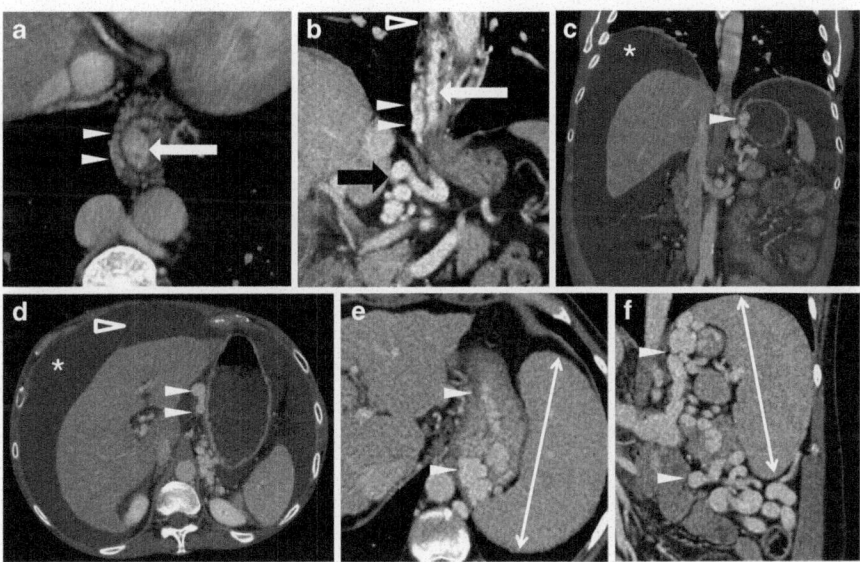

Fig. 13.2 Portal hypertension features on CT. Portal venous phase CT scan shows (**a**) and (**b**). Multiplanar reformated in the axial and coronal plans with communications between esophageal mucosal varices (white arrow), peri-esophagal varices (white arrowheads) and azygos vein (empty arrowhead) in continuity with a dilated and tortuous left gastric vein (black arrow); (**c**) and (**d**). Multiplanar reformated in the coronal and axial plans with an abundant ascites (asterisk) and a dilated left gastric vein. Note the falciform ligament (white arrowhead); (**e**) Mucosal gastric and peri-gastric varices (arrowheads) and splenomegaly (on a single axial measurement); (**f**) Indirect spleno-renal collaterals and splenomegaly (on a single coronal measurement)

Table 13.2 Performance of CT for the detection and grading of esophageal and gastric varices

Statistical characteristics	Se (%)	Sp (%)
Any size esophageal varices [8, 76]	92–87	84–80
High-risk esophageal varices (large >3 mm) [75]	91.9	92
Gastric varices [78]	83–89	75–79

Se sensitivity, *Sp* specificity

vein and a set of engorged and tortuous collateral vessels between the portal venous drainage (stomach, spleen, small bowel and large bowel) and systemic venous drainage (esophagus, distal rectum, retroperitoneal veins or para-umbilical vein or persistant ductus venosus) [60, 61]. Endoscopy is the reference standard method for the diagnosis of esophagal varices, but the accuracy of CT in detecting and grading varices in cirrhotic patients is now recognized [62]. Advantages of CT include capability of visualizing extra-mucosal varices, ectopic varices (Table 13.2), and detecting other complications of cirrhosis, being cheaper and less invasive than endoscopy [63, 64]. Furthermore, CT has been shown to be a cost-effective method for initial screening [65, 66].

13.4.1 Gastro-Esophageal and Splenorenal Collaterals

Because nearly 95% of the variceal bleeding arises from gastro-esophageal varices, their screening is crucial. The left gastric vein that drains the distal esophagus and stomach is dilated (diameter > 7 mm) and presents retrograde flow in the case of PHT [67].

The left gastric varix is considered one of the commonest collaterals, present in 80% of patients with PHT [62]. The anterior and posterior esophageal venous tributaries of the left gastric vein dilate and form the esophageal (submucosal) and para-esophageal (peri-adventitial) varices. These varices drain into the azygos and hemiazygos venous systems when the varices are located in the lower to mid-esophagus. If they extend into the upper esophagus, these varices drain into the subclavian/brachiocephalic system. CT shows submucosal varices as nodular thickening of the esophageal wall and enhancing nodular lesions protruding into the esophageal lumen.

Gastric varices result from dilatation of peripheral venous tributaries of the left gastric, short gastric and gastro-epiploic veins [59]. Isolated gastric varices without esophageal varices occur in the presence of splenic vein occlusion and may occur around the fundus or other portions of the stomach. The gastric and gastro-esophageal veins can communicate either with the azygos and hemiazygos systems or with the phrenic veins which join the adrenal veins, then the left renal vein to form the gastro-phrenico-renal shunt that drains into the inferior vena cava [68]. Gastric varices are not as frequently the source of bleeding as esophageal varices. However, it is important to recognize them because if there is bleeding, treatment options are limited and morbidity and mortality are higher [69]. CT provides an understanding of the physiology of gastric varices with regard to the pathways of drainage and the implications for therapy [70]. Indeed, gastric varices that drain via the esophageal-azygos shunt tend to have hemodynamics similar to those of esophageal varices, whereas gastric varices that drain via the gastro-phrenico-renal shunt often have large spleno-renal shunts that decompress the system, resulting in lower portal venous pressures than those seen in patients with gastro-esophageal varices [71]. This difference has direct clinical implications since the use of transjugular intrahepatic portosystemic shunt (TIPS) without concomitant gastric variceal embolization may not be as effective in controlling or preventing future variceal bleeding. CT is also accurate for planning interventions against portal hypertension-related events, using real-time 3D guidance with the use of preoperative CT for assisting in a TIPS procedure [72].

Endoscopy is the reference standard method for the detection and grading of esophagal varices. In general, the estimation of the risk of variceal bleeding is made by using endoscopic findings such as the size, color, and location of varices [73]. Yet, the presence of portosystemic shunts, such as esophageal, para-esophageal and gastric varices, can be depicted with CT [74]. Kim et al. have evaluated the performance of CT in the detection and grading of esophageal varices in cirrhotic patients, using endoscopy as the reference technique. They found that the overall detection rate of esophageal varices ranged between 64% and 69%. The detection rate for large varices was 92%. When the threshold value for varix diameter was accepted as 3 mm, sensitivity, specificity and accuracy of CT were 92%, 84% and 85%, respectively. CT variceal grading showed a strong correlation with endoscopic grading, with a high interobserver agreement [8]. This 3 mm threshold value is the most accepted [75]. It seems that the limitation of the ability of CT to detect esophageal varices (EV) results from the collapsed esophageal lumen on CT. Esophageal preparation and air lumen dilatation improve the ability of CT to detect EV. Cansu et al. found sensitivity and specificity of 100% and 88.2% to detect the presence of EV using an effervescent powder whereas without using effervescent powder, sensitivity and specificity were 75% and 66% respectively [7].

Kim et al. also showed that CT was able to differentiate low and high-risk varices. They performed CT with the injection of 10 mg of butyl scopolamine to facilitate hypotonia and with esophageal air insufflation. They demonstrated that CT was able to differentiate EV low/high grade and that CT was better tolerated by patients than upper gastrointestinal endoscopy. Perri et al. considered the size of varices at high risk of bleeding as ≥5 mm, and found a specificity of CT to exclude large varices as 82–90% for two readers. CT screening of varices was more cost-effective than endoscopy screening and than CT followed by endoscopy in patients with small varices on CT [65].

A recent meta-analysis from Deng et al. confirmed a high accuracy of CT for the diagnosis of varices in liver cirrhosis with a sensitivity, specificity and area under the summary receiver operating characteristic curve (AUSROC) of 87%/80%/0.8975 for any size, and 87%/88%/0.9494 for high-risk varices [76].

If the association between platelet count ($>150 \times 10^9$ cells/L) and liver stiffness measurement (<20 kPa) has been proposed by the Baveno VI conference to exclude patients with esophageal varices, CT can be seen as a good complement to evaluate the grade of EV and to select patients with a high risk of bleeding varices.

13.4.2 Para-Umbilical Collaterals

These veins are anterior abdominal varices around the umbilicus resulting from dilatation of the para-umbilical vein in the falciform ligament. The para-umbilical vein is a branch of the left portal vein in communication with the superior epigastric veins of the internal thoracic veins and the inferior epigastric veins that usually drain into the external iliac veins (Fig. 13.3) [59]. The para-umbilical vein is the only collateral with hepatofugal flow, thus acting as a physiological TIPS [77].

13.4.3 Others Collaterals

Others porto-systemic collaterals can be visualized by abdomino-pelvic CT (Fig. 13.4). Rectal varices are secondary to the communication between the superior haemorrhoidal veins of the inferior mesenteric vein and the middle and inferior haemorrhoidal veins of the internal iliac veins [59]. Physiological communications

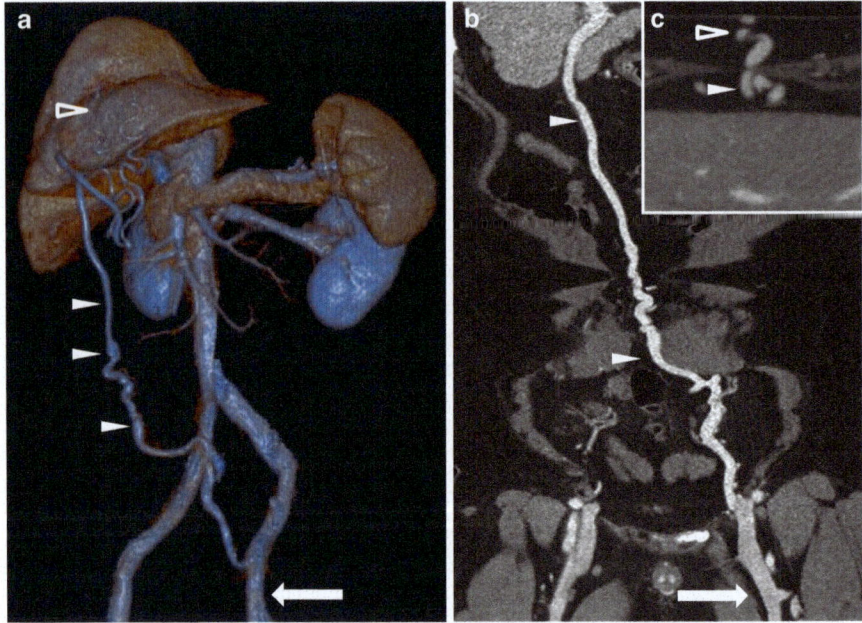

Fig. 13.3 Para-umbilical vein secondary to portal hypertension. 3D volume rendering (**a**) and portal venous phase CT scan with curvilinear vein reconstruction in the coronal plane (**b**) shows two para-umbilical veins (white arrowheads) in the same patient in communication with the superior vena cava via internal thoracic veins (empty arrowhead) and the inferior veina cava via external iliac vein (white arrow). Portal venous phase CT in axial plan shows intra-peritoneal (white arrowhead) and then extra-peritoneal (empty arrowhead) component of the para-umbilical vein separated by the anterior abdominal wall (**c**)

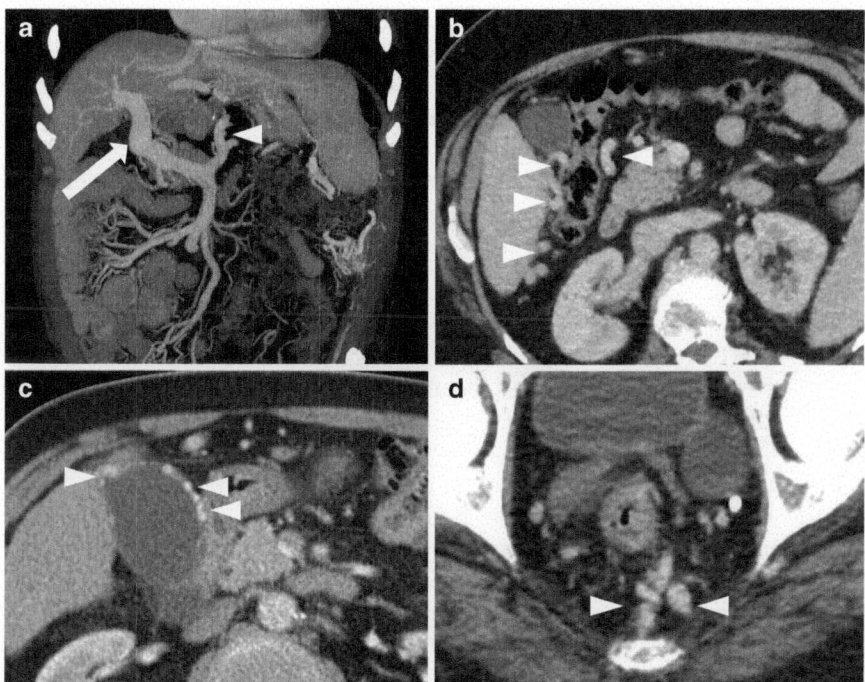

Fig. 13.4 Portal hypertension features on CT. Portal venous phase CT shows (**a**). Coronal maximum intensity projection (MIP) with an enlarged portal vein (white arrow) and a dilated left gastric vein (white arrowhead); Other porto-systemic collaterals, such as dilated right colic vein (white arrowheads) drained into the right renal vein (**b**); Peri-cholecystic varices (white arrowheads) (**c**) and perirectal varices (white arrowheads) (**d**)

of peritoneal (mesenteric) and retroperitoneal (paraduodenal, gonadal or lumbar) veins explain retroperitoneal varices. Paraduodenal varices form a distinct entity wherein the efferent venules from the descending and transverse portion of the duodenum drain into the IVC through veins of Retzius [78]. Other collaterals with lesser clinical interest are less frequently encountered, such as stomal and parastomal varices [59], vesical varices [79] or omental and superficial abdominal wall varices.

13.4.4 Ascites

Sodium and water retention compounded by low albumin levels, as well as increased portal hydrostatic pressure, lead to ascites, one of the most common complications of PHT [80]. Ascites is not a specific sign of PHT and may be present in patients with hepatic impairment or hypoalbuminemia. CT is more sensitive than ultrasound to detect small amounts of fluid in the peritoneum, which collects preferentially in the dependent regions, such as Morison's pouch and the pelvis. Assessment of the density of intraperitoneal fluid may provide a clue about the underlying etiology of ascites on CT. In decompensated cirrhosis, ascites is classically a "transudative fluid" with a density equivalent to that of water (between -10 and $+10$ Hounsfield Units UH), different from other causes of peritoneal effusion such as hemoperitoneum (density between 40 and 60 HU). Although the role of CT is minor in the diagnosis of ascites (based on clinical history, physical examination and ascitic fluid analysis), CT is essential for the planning of a TIPS procedure in the setting of refractory ascites [81].

13.5   Part III: Assessment of the Severity of Disease, Prediction of Related Events, and Detection of Complications

CT, as a non-invasive prognostic tool for predicting the severity of cirrhosis, portal hypertension, and liver-related events is an active research field. Indeed, CT represents a promising modality for the assessment of complications, such as hemorrhage, decompensation of cirrhosis, and death.

Many intercurrent events can occur during the course of the disease. CT plays an important role in the diagnosis and prognostic evaluation of these complications, including abdominal (portal vein thrombosis, portal hypertensive enteropathy or portal biliopathy) and thoracic (hepatic hydrothorax, hepatopulmonary syndrome or portopulmonary hypertension) complications.

13.5.1 Prediction of Portal Hypertension Severity

CT can be a good non-invasive tool to diagnose clinically significant portal hypertension, as it can easily show associated features such as ascites, porto-systemic shunts, and increased spleen size (see part II). Iranmanesh et al. [82] proposed a CT-based model with a high accuracy in prediction of HVPG >10 mmHg. Their model includes the liver/spleen volume ratio and the presence of peri-hepatic ascites, and showed an area under the ROC curve of 0.911 in cirrhotic patients with hepatocellular carcinoma. Kihira et al. [83] tried to retrospectively correlate CT features to HVPG, and built a composite score including the number of variceal sites, the volume of ascites and the maximum cranio-caudal diameter of the spleen. They observed an AUC of their score of 0.77 and 0.83 to diagnose PHT and clinically significant PHT, respectively. Yet, thus far, no prospective study has validated any CT score to evaluate the severity of portal hypertension. The value of CT is probably underestimated. Recently, portal venous mapping from CT angiography and measurement of virtual portal pressure gradient, an equivalent assessment of hepatic venous pressure gradient, has been investigated and showed good performance at grading portal hypertension with an area under the ROC curve of 0.98 [84].

13.5.2 Prediction of GI Hemorrhage, Cirrhosis Decompensation and Death

It is very important to identify cirrhotic patients with a high risk of esophageal variceal bleeding, because they require effective therapy to reduce the incidence of a first bleed [85]. Studies tried to assess the relation between features of portal hypertension on CT scan and the risk of a first episode of bleeding. CT allows the visualization of the portal venous system and almost all of the porto-systemic shunts. Among them, the paraumbilical vein may play a more important role due its unique anatomic features. This vein is the only one with hepatofugal flow, thus acting as a physiological TIPS, explaining why its size has a particular prognostic value to predict variceal bleeding. We demonstrated that the size of the paraumbilical vein was associated with a first episode of hemorrhage, and in association with the spleen size and the presence of ascites, could help predict a first episode of variceal bleeding [77]. We observed that the protective effect of a para-umbilical vein was maximal in patients with a vein larger than 10 mm in diameter. Ge et al. [86] proposed another imaging score including the diameter of the inferior mesenteric vein, posterior gastric vein, and esophageal varices in patients with HBV-related cirrhosis.

The size of the left gastric vein, feeding esophageal varices, is associated with variceal bleeding. For this purpose, Kodama et al. showed that the decreased size of the left gastric vein and para-esophageal vein after ligation treatment for a first variceal hemorrhage was associated with a lower incidence of re-bleeding. All these findings indicate that the size of portosystemic shunts plays a significant role in portal flow and therefore, in variceal hemorrhage [87].

Recently, Smith et al. have proposed a quantitative biomarker derived from routine CT scan images, the liver surface nodularity score, for prediction of cirrhosis decompensation and death in adult patients with cirrhosis. A risk model combining liver surface nodularity and MELD scores was created for predicting liver-related events. The liver surface nodularity score was independently predictive of hepatic decompensation (HR 1.38; 95% CI: 1.06, 1.79) and death (HR 1.22; 95% CI: 1.11, 1.33) [88].

13.5.3 Portal Vein Thrombosis

Portal vein thrombosis (PVT), whether cruoric or neoplastic (invasion of the vein), has a reported prevalence of 1% in autopsy-based series [89, 90], and is a major cause of non-cirrhotic presinusoidal portal hypertension. The role of CT in the management of portal thrombosis is fivefold: diagnose PVT, assess the type of obstruction (bland or tumoral), evaluate PVT extension, search for local or distant cofactors, and evaluate the stage (acute or chronic) (Fig. 13.5) [91]. Most of the time, hepatic Doppler ultrasound is the first examination in the case of suspected portal vein thrombosis [91]. Clinical consequences of PVT mainly depend on the number of vessels completely occluded and its age. Unenhanced CT provides information on

198   M. Ronot et al.

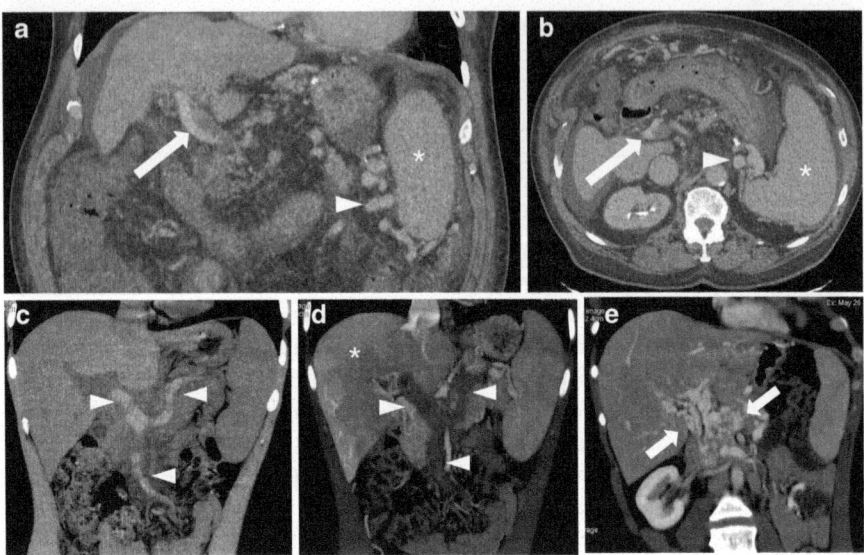

Fig. 13.5 Portal vein thrombosis on CT in a cirrhotic (**a**, **b**) and a non-cirrhotic (**c–e**) patients. In a 54 yo cirrhotic male patient, portal venous phase CT with multiplanar reformated in the coronal (**a**) and axial (**b**) plans shows chronic partial portal vein thrombosis, without cavernomatous transformation (arrows). Note the splenomegaly (asterisk) and splenorenal collaterals (white arrowhead). In a 57 yo non-cirrhotic male patient, acute splanchnic thrombosis appears spontaneously hyperattenuating (white arrowheads) on unenhanced CT (**c**), and hypoattenuating (white arrowheads) on arterial phase images (**d**). Note the peripheral hetetogenous hyperenhancement of the liver on arterial phase images (asterisk) corresponding to the hyperarterialization compensating the significant decrease of portal blood perfusion. A few weeks later, the cavernomatous transformation is depicted on portal venous phase CT (white arrows) (**e**)

the stage, as the thrombus is spontaneously hyperattenuating in acute cases [92]. On portal venous phase CT, PVT appears as a complete or partial luminal filling defect. Furthermore, CT can also show enhancement of the walls of the portal vein in relation to dilated vasa vasorum or a thin peripheral lumen remaining patent. Transient hepatic attenuation differences of the lobe or segment ipsilateral to the portal venous obstruction are mostly seen in the arterial phase, showing increased enhancement compared to normally perfused liver due to hepatic arterial compensatory flow. Cavernous portal venous transformation occurs several days after the obstruction and develops over time. It corresponds to the development of multiple small periportal veins around the common bile duct. At a chronic stage, the obstructed portal vein may disappear or calcify. Any enhancement of the thrombus is suggestive of tumoral venous invasion, classically associated with HCC. Yet, the differentiation between bland PVT and neoplastic portal vein obstruction in patients seems to be more difficult with CT than US or MR imaging [93, 94]. Differentiation may be improved by software-based texture analysis [95] or iodine quantification analysis [96].

13.5.4 Portal Hypertensive Gastropathy, Enteropathy and Colopathy

Chronic portal venous congestion leads to dilatation and ectasia of the submucosal vessels in the stomach (portal hypertensive gastropathy), small bowel (portal hypertensive enteropathy) and/or large bowel (portal hypertensive colopathy). This may result in upper or lower gastrointestinal bleeding, even in the absence of varices. CT shows gastric or bowel wall thickening [97], and enhancement of the inner layer of the gastric wall [98]. Rarely, marked thickening of the large bowel wall, in the context of sepsis in cirrhotic patients with portal hypertensive colopathy, may be suggestive of phlegmonous colitis [99]. However, the diagnosis of portal hypertensive gastropathy or colopathy is preferentially made at the time of endoscopic evaluation [100].

13.5.5 Portal Biliopathy

Portal biliopathy refers to abnormalities of the bile ducts observed in patients with portal hypertension, including extra- and intrahepatic bile duct narrowing and dilatation, biliary stones and choledochal varices. Compression of the common bile duct by dilated veins plays a central role, and is secondary to a mass effect directly related to cavernous transformation of the portal vein. Extension of a thrombotic process may also lead to ischemia of the bile duct wall with subsequent stricture formation. CT (and MR cholangiography with MR portography) should be part of the initial workup [101]. The role of CT is to elucidate the mechanisms of biliary obstruction, to delineate portal venous anatomy and to search for biliary abnormalities. CT may show bile duct dilatation, stenosis and/or angulation of the common bile duct, but MR cholangiography is more accurate in this setting [102].

13.5.6 Hepatic Hydrothorax

Hepatic hydrothorax is an uncommon pleural manifestation of cirrhosis with portal hypertension and ascites. Its estimated prevalence among cirrhotic patients is around 5–10% [103]. It is characterized by formation of pleural effusions usually abundant in patients without any other underlying primary cardiopulmonary cause [104]. It is thought to occur when ascitic fluid moves through diaphragmatic defects that have been opened by increased peritoneal pressure. CT identifies a pleural effusion with the same attenuation as ascites, and can quantify the volume of the effusion and guide thoracocentesis. The pleural effusion is right-sided in the majority of cases (between 73% and 85% of cases) and less frequently bilateral (maximum 10% of cases) [105].

13.5.7 Hepatopulmonary Syndrome

Hepatopulmonary syndrome is a combination of hepatic dysfunction, hypoxemia and pulmonary vascular dilatation. It is estimated to be present in 15% of adults with liver cirrhosis [106, 107]. Physiologically, arterial hypoxemia in patients with hepatopulmonary syndrome is thought to occur because of ventilation-perfusion mismatch, limitations in oxygen diffusion due to vascular dilatation and in some patients, intrapulmonary shunting through dilated vascular malformations. The radiologic manifestations of this disease include distal vascular dilatation associated with an abnormally large number of visible terminal vessel branches, which are often concentrated in the lower lung areas. CT may show peripheral arteriolar dilatation with an increased number of terminal branches extending towards the pleura [103]. Two patterns are described. The first type is most common (85%) and manifests as distal vascular dilatation with subpleural telangiectasia. Features include multiple, slightly dilated subpleural vessels that do not taper normally and therefore extend to the pleural surface. The second type, less common (15%), is seen as individual arteriovenous malformations on angiograms and nodular dilatation of peripheral pulmonary vessels [103]. When used in a diagnostic algorithm with echocardiography, CT contributes to the non-invasive detection of portopulmonary hypertension and may have a role in the pre-liver transplantation triage of patients with portopulmonary hypertension for right-sided heart catheterization [108].

13.5.8 Portopulmonary Hypertension

Portopulmonary hypertension corresponds to a pulmonary hypertension in patients with liver disease or portal hypertension, because of excessive pulmonary vasoconstriction [109]. It occurs in less than 1% of patients with cirrhosis [110] and the risk of developing porto-pulmonary hypertension has been estimated as 2–10% in cirrhotic patients [111, 112]. According to the current World Health Organization classification, porto-pulmonary hypertension is classified as pulmonary arterial hypertension [113]. It is almost exactly the opposite of hepatopulmonary syndrome. Portosystemic shunts contribute to diffuse pulmonary vessel vasoconstriction and to portopulmonary hypertension. Most patients are asymptomatic. Dyspnoea on exertion, fatigue, orthopnoea, chest pain, peripheral oedema, syncope and then dyspnoea at rest may appear in advanced forms. The diagnosis requires objective measurement of increased pulmonary arterial pressure and resistance (defined by invasive right-heart catheterisation showing an elevated mean pulmonary artery pressure >25 mmHg at rest, a pulmonary capillary pressure <15 mmHg and a pulmonary vascular resistance >120 dynes s cm^{-2}) combined with exclusion of other causes of pulmonary hypertension. CT features of pulmonary hypertension also have to be carefully identified. Enlargement of the pulmonary artery up to 30 mm or an increased PA/Aorta ratio >1, dilatation of the right heart chambers and right ventricular hypertrophy, straightening or bowing of the interventricular septum could be depicted on a routine chest CT [103, 114, 115]. In severe and chronic pulmonary hypertension, in situ thrombus may develop in small or large vessels because of slow flow. It is neither a pulmonary embolism nor a chronic thrombo-embolic pulmonary disease *per se*. CT also helps to exclude other common causes of pulmonary hypertension, such as left-heart disease, lung disease, or chronic thromboembolic pulmonary hypertension, before the diagnosis can be made.

13.5.9 Hepatic Encephalopathy

Hepatic encephalopathy is a neuropsychiatric syndrome due to enlarged porto-systemic collaterals and underlying liver disease [116]. This metabolic encephalopathy is a clinical diagnosis that can be assisted by neuropsychology and neurophysiology. The imaging diagnosis relies on MR imaging, as CT is not sensitive enough to highlight the rearrangements of the metabolic encephalopathy [117]. Yet, in most patients with hepatic encephalopathy, CT shows large portosystemic collaterals, often splenorenal [118].

13.5.10 Hepatic Tumors

Contrast-Enhanced CT is one of the imaging modalities that are considered to be standard methods for the characterization of hepatic nodules on a background of chronic liver disease. The cirrhotic liver is a permanent regenerative process. This explains why the occurrence of nodules in such an environment is a frequent event, constituting a diagnostic challenge, in particular for the diagnosis of hepatocellular carcinoma. This subject will not be developed here, as it is beyond the scope of the present chapter.

13.6 Part IV: Future Technical Perspectives

Over the past decades, technological advances in the field of CT have led to a new physiological and diagnostic approach to hepatic fibrosis, cirrhosis and portal hypertension. These advances include perfusion CT, Dual-Energy CT, assessment of Extracellular Volume Fraction CT and texture analysis.

13.6.1 Perfusion CT

Perfusion imaging provides information about tissue microcirculation or the movement of water and solutes at levels far below the spatial resolution of conventional imaging techniques. Thus, perfusion imaging is not the dynamic, qualitative analysis commonly obtained with tissue enhancement, but a quantitative extraction of physiological perfusion parameters of the liver. It requires the injection of a tracer and the acquisition by rapid temporal sampling of signal intensity/time curves that provide information on variations in tracer concentrations over time. The physiological parameters are extracted from these curves by adjusting them to mathematical perfusion models.

Many studies showed that increased arterial flow and arterial fractional flow were correlated with portal hypertension and hepatic fibrosis [41, 42, 119]. Hepatic microcirculation is modified by fibrogenesis and it results in increased total hepatic resistance with altered portal venous blood flow, compensated by increased hepatic arterial flow [120, 121]. Therefore, arterial enhancement fraction is higher in patients with cirrhosis compared with those without liver disease, and is also significantly different between moderate and severe stage fibrosis, or hepatic cirrhosis [41, 42, 119]. Yet, the large overlap between fibrosis groups prevents from using this for individual assessment.

Research has also focused on venous flow such as splenic perfusion as a dynamic marker of PHT, since portal vein congestion causes a decrease in splenic venous perfusion [122]. Talakic et al. showed a strong correlation between splenic clearance (corresponding to total flow from the intravascular to the extravascular space) and hepatic venous pressure gradient [123]. Fischer et al. showed that peak-splenic enhancement was decreased and delayed in patients with PHT. Splenic flow was directly modified by PHT contrary to peak-renal enhancement that appeared insensitive to PHT. The use of the latter as a perfusion reference might improve perfusion modeling. Finally, the difference between peak-splenic enhancement and peak-renal enhancement might serve as a noninvasive biomarker for PHT [124]. As a sensitive, reproducible and non-invasive method in the assessment of PHT, perfusion CT may be used more routinely in years to come. Though promising, such techniques require higher radiation dose than routine CT, and significant post-processing. Moreover, post-processing significantly differs from one manufacturer to another and leads to substantial variations of results for the same patient.

13.6.2 Dual-Energy CT and Extracellular Volume Fraction

Dual-energy CT (DECT) is a new CT technique that has the ability to discriminate between different tissue types. It uses high and low X-ray energy datasets to generate qualitative and quantitative material-specific (named material density) imaging information [125]. One of the most important components is the iodine map. Research suggests a correlation between iodine concentrations on delayed phase images and higher stages of fibrosis, enabling the computation of a fibrosis score and a quantitative map showing the spatial distribution of liver fibrosis for each patient [126]. Indeed, a normalized iodine concentration (liver/aorta) may be used to estimate the severity of disease. Lv et al. reported that, the combination of normalized iodine concentration and iodine concentration ratio showed 77% sensitivity and 87% specificity for differentiating quantitatively normal and cirrhotic livers [127]. Another study confirmed that the arterial iodine fraction was statistically significantly different between patients with and without chronic liver disease, but also among different Child–Pugh grades of patients with cirrhosis [128].

The liver is generally considered to be composed of three distinct spaces: fractional intravascular, fractional intracellular and fractional extravascular extracellular spaces [129]. In chronic liver disease, the latter fractional extravascular extracellular space expands with the progressive deposition of collagen. This creates a larger volume of distribution within the parenchyma for contrast agent that diffuses into the liver leading to abnormally high liver attenuation. Therefore, quantification of fractional extravascular extracellular spaces may be a good biomarker of fibrosis stage. Using conventional CT, quantification of fractional extravascular extracellular spaces requires an unenhanced CT scan and a delayed/equilibrium phase scan (5 min or more) [130]. Zissen et al. showed that such non-invasive contrast-enhanced CT quantification of the fractional extracellular space correlated with the MELD score. Fractional extracellular space quantification has also been shown to be significantly more efficient at predicting cirrhosis than conventional perfusion CT [131]. An expanded fractional extracellular space greater than 30% had 92% sensitivity and 83% specificity for the prediction of cirrhosis [131]. Yet, other studies investigating the ability of fractional extravascular extracellular spaces quantification for the assessment of liver fibrosis showed more modest results [132–134]. Using iodine maps, DECT may be used in years to come to estimate the fractional extracellular space without the need for an additional unenhanced CT scan.

13.6.3 Texture Analysis

Texture analysis of the liver parenchyma is a new area of imaging research, and may have a role in assessing liver fibrosis. Texture analysis is a type of computer-aided image analysis whereby mathematical transformations and statistical analysis are applied to the distribution of grayscale values in an image [20], which can be applied on US, MRI or CT images [135]. CT could be used for the quantification of texture features correlated with hepatic fibrosis [135, 136].

Conclusion

In patients with hepatic fibrosis and portal hypertension, early and non-invasive diagnosis is the main challenge because it allows for the fastest possible management when pathological changes are potentially, at least partially, reversible. Non-invasive diagnosis is a major trend of contemporary medicine, with better tolerance and acceptance of the diagnostic process by patients. CT is routinely used for the diagnosis of chronic liver disease and its complications, especially portal hypertension. Routine CT allows for the assessment of morphological and functional changes in cirrhosis, such as liver morphologic changes, liver heterogeneity secondary to nodules and fibrosis, and liver perfusion anomalies. It can also evaluate the presence and severity of portal hypertension by mapping portosystemic collaterals, depicting organomegaly and abdominal and thoracic complications. It is now used for the non-invasive assessment of the severity of portal hypertension, with an excellent correlation with more invasive methods, and for event-related prediction, such as hemorrhage caused by gastro-esophageal varices, cirrhosis decompensation or death. New CT techniques, including perfusion, dual-energy, fractional extracellular space quantification, and texture analysis, are expected to refine diagnosis and prognostication of hepatic fibrosis and portal hypertension.

References

1. Viallet A, Huet PM, Marleau D, Villeneuve JP. Assessment of portal hemodynamics. Gastroenterology. 1980;79(3):603–5.
2. Bosch J, Garcia-Pagan JC, Berzigotti A, Abraldes JG. Measurement of portal pressure and its role in the management of chronic liver disease. Semin Liver Dis. 2006;26(4):348–62.
3. Kim MY, Jeong WK, Baik SK. Invasive and non-invasive diagnosis of cirrhosis and portal hypertension. World J Gastroenterol. 2014;20(15):4300–15.
4. Park HS, Kim YJ, Choe WH, Ko SY, Bak SH, Il Jung S, Jeon HJ. Diagnosis of esophageal varices on liver CT: is thin-section reconstruction necessary? Hepato-Gastroenterology. 2015;62(138):333–40.
5. Yu NC, Margolis D, Hsu M, Raman SS, Lu DS. Detection and grading of esophageal varices on liver CT: comparison of standard and thin-section multiplanar reconstructions in diagnostic accuracy. AJR Am J Roentgenol. 2011;197:643–9.
6. Mazzeo S, Caramella D, Gennai A, Giusti P, Neri E, Melai L, Cappelli C, Bertini R, Capria A, Rossi M, Bartolozzi C. Multidetector CT and virtual endoscopy in the evaluation of the esophagus. Abdom Imaging. 2004;29(1):2–8.
7. Cansu A, Ahmetoglu A, Kul S, Yukunc G, Fidan S, Arslan M, Topbas M. Diagnostic performance of using effervescent powder for detection and grading of esophageal varices by multidetector computed tomography. Eur J Radiol. 2014;83(3):497–502.
8. Kim SH, Kim YJ, Lee JM, Choi KD, Chung YJ, Han JK, Lee JY, Lee MW, Han CJ, Choi JI, Shin KS, Choi BI. Esophageal varices in patients with cirrhosis: multidetector CT esophagography – comparison with endoscopy. Radiology. 2007;242(3):759–68.
9. Torres WE, Whitmire LF, Gedgaudas-McClees K, Bernardino ME. Computed tomography of hepatic morphologic changes in cirrhosis of the liver. J Comput Assist Tomogr. 1986;10(1):47–50.
10. Brancatelli G, Federle MP, Ambrosini R, Lagalla R, Carriero A, Midiri M, Vilgrain V. Cirrhosis: CT and MR imaging evaluation. Eur J Radiol. 2007;61(1):57–69.
11. Lafortune M, Matricardi L, Denys A, Favret M, Déry R, Pomier-Layrargues G. Segment 4 (the quadrate lobe): a barometer of cirrhotic liver disease at US. Radiology. 1998;206(1):157–60.
12. Harbin WP, Robert NJ, Ferrucci JT Jr. Diagnosis of cirrhosis based on regional changes in hepatic morphology: a radiological and pathological analysis. Radiology. 1980;135(2):273–83.
13. Awaya H, Mitchell DG, Kamishima T, Holland G, Ito K, Matsumoto T. Cirrhosis: modified caudate-right lobe ratio. Radiology. 2002;224:769–74.
14. Ito K, Mitchell DG, Gabata T. Enlargement of hilar peri-portal space: a sign of early cirrhosis at MR imaging. J Magn Reson Imaging. 2000;11(2):136–40.
15. Tan KC. Enlargement of the hilar periportal space. Radiology. 2008;248(2):699–700.
16. Zhang Y, Zhang XM, Prowda JC, Zhang HL, Sant'anna Henry C, Shih G, Emond JC, Prince MR. Changes in hepatic venous morphology with cirrhosis on MRI. J Magn Reson Imaging. 2009;29(5):1085–92.
17. Ito K, Mitchell DG, Kim MJ, Awaya H, Koike S, Matsunaga N. Right posterior hepatic notch sign: a simple diagnostic MR sign of cirrhosis. J Magn Reson Imaging. 2003;18:561–6.
18. Tan KC. The right posterior hepatic notch sign. Radiology. 2008;248(1):317–8.
19. Ito K, Mitchell DG, Gabata T, Hussain SM. Expanded gallbladder fossa: simple MR imaging sign of cirrhosis. Radiology. 1999;211:723–6.

20. Horowitz JM, Venkatesh SK, Ehman RL, Jhaveri K, Kamath P, Ohliger MA, Samir AE, Silva AC, Taouli B, Torbenson MS, Wells ML, Yeh B, Miller FH. Evaluation of hepatic fibrosis: a review from the society of abdominal radiology disease focus panel. Abdom Radiol (NY). 2017;42(8):2037–53.
21. Rustogi R, Horowitz J, Harmath C, Wang Y, Chalian H, Ganger DR, Chen ZE, Bolster BD Jr, Shah S, Miller FH. Accuracy of MR elastography and anatomic MR imaging features in the diagnosis of severe hepatic fibrosis and cirrhosis. J Magn Reson Imaging. 2012;35(6): 1356–64.
22. Venkatesh SK, Yin M, Takahashi N, Glockner JF, Talwalkar JA, Ehman RL. Non-invasive detection of liver fibrosis: MR imaging features vs. MR elastography. Abdom Imaging. 2015;40(4):766–75.
23. Krinsky GA, Lee VS. MR imaging of cirrhotic nodules. Abdom Imaging. 2000;25:471–82.
24. Ito K, Mitchell DG, Gabata T, Hann HW, Kim PN, Fujita T, Awaya H, Honjo K, Matsunaga N. Hepatocellular carcinoma: association with increased iron deposition in the cirrhotic liver at MR imaging. Radiology. 1999;212(1):235–40.
25. Berzigotti A, Abraldes JG, Tandon P, Erice E, Gilabert R, García-Pagan JC, Bosch J. Ultrasonographic evaluation of liver surface and transient elastography in clinically doubtful cirrhosis. J Hepatol. 2010;52(6):846–53.
26. Smith AD, Branch CR, Zand K, Subramony C, Zhang H, Thaggard K, Hosch R, Bryan J, Vasanji A, Griswold M, Zhang X. Liver surface nodularity quantification from routine CT images as a biomarker for detection and evaluation of cirrhosis. Radiology. 2016;280(3):771–81.
27. Dodd GD III, Baron RL, Oliver JH III, Federle MP. Spectrum of imaging findings of the liver in end-stage cirrhosis. Part I. Gross morphology and diffuse abnormalities. AJR. 1999;173:1031–6.
28. Ichikawa T, Nakajima H, Nanbu A, Hori M, Araki T. Effect of injection rate of contrast material on CT of hepatocellular carcinoma. AJR. 2006;186:1413–8.
29. Brancatelli G, Baron RL, Peterson MS, Marsh W. Helical CT screening for hepatocellular carcinoma in patients with cirrhosis: frequency and causes of false-positives interpretation. AJR. 2003;180:1007–14.
30. Itai Y, Hachiya J, Makita K, Ohtomo K, Kokubo T, Yamauchi T. Transient hepatic attenuation differences on dynamic computed tomography. J Comput Assist Tomogr. 1987;11:461–5.
31. Ahn JH, Yu JS, Hwang SH, Chung JJ, Kim JH, Kim KW. Non-tumorous arterio-portal shunts in the liver: CT and MRI findings considering mechanisms and fate. Eur Radiol. 2010;20:385–94.
32. Itai Y, Matsui O. Blood flow and liver imaging. Radiology. 1997;202(2):306–14.
33. Nishida O, Moriyasu F, Nakamura T, Ban N, Miura K, Sakai M, Uchino H, Miyake T. Hemodynamics of splenic artery aneurysm. Gastroenterology. 1986;90(4):1042–6.
34. Kóbori L, van der Kolk MJ, de Jong KP, Peeters PM, Klompmaker IJ, Kok T, Haagsma EB, Slooff MJ. Splenic artery aneurysms in liver transplant patients. Liver Transplant Group J Hepatol. 1997;27(5):890–3.
35. Heestand G, Sher L, Lightfoote J, Palmer S, Mateo R, Singh G, Moser J, Selby R, Genyk Y, Jabbour N. Characteristics and management of splenic artery aneurysm in liver transplant candidates and recipients. Am Surg. 2003;69(11):933–40.
36. Asthana S, Toso C, McCarthy M, Shapiro AM. The management of splenic artery aneurysm in patients awaiting liver transplantation. Clin Transpl. 2010;24(5):691–4.
37. Kaya M, Baran Ş, Güya C, Kaplan MA. Prevalence and predictive factors for development of splenic artery aneurysms in cirrhosis. Indian J Gastroenterol. 2016;35(3):201–6.
38. Esen K, Balci Y, Tok S, Ucbilek E, Kara E, Kaya O. The evaluation of the right inferior phrenic artery diameter in cirrhotic patients. Jpn J Radiol. 2017 Jun 24. https://doi.org/10.1007/s11604-017-0662-7.
39. Miles KA, Hayball MP, Dixon AK. Functional images of hepatic perfusion obtained with dynamic CT. Radiology. 1993;188(2):405–11.
40. Blomley MJ, Coulden R, Dawson P, Kormano M, Donlan P, Bufkin C, Lipton MJ. Liver perfusion studied with ultrafast CT. J Comput Assist Tomogr. 1995;19(3):424–33.

41. Van Beers BE, Leconte I, Materne R, Smith AM, Jamart J, Horsmans Y. Hepatic perfusion parameters in chronic liver disease: dynamic CT measurements correlated with disease severity. AJR Am J Roentgenol. 2001;176(3):667–73.
42. Ronot M, Asselah T, Paradis V, Michoux N, Dorvillius M, Baron G, Marcellin P, Van Beers BE, Vilgrain V. Liver fibrosis in chronic hepatitis C virus infection: differentiating minimal from intermediate fibrosis with perfusion CT. Radiology. 2010;256(1):135–42.
43. Suzuki T, Yamada A, Komatsu D, Kurozumi M, Fujinaga Y, Ueda K, Miyagawa S, Kadoya M. Evaluation of splenic perfusion and spleen size using dynamic computed tomography: usefulness in assessing degree of liver fibrosis. Hepatol Res. 2017 Apr 1. https://doi.org/10.1111/hepr.12900.
44. Gibson PR, Gibson RN, Ditchfield MR, Donlan JD. Splenomegaly—an insensitive sign of portal hypertension. Aust N Z J Med. 1990;20(6):771–4.
45. Bolognesi M, Merkel C, Sacerdoti D, Nava V, Gatta A. Role of spleen enlargement in cirrhosis with portal hypertension. Dig Liver Dis. 2002;34(2):144–50.
46. Yanaga K, Tzakis AG, Shimada M, Campbell WE, Marsh JW, Stieber AC, Makowka L, Todo S, Gordon RD, Iwatsuki S, et al. Reversal of hypersplenism following orthotopic liver transplantation. Ann Surg. 1989;210(2):180–3.
47. Pickhardt PJ, Malecki K, OF H, Beaumont C, Kloke J, Ziemlewicz TJ, Lubner MG. Hepatosplenic volumetric assessment at MDCT for staging liver fibrosis. Eur Radiol. 2017;27(7):3060–8.
48. Prassopoulos P, Daskalogiannaki M, Raissaki M, Hatjidakis A, Gourtsoyiannis N. Determination of normal splenic volume on computed tomography in relation to age, gender and body habitus. Eur Radiol. 1997;7(2):246–8.
49. Bezerra AS, D'Ippolito G, Faintuch S, Szejnfeld J, Ahmed M. Determination of splenomegaly by CT: is there a place for a single measurement? AJR Am J Roentgenol. 2005;184(5):1510–3.
50. Ikegami T, Shimada M, Imura S. Recent role of splenectomy in chronic hepatic disorders. Hepatol Res. 2008;38(12):1159–71.
51. Tarao K, Hoshino H, Motohashi I, Iimori K, Tamai S, Ito Y, Takagi S, Oikawa Y, Unayama S, Fujiwara T, et al. Changes in liver and spleen volume in alcoholic liver fibrosis of man. Hepatology. 1989;9(4):589–93.
52. Ozaki K, Matsui O, Kobayashi S, Minami T, Kitao A, Gabata T. Morphometric changes in liver cirrhosis: aetiological differences correlated with progression. Br J Radiol. 2016;89(1059):20150896.
53. Park SH, Kim PN, Kim KW, Lee SW, Yoon SE, Park SW, Ha HK, Lee MG, Hwang S, Lee SG, Yu ES, Cho EY. Macrovesicular hepatic steatosis in living liver donors: use of CT for quantitative and qualitative assessment. Radiology. 2006;239(1):105–12.
54. Howard JM, Ghent CN, Carey LS, Flanagan PR, Valberg LS. Diagnostic efficacy of hepatic computed tomography in the detection of body iron overload. Gastroenterology. 1983;84:209–15.
55. Queiroz-Andrade M, Blasbalg R, Ortega CD, Rodstein MA, Baroni RH, Rocha MS, Cerri GG. MR imaging findings of iron overload. Radiographics. 2009;29(6):1575–89.
56. Oelckers S, Graeff W. In situ measurement of iron overload in liver tissue by dual-energy methods. Phys Med Biol. 1996;41(7):1149–65.
57. Dodd GD III, Baron RL, Oliver JH III, Federle MP. End-stage primary sclerosing cholangitis: CT findings of hepatic morphology in 36 patients. Radiology. 1999;211:357–62.
58. Blachar A, Federle M, Brancatelli G. Primary biliary cirrhosis: clinical, pathologic, and helical CT findings in 53 patients. Radiology. 2001;220:329–36.
59. Pillai AK, Andring B, Patel A, Trimmer C, Kalva SP. Review of portosystemic collateral pathways and endovascular interventions. Clin Radiol. 2015;70(10):1047–59.
60. Kim M, Mitchell DG, Ito K. Portosystemic collaterals of the upper abdomen: review of anatomy and demonstration on MR imaging. Abdom Imaging. 2000;25:462e70.
61. Ito K, Fujita T, Shimizu A, Sasaki K, Tanabe M, Matsunaga N. Imaging findings of unusual intra- and extrahepatic portosystemic collaterals. Clin Radiol. 2009;64(2):200–7.

62. Cho KC, Patel YD, Wachsberg RH, Seeff J. Varices in portal hypertension: evaluation with CT. Radiographics. 1995;15(3):609–22.
63. Kang HK, Jeong YY, Choi JH, Choi S, Chung TW, Seo JJ, Kim JK, Yoon W, Park JG. Three-dimensional multi-detector row CT portal venography in the evaluation of portosystemic collateral vessels in liver cirrhosis. Radiographics. 2002;22(5):1053–61.
64. Henseler KP, Pozniak MA, Lee FT Jr, Winter TC 3rd. Three-dimensional CT angiography of spontaneous portosystemic shunts. Radiographics. 2001;21:691–704.
65. Perri RE, Chiorean MV, Fidler JL, Fletcher JG, Talwalkar JA, Stadheim L, Shah ND, Kamath PS. A prospective evaluation of computerized tomographic (CT) scanning as a screening modality for esophageal varices. Hepatology. 2008;47(5):1587–94.
66. Lotfipour AK, Douek M, Shimoga SV, Sayer JW, Han SB, Jutabha R, Lu DS. The cost of screening esophageal varices: traditional endoscopy versus computed tomography. J Comput Assist Tomogr. 2014;38(6):963–7.
67. Lafortune M, Marleau D, Breton G, Viallet A, Lavoie P, Huet PM. Portal venous system measurements in portal hypertension. Radiology. 1984;151(1):27–30.
68. Saad WE. Vascular anatomy and the morphologic and hemodynamic classifications of gastric varices and spontaneous portosystemic shunts relevant to the BRTO procedure. Tech Vasc Interv Radiol. 2013;16:60e100.
69. Ryan BM, Stockbrugger RW, Ryan JM. A pathophysiologic, gastroenterologic, and radiologic approach to the management of gastric varices. Gastroenterology. 2004;126(4):1175–89.
70. Lopera JE. Gastric varices. Radiographics. 2013;33(1):100–1.
71. Kiyosue H, Ibukuro K, Maruno M, Tanoue S, Hongo N, Mori H. Multidetector CT anatomy of drainage routes of gastric varices: a pictorial review. Radiographics. 2013;33(1):87–100.
72. Luo X, Wang X, Zhao Y, Ma H, Ye L, Yang L, Tsauo J, Jiang M, Li X. Real-time 3D CT image guidance for transjugular intrahepatic portosystemic shunt creation using preoperative CT: a prospective feasibility study of 20 patients. AJR Am J Roentgenol. 2017;208(1):W11–6.
73. Sarin SK, Lahoti D, Saxena SP, Murthy NS, Makwana UK. Prevalence, classification and natural history of gastric varices: a long-term follow-up study in 568 portal hypertension patients. Hepatology. 1992;16:1343–9.
74. Dell'era A, Bosch J. Review article: The relevance of portal pressure and other risk factors in acute gastro-oesophageal variceal bleeding. Aliment Pharmacol Ther. 2004;20(Suppl 3):8–15. discussion 16–7
75. Kim H, Choi D, Gwak GY, Lee JH, Lee SJ, Kim SH, Lee JY, Park Y, Chang I, Lim HK. High-risk esophageal varices in patients treated with locoregional therapies for hepatocellular carcinoma: evaluation with regular follow-up liver CT. Dig Dis Sci. 2009;54(10):2247–52.
76. Deng H, Qi X, Guo X. Computed tomography for the diagnosis of varices in liver cirrhosis: a systematic review and meta-analysis of observational studies. Postgrad Med. 2017;129(3):318–28.
77. Calame P, Ronot M, Bouveresse S, Cervoni JP, Vilgrain V, Delabrousse E. Predictive value of CT for first esophageal variceal bleeding in patients with cirrhosis: value of para-umbilical vein patency. Eur J Radiol. 2017;87:45–52.
78. Kim M, Mitchell DG, Ito K. Portosystemic collaterals of the upper abdomen: review of anatomy and demonstration on MR imaging. Abdom Imaging. 2000;25:462–70.
79. Kim M, Al-Khalili R, Miller J. Vesical varices: an unusual presentation of portal hypertension. Clin Imaging. 2015;39(5):920–2.
80. Gines P, Quintero E, Arroyo V, Terés J, Bruguera M, Rimola A, Caballería J, Rodés J, Rozman C. Compensated cirrhosis: natural history and prognostic factors. Hepatology. 1987;7(1):122–8.
81. Thoeni RF. The role of imaging in patients with ascites. AJR Am J Roentgenol. 1995;165(1):16–8.
82. Iranmanesh P, Vazquez O, Terraz S, Majno P, Spahr L, Poncet A, Morel P, Mentha G, Toso C. Accurate computed tomography-based portal pressure assessment in patients with hepatocellular carcinoma. J Hepatol. 2014;60(5):969–74.

83. Kihira S, Kagen AC, Vasudevan P, Jajamovich GH, Schiano TD, Andrle AF, Babb JS, Fischman A, Taouli B. Non-invasive prediction of portal pressures using CT and MRI in chronic liver disease. Abdom Radiol (NY). 2016;41(1):42–9.

84. Qi X, Li Z, Huang J, Zhu Y, Liu H, Zhou F, Liu C, Xiao C, Dong J, Zhao Y, Xu M, Xing S, Xu W, Yang C. Virtual portal pressure gradient from anatomic CT angiography. Gut. 2015;64(6):1004–5.

85. Carbonell N, Pauwels A, Serfaty L, Fourdan O, Lévy VG, Poupon R. Improved survival after variceal bleeding in patients with cirrhosis over the past two decades. Hepatology. 2004;40(3):652–9.

86. Ge W, Wang Y, Cao YJ, Xie M, Ding YT, Zhang M, Yu DC. Radiological score for hemorrhage in the patients with portal hypertension. Int J Clin Exp Pathol. 2015;8(9):11517–23.

87. Kodama H, Aikata H, Takaki S, Azakami T, Katamura Y, Kawaoka T, Hiramatsu A, Waki K, Imamura M, Kawakami Y, Takahashi S, Toyota N, Ito K, Chayama K. Evaluation of portosystemic collaterals by MDCT-MPR imaging for management of hemorrhagic esophageal varices. Eur J Radiol. 2010;76(2):239–45.

88. Smith AD, Zand KA, Florez E, Sirous R, Shlapak D, Souza F, Roda M, Bryan J, Vasanji A, Griswold M, Lirette ST. Liver surface nodularity score allows prediction of cirrhosis decompensation and death. Radiology. 2017;283(3):711–22.

89. Ogren M, Bergqvist D, Bjorck M, Acosta S, Eriksson H, Sternby NH. Portal vein thrombosis: prevalence, patient characteristics and lifetime risk: a population study based on 23,796 consecutive autopsies. World J Gastroenterol. 2006;12(13):2115–9.

90. Rajani R, Bjornsson E, Bergquist A, Danielsson A, Gustavsson A, Grip O, Melin T, Sangfelt P, Wallerstedt S, Almer S. The epidemiology and clinical features of portal vein thrombosis: a multicentre study. Aliment Pharmacol Ther. 2010;32(9):1154–62.

91. Margini C, Berzigotti A. Portal vein thrombosis: the role of imaging in the clinical setting. Dig Liver Dis. 2017;49(2):113–20.

92. Mori H, Hayashi K, Uetani M, Matsuoka Y, Iwao M, Maeda H. High-attenuation recent thrombus of the portal vein: CT demonstration and clinical significance. Radiology. 1987;163(2):353–6.

93. Rossi S, Rosa L, Ravetta V, Cascina A, Quaretti P, Azzaretti A, Scagnelli P, Tinelli C, Dionigi P, Calliada F. Contrast-enhanced versus conventional and color Doppler sonography for the detection of thrombosis of the portal and hepatic venous systems. AJR Am J Roentgenol. 2006;186(3):763–73.

94. Li C, Hu J, Zhou D, Zhao J, Ma K, Yin X, Wang J. Differentiation of bland from neoplastic thrombus of the portal vein in patients with hepatocellular carcinoma: application of susceptibility-weighted MR imaging. BMC Cancer. 2014;14:590.

95. Canellas R, Mehrkhani F, Patino M, Kambadakone A, Sahani D. Characterization of portal vein thrombosis (neoplastic versus bland) on CT images using software-based texture analysis and thrombus density (Hounsfield units). AJR Am J Roentgenol. 2016;207(5):W81–7.

96. Ascenti G, Sofia C, Mazziotti S, Silipigni S, D'Angelo T, Pergolizzi S, Scribano E. Dual-energy CT with iodine quantification indistinguishing between bland and neoplastic portal vein thrombosis in patients with hepatocellular carcinoma. Clin Radiol. 2016;71(9): 938.e1–9.

97. Chang D, Levine MS, Ginsberg GG, Rubesin SE, Laufer I. Portal hypertensive gastropathy: radiographic findings in eight patients. AJR Am J Roentgenol. 2000;175(6):1609–12.

98. Ishihara K, Ishida R, Saito T, Teramoto K, Hosomura Y, Shibuya H. Computed tomography features of portal hypertensive gastropathy. J Comput Assist Tomogr. 2004;28(6):832–5.

99. Holzer T, Gervaz P, Spahr L, McKee T, Bucher P, Morel P. Phlegmonous colitis: another source of sepsis in cirrhotic patients? BMC Gastroenterol. 2009;9:94.

100. Urrunaga NH, Rockey DC. Portal hypertensive gastropathy and colopathy. Clin Liver Dis. 2014;18(2):389–406.

101. Le Roy B, Gelli M, Serji B, Memeo R, Vibert E. Portal biliopathy as a complication of extrahepatic portal hypertension: etiology, presentation and management. J Visc Surg. 2015;152(3):161–6.

102. Condat B, Vilgrain V, Asselah T, O'Toole D, Rufat P, Zappa M, Moreau R, Valla D. Portal cavernoma-associated cholangiopathy: a clinical and MR cholangiographycoupled with MR portography imaging study. Hepatology. 2003;37(6):1302–8.

103. Kim YK, Kim Y, Shim SS. Thoracic complications of liver cirrhosis: radiologic findings. Radiographics. 2009;29(3):825–37.

104. Krok KL, Cárdenas A. Hepatic hydrothorax. Semin Respir Crit Care Med. 2012;33(1): 3–10.

105. Lazaridis KN, Frank JW, Krowka MJ, Kamath PS. Hepatic hydrothorax: pathogenesis, diagnosis, and management. Am J Med. 1999;107:262–7.

106. Noli K, Solomon M, Golding F, Charron M, Ling SC. Prevalence of hepatopulmonary syndrome in children. Pediatrics. 2008;121(3):e522–7.

107. Rodríguez-Roisin R, Krowka MJ. Hepatopulmonary syndrome—a liver- induced lung vascular disorder. N Engl J Med. 2008;358(22):2378–87.

108. Devaraj A, Loveridge R, Bosanac D, Stefanidis K, Bernal W, Willars C, Wendon JA, Auzinger G, Desai SR. Portopulmonary hypertension: improved detection using CT and echocardiography in combination. Eur Radiol. 2014;24(10):2385–93.

109. Rodriquez-Roisin R, Krowka MJ, Herve P, Fallon MB, Committee ERSTF-PS. Highlights of the ERS Task Force on pulmonary-hepatic vascular disorders (PHD). J Hepatol. 2005;42(6):924–7.

110. McDonnell PJ, Toye PA, Hutchins GM. Primary pulmonary hypertension and cirrhosis: are they related? Am Rev Respir Dis. 1983;127(4):437–41.

111. Hadengue A, Benhayoun MK, Lebrec D, Benhamou JP. Pulmonary hypertension complicating portal hypertension: prevalence and relation to splanchnic hemodynamics. Gastroenterology. 1991;100(2):520–8.

112. Herve P, Lebrec D, Brenot F, Simonneau G, Humbert M, Sitbon O, Duroux P. Pulmonary vascular disorders in portal hypertension. Eur Respir J. 1998;11(5):1153–66.

113. Simonneau G, Gatzoulis MA, Adatia I, Celermajer D, Denton C, Ghofrani A, Gomez Sanchez MA, Krishna Kumar R, Landzberg M, Machado RF, Olschewski H, Robbins IM, Souza R. Updated clinical classification of pulmonary hypertension. J Am Coll Cardiol. 2013;62(25 Suppl):D34–41.

114. Tan RT, Kuzo R, Goodman LR, Siegel R, Haasler GB, Presberg KW. Utility of CT scan evaluation for predicting pulmonary hypertension in patients with parenchymal lung disease. Medical College of Wisconsin Lung Transplant Group. Chest. 1998;113(5):1250–6.

115. Ng CS, Wells AU, Padley SP. A CT sign of chronic pulmonary arterial hypertension: the ratio of main pulmonary artery to aortic diameter. J Thorac Imaging. 1999;14(4):270–8.

116. Leise MD, Poterucha JJ, Kamath PS, Kim WR. Management of hepatic encephalopathy in the hospital. Mayo Clin Proc. 2014;89(2):241–53.

117. Ellul MA, Gholkar SA, Cross TJ. Hepatic encephalopathy due to liver cirrhosis. BMJ. 2015;351:h4187.

118. Ohnishi K, Saito M, Sato S, Nakayama T, Takashi M, Iida S, Nomura F, Koen H, Okuda K. Direction of splenic venous flow assessed by pulsed Doppler flowmetry in patients with a large splenorenal shunt. Relation to spontaneous hepatic encephalopathy. Gastroenterology. 1985;89(1):180.

119. Bonekamp D, Bonekamp S, Geiger B, Kamel IR. An elevated arterial enhancement fraction is associated with clinical and imaging indices of liver fibrosis and cirrhosis. J Comput Assist Tomogr. 2012;36(6):681–9.

120. Richter S, Mucke I, Menger MD, Vollmar B. Impact of intrinsic blood flow regulation in cirrhosis: maintenance of hepatic arterial buffer response. Am J Physiol Gastrointest Liver Physiol. 2000;279(2):G454–G62.

121. Gulberg V, Haag K, Rossle M, Gerbes AL. Hepatic arterial buffer response in patients with advanced cirrhosis. Hepatology. 2002;35(3):630–4.

122. Tsushima Y, Koizumi J, Yokoyama H, Takeda A, Kusano S. Evaluation of portal pressure by splenic perfusion measurement using dynamic CT. AJR Am J Roentgenol. 1998;170(1): 153–5.

123. Talakić E, Schaffellner S, Kniepeiss D, Mueller H, Stauber R, Quehenberger F, Schoellnast H. CT perfusion imaging of the liver and the spleen in patients with cirrhosis: Is there a correlation between perfusion and portal venous hypertension? Eur Radiol. 2017 Mar 20. https://doi.org/10.1007/s00330-017-4788-x.
124. Fischer MA, Brehmer K, Svensson A, Aspelin P, Brismar TB. Renal versus splenic maximum slope based perfusion CT modeling in patients with portal hypertension. Eur Radiol. 2016;26(11):4030–6.
125. Silva AC, Morse BG, Hara AK, Paden RG, Hongo N, Pavlicek W. Dual-energy (spectral) CT: applications in abdominal imaging. Radiographics. 2011;31(4):1031–46. discussion 1047–50
126. Lamb P, Sahani DV, Fuentes-Orrego JM, Patino M, Ghosh A, Mendonça PR. Stratification of patients with liver fibrosis using dual-energy CT. IEEE Trans Med Imaging. 2015;34(3):807–15.
127. Lv P, Lin X, Gao J, Chen K. Spectral CT: preliminary studies in the liver cirrhosis. Korean J Radiol. 2012;13(4):434–42.
128. Zhao LQ, He W, Yan B, Wang HY, Wang J. The evaluation of haemodynamics in cirrhotic patients with spectral CT. Br J Radiol. 2013;86(1028):20130228.
129. Villeneuve JP, Dagenais M, Huet PM, Roy A, Lapointe R, Marleau D. The hepatic microcirculation in the isolated perfused human liver. Hepatology. 1996;23(1):24–31.
130. Varenika V, Fu Y, Maher JJ, Gao D, Kakar S, Cabarrus MC, Yeh BM. Hepatic fibrosis: evaluation with semiquantitative contrast-enhanced CT. Radiology. 2013;266(1):151–8.
131. Zissen MH, Wang ZJ, Yee J, Aslam R, Monto A, Yeh BM. Contrast-enhanced CT quantification of the hepatic fractional extracellular space: correlation with diffuse liver disease severity. Am J Roentgenol. 2013;201(6):1204–10.
132. Yoon JH, Lee JM, Klotz E, Jeon JH, Lee KB, Han JK, Choi BI. Estimation of hepatic extracellular volume fraction using multiphasic liver computed tomography for hepatic fibrosis grading. Investig Radiol. 2015;50(4):290–6.
133. Bandula S, Punwani S, Rosenberg WM, Jalan R, Hall AR, Dhillon A, Moon JC, Taylor SA. Equilibrium contrast-enhanced CT imaging to evaluate hepatic fibrosis: initial validation by comparison with histopathologic sampling. Radiology. 2015;275(1):136–43.
134. Guo SL, Su LN, Zhai YN, Chirume WM, Lei JQ, Zhang H, Yang L, Shen XP, Wen XX, Guo YM. The clinical value of hepatic extracellular volume fraction using routine multiphasic contrast-enhanced liver CT for staging liver fibrosis. Clin Radiol. 2017;72(3):242–6.
135. Zhang X, Gao X, Liu BJ, Ma K, Yan W, Liling L, Yuhong H, Fujita H. Effective staging of fibrosis by the selected texture features of liver: which one is better, CT or MR imaging? Comput Med Imaging Graph. 2015;46(Pt 2):227–36.
136. Daginawala N, Li B, Buch K, Yu H, Tischler B, Qureshi MM, Soto JA, Anderson S. Using texture analyses of contrast enhanced CT to assess hepatic fibrosis. Eur J Radiol. 2016;85(3):511–7.

Magnetic Resonance Imaging Methods for Assessing Cirrhosis and Portal Hypertension

14

Naaventhan Palaniyappan, Indra Neil Guha, and Guruprasad Padur Aithal

14.1 Introduction

Magnetic resonance imaging (MRI) has been widely used for the detection and characterisation of focal lesions of the liver. Its ability to distinguish the physical properties of the tissue as well as the vasculature with contrast enhancement has made MRI the gold-standard test for the diagnosis of hepatocellular carcinoma. Both of these properties should make MRI an attractive imaging modality in assessing chronic liver disease and hence, MRI methodologies for the evaluation and stratification of chronic liver disease are being developed recently. MRI permits assessment of the whole liver in contrast to the 1 /50,000th portion of the organ obtained by liver biopsy, the current gold standard for the evaluation of the degree of liver injury, inflammation or scarring. Routine liver biochemistry or ultrasound examinations that have been used for decades lack sensitivity to estimate the degree of liver pathology, therefore are not useful in patient stratification, prognostication or monitoring. MRI is non-invasive, widely available technology with the most potential to develop further in the future. MRI does not involve ionising radiation, which makes it a preferable, especially for repeated assessments in surveillance. In this chapter, we discuss the advances in MRI in diagnosing and assessing cirrhosis and portal hypertension. The role of magnetic resonance elastography (MRE) is discussed separately.

N. Palaniyappan • I.N. Guha • G.P. Aithal, M.B.B.S., M.D., F.R.C.P., Ph.D. (✉)
Nottingham Digestive Diseases Centre, University of Nottingham, NIHR Nottingham
Biomedical Research Centre, Nottingham University Hospitals NHS Trust and University of
Nottingham, Nottingham, UK
e-mail: guru.aithal@nuh.nhs.uk; guru.aithal@nottingham.ac.uk

© Springer International Publishing AG, part of Springer Nature 2018
A. Berzigotti, J. Bosch (eds.), *Diagnostic Methods for Cirrhosis and Portal
Hypertension*, https://doi.org/10.1007/978-3-319-72628-1_14

14.2   Cirrhosis

14.2.1 Conventional MRI

Evaluation of the morphological changes in the cirrhotic liver using MRI has been described for the diagnosis of cirrhosis. The key imaging features studied include: liver surface nodularity, atrophy of the right lobe, hypertrophy of the caudate lobe, expansion of gallbladder fossa and splenomegaly.

In a recent study, the parenchymal texture on MRI was reported to have the highest accuracy among all other studied morphological changes in diagnosing cirrhosis but the sensitivity and specificity was suboptimal (76.5% and 84.4% respectively) [1]. The description of these morphological changes is subjective and the reported interobserver agreement for the MRI changes in liver parenchymal texture was modest (kappa, κ statistic = 0.28) [1]. Awaya et al. attempted to quantify the morphological change in cirrhosis by calculating the ratio of caudate-to-right lobe of the liver [2]. However, it was of limited value in diagnosing cirrhosis as the cut-off of caudate-to-right-lobe ratio of >0.9 only had sensitivity of 71.7% and specificity of 77.4%.

14.2.2 Contrast Enhanced MRI

Administration of contrast agents can improve the visualisation of liver fibrosis. Gadolinium-based contrast agents results in enhancement of the T_1-weighted images. The peak enhancement is noticed during the late venous phase after intravenous injection of the contrast. Superparamagnetic iron oxide (SPIO) is a contrast agent specific to the reticuloendothelial system. After intravenous injection, the iron oxide particles are cleared from the blood through phagocytosis and accumulate in the reticuloendothelial system of the liver, spleen and bone marrow. Approximately 80% of this is taken up by the liver [3]. Accumulation of iron cores causes local magnetic field inhomogeneities which results in shortening of the T_2* and consequently signal loss on the MR images. These signal losses are seen best on gradient-echo images and T_2-weighted spin echo images. Therefore, in SPIO-enhanced liver imaging, the hepatic parenchyma has low signal intensity. In fibrosis and cirrhosis, less iron particle is accumulated and hence, the signal loss is minimised [4]. Double contrast-enhanced MRI involves sequential administration of SPIO and gadolinium based contrast. As both these contrast agents enhance visualisation of fibrosis via differing mechanisms, they can potentially act synergistically to improve detection of liver fibrosis and cirrhosis. MRI acquisition parameters are chosen to optimise both T_1-weighting (to increase sensitivity of signal augmentation from gadolinium) and T_2*-weighting (to increase sensitivity of the signal loss mediated by SPIO). Aguirre et al. reported an improved diagnostic performance in detecting cirrhosis using double contrast-enhanced MRI compared to SPIO [5] (Fig. 14.1).

Perfusion-weighted MRI can be performed by measuring the signal intensity in the tissue of interest after the injection of contrast against time. Initial assumption of a linear relationship between the signal intensity and the concentration of gadolinium in

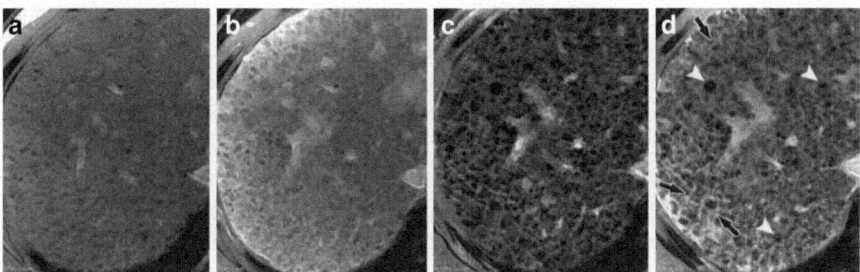

Fig. 14.1 MR images of (**a**) Unenhanced, (**b**) Gadolinium-enhanced, (**c**) SPIO-enhanced, and (**d**) double-contrast enhanced (with SPIO and gadolinium) liver parenchyma in a patient with HCV-related cirrhosis. The combination of contrast agents acts synergistically and depicts fibrotic reticulations (black arrows in (**d**)) and regenerative nodules (white arrowheads in (**d**)) (adapted from Faria et al. [6])

the liver using a single-input single-compartment model is simplistic and inaccurate, as it does not take into account the separate portal venous and hepatic arterial contributions [7]. Subsequent analysis of signal intensity over the portal vein, aorta and liver parenchyma against time can be fitted to a dual-input single-compartment model [8]. The parameters that can be obtained during the MR perfusion imaging include absolute portal venous and hepatic arterial perfusions, portal venous and hepatic arterial fractions, distribution volume of gadolinium through the liver and mean transit time (MTT). In animal studies, increase in liver MTT and decrease in distribution volume correlated with accumulation of collagen in the liver [9]. In humans, decreased portal fraction and total liver perfusion and increased arterial fraction as well as increased MTT was associated with cirrhosis [10]. Subsequent prospective study of the MR liver perfusion parameters showed that the distribution volume of the contrast in the liver had the best diagnostic performance (Area Under the Receiver Operator Curve, AUROC = 0.824) in detecting advanced fibrosis and cirrhosis [11]. However, the sample size was small in this (27 patients) study. While promising, these contrast-enhanced MR perfusion imaging methodology needs further validation.

The adverse events associated with the use of contrast agents limits the use of contrast-enhanced MR in patients with chronic liver disease. Gadolinium based contrast agents are reported to cause nephrogenic systemic fibrosis in patients with renal failure [12]. The U.S. Food and Drug Administration (FDA) has issued an alert in 2015 on the risk of brain deposits of gadolinium-based contrast agents in patients undergoing contrast MRI scans. Although the review to date has not confirmed any harmful effects from the gadolinium retained in the brain, the investigation regarding the potential risk of gadolinium-based contrast agents hasn't yet concluded (https://www.fda.gov/Drugs/DrugSafety/ucm559007.htm).

14.2.3 Diffusion-Weighted Imaging

Diffusion weighted imaging (DWI) is based on intravoxel incoherent Brownian motion of the water molecules, mainly in the extracellular space. This motion is quantified by calculating the apparent diffusion coefficient (ADC), which is dependent on the tissue structure. It was hypothesised that the ADC of the liver would be reduced in cirrhosis, which would reflect the restriction of the diffusion of water molecules in the fibrotic liver tissue. This has been confirmed by several studies [13, 14] with the technique achieving an AUROC of 0.92 in detecting advanced fibrosis. The ADC of the spleen has been reported to be higher in cirrhosis compared to healthy subjects [15], and correlated with the Child-Pugh grade. However, DWI is significantly influenced by the technical parameters especially the level of diffusion weighting (b-value). The selection of the b-values is a compromise between the image quality, acquisition time and adequate diffusion-weighting. These technical factors lead to poor reproducibility of this methodology, and a lack of standardised cut-off values for the ADC [16].

The underlying mechanism of the restriction of diffusion in the cirrhotic livers is poorly understood. It is likely related to the increased connective tissue in the liver and decreased hepatic perfusion related to microvascularisation. The latter observation led to the intravoxel incoherent motion (IVIM) MRI technique. This method is based on DWI with multiple b values, which allows for analysis of the different components of the restriction of random water motion in the tissue. Perfusion-related diffusion coefficient (D*) and perfusion fraction (f) reflect the diffusion restriction due to blood perfusion, while pure molecular diffusion (D) is related to water diffusion. In a recent meta-analysis, D* and f were found to be significantly lower in cirrhosis [17]. Although it has been suggested that these IVIM-based parameters could be superior to conventional ADC in diagnosing cirrhosis, the measurement repeatability of IVIM parameters appears to be worse. Within-subject coefficient of variation (CoV) of D* of up to 156% has been reported [18]. This precludes the routine use of this complex technique in clinical practice.

14.2.4 Longitudinal Relaxation Time (T_1)

The tissue T_1 relaxation time has been shown to be related to the degree of fibrosis in the tissue of interest. T_1 of the myocardial tissue reflects specific cardiac diseases such as acute coronary syndrome, myocarditis, diffuse fibrosis and cardiac amyloid [19]. In the liver, Thomsen et al. reported significantly higher hepatic T_1 relaxation time in patients with cirrhosis compared to healthy volunteers in 1990 [20]. The liver T_1 was measured from a ROI placed centrally in the liver. However, no correlation was found between histopathology and the relaxation time. Heye et al. confirmed the earlier finding with significantly increased liver T_1 in patients with cirrhosis compared to age-matched healthy control group [21]. Furthermore, in patients with cirrhosis, the liver T_1 was seen to correlate with disease severity as classified by Child-Pugh stages; the liver T_1 of patients with Child-Pugh stages A and B were significantly lower than patients with Child-Pugh stage C. The T_1 relaxation time was acquired on a single MR slice during a single breath-hold and a 'region of interest' (ROI) was drawn over the liver avoiding any blood vessels. Banerjee et al. reported a significant relationship between liver T_1 and histological stages of liver fibrosis in patients investigated with a liver biopsy [22]. The T_1 relaxation map was acquired on a single transverse slice through the right lobe of the liver during expiratory breath-hold using shortened Modified Look Locker Inversion (shMOLLI) recovery sequence. A ROI was placed in segment 8 of the liver and the tissue volume assessed in each ROI ranged between 25 and 30 ml. However, the shMOLLI sequence is susceptible to hepatic fat interference and therefore T_1 values are affected by steatosis [23]. The liver T_1 has also been reported to predict liver-related clinical outcomes [24]. This data has to be interpreted with caution as the report included only six decompensation event among 112 patients over the period of follow-up.

Hoad et al. have recently shown that liver T_1 relaxation time is independently associated with the degree of fibrosis and inflammation in the liver [25]. In consecutive patients investigated for chronic liver disease with a liver biopsy core length of at least 25 mm, liver T_1 increased with increasing stages of fibrosis. Inflammation was also found to independently increase liver T_1 in patients without significant fibrosis. In patients with advanced fibrosis, the liver T_1 correlated significantly with percentage fibrosis on visual morphometry [26]. This allows quantitative assessment of fibrosis as a continuous variable which can be useful in monitoring progression or regression of fibrosis; a continuous measure of fibrosis can be superior to histological staging which has a 'ceiling effect' in cirrhosis. The technique for T_1 data acquisition in this study had a number of advantages. A respiratory-triggered multi-slice echo planar imaging (EPI) readout allowed sampling of the whole liver in a reasonable imaging time. The sequence was also fat suppressed and therefore the T_1 values were independent of the degree of hepatic steatosis. The histogram analysis provided a quick and user-friendly method to exclude signals from blood vessels in the liver without having to draw a ROI. The liver T_1 measurement was highly reproducible; the coefficient of variation of liver T_1 in 14 healthy subjects scanned on 2 separate days was less than 2%. The inter- and intra-observer variability was also low (less than 1%) (Fig. 14.2).

The degree of hepatic fibrosis and inflammation have independent effects on liver T_1 relaxation time and at present, it is not possible to dissect the precise contribution of these distinct disease processes. Therefore, liver T_1 cannot be assumed to reflect purely the degree of fibrosis.

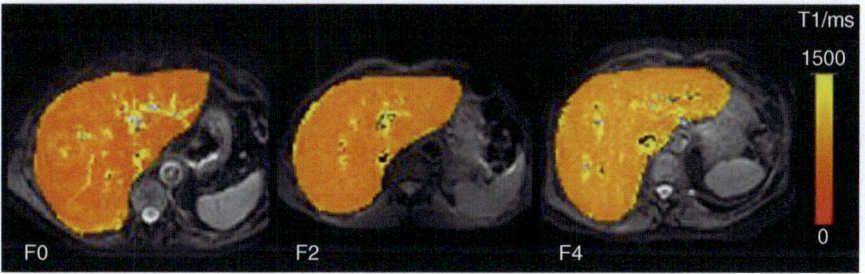

Fig. 14.2 Example of T_1 relaxation map with increasing T_1 relaxation time with worsening degree of liver fibrosis

Table 14.1 MRI methodologies used in the assessment of fibrosis and cirrhosis

MRI technique	Advantages	Limitations
Conventional MRI	• Can be implemented on routine clinical liver MRI scans	• Description of morphological changes are subjective • Morphological changes are qualitative and lack quantitative values
Contrast-enhanced perfusion weighted MRI	• Takes into account the haemodynamic changes in cirrhosis	• Intravenous contrast contraindicated in the presence of acute kidney injury or chronic kidney disease • Small sample size in the studies
Diffusion-weighted imaging	• Non-invasive assessment of tissue perfusion	• Poor reproducibility due to lack of standardisation of the technical parameters
T_1 relaxation time	• Correlates with degree of fibrosis assessed on morphometry • Continuous variable and therefore the is no 'ceiling effect' in cirrhosis • Reproducible with low coefficient of variation	• Influenced by degree of inflammation in the liver • Multiple acquisition methodologies with significant differences in the results obtained

Table 14.1 summarises the key advantages and limitations of the different MRI techniques in evaluating cirrhosis.

14.3 Portal Hypertension

The development and progression of portal hypertension is characterised by an increased intrahepatic resistance and progressive splanchnic vasodilation with formation of porto-systemic collaterals. Distortion of hepatic architecture resulting from fibrogenesis and nodule formation results in 'static' hepatic vascular resistance, while a 'dynamic' component is contributed by an active contraction of myofibroblast and increased hepatic vascular tone [27]. The rise of portal pressure is perpetuated by the excessive release of endogenous vasodilators in the systemic and splanchnic circulation resulting in splanchnic vasodilation and increased porto-collateral blood flow (hyperdynamic circulation).

14.3.1 Assessment of Blood Flow

Phase contrast (PC)-MRI is a non-invasive technique to measure flow in a blood vessel without the use of any intravenous contrast agents. PC-MR is based on the fact that MR signal from spins that move in a magnetic field is at a different phase to that of static spins. The phase shift of the flowing blood is proportional to its velocity. PC-MRI provides velocity measurement for every voxel in the ROI and the

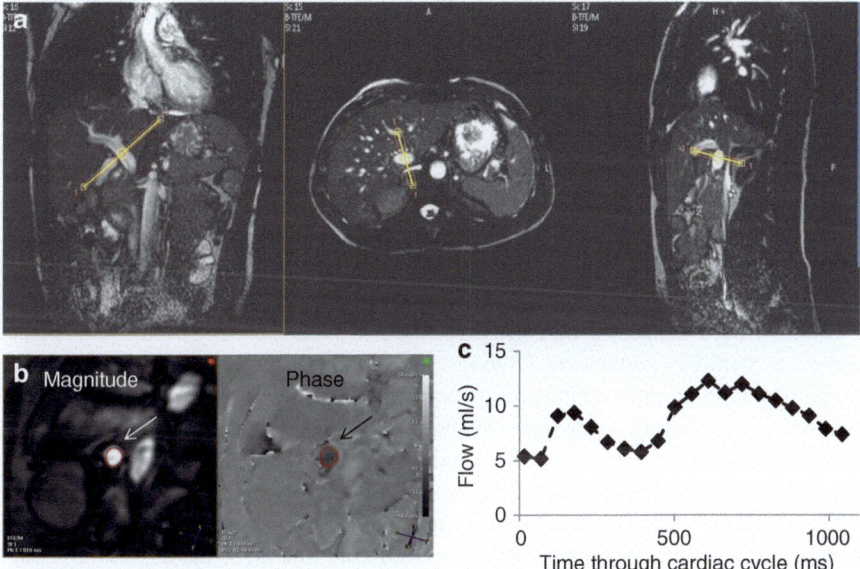

Fig. 14.3 Phase contrast (PC)-MRI measurement of portal venous flow. The identification of the portal vein in the three planes is shown in (**a**). The resulting phase contrast image is shown in (**b**), which quantifies the flow in the vessel through the cardiac cycle in (**c**)

average velocity over the measured vessel area can be obtained. The flow rate is the product of the measured velocity and the pixel area of the vessel (Fig. 14.3).

PC-MRI is able to measure blood flow with high accuracy and this was confirmed in comparative studies using flow phantoms [28, 29] and *in vivo* studies with direct measurement in deep canine arteries and veins [30]. Measurement of portal venous flow using PC-MRI was first reported by Burkart et al. in 1993 [28]; the portal venous flow rates measured with PC-MRI correlated very well with US Doppler measurements. Consecutive PC-MRI measurements at the same location of main portal vein in 12 healthy subjects revealed that mean variability of portal vein flow is 11 ± 5% [31]. The feasibility of the PC-MRI measurement of hepatic artery flow was reported much later by Wilson et al. in 2009 [32] despite earlier studies on other arterial systems including renal arteries [33–35] and superior mesenteric artery [36, 37]. This was likely due to the difficulties in localising the hepatic arteries, the anatomic variations and its sensitivity to respiratory motion. Yzet et al. measured hepatic artery flow in 20 healthy subjects and reported that it formed 19.1% of total hepatic blood flow, which is in agreement with the literature [38]. In a direct comparison with Doppler US, PC-MRI largely underestimated hepatic artery blood flow with a lower variability and higher reproducibility [39].

The continuous thermodilution technique has been accepted as the gold standard in the measurement of azygous vein flow [40, 41]. This technique involves retrograde catheterisation of the azygous vein with a double thermistor catheter. The catheter also has a thermally insulated injection channel through which an indicator

(5% dextrose in water) is infused against the blood flow at a constant rate. The temperature of the indicator, blood and mixture of blood plus indicator are measured; subsequently the blood flow is derived from these measured values. Endoscopic ultrasound (EUS) has also been used to study azygous vein flow [42, 43]. However, the uses of these techniques have been limited by the invasive nature of the procedures. PC-MRI is an attractive non-invasive modality to study azygous vein flow [44]. The PC-MRI measured azygous vein flow has been shown to be significantly higher in patients with cirrhosis compared to healthy subjects. A low intra-subject variability has been reported in three repeat measurements of azygous vein flow within 72 h in healthy subjects [45].

The PC-MRI measured azygous vein flow has been shown to correlate with the degree of portal hypertension. Gouya et al. reported the correlation between the azygous vein flow and oesophageal varices grade [29], but portal pressure was not measured in this study. Subsequent studies have shown that azygous vein flow correlated with hepatic venous pressure gradient (HVPG) [46, 47], but the correlation was absent in patients with clinically significant portal hypertension (HVPG ≥10 mmHg) [47]. The correlation between hepatic inflow and portal pressure is less well established. Portal venous flow does not correlate with the degree of portal hypertension [46, 47]. In a recent study, the hepatic arterial fraction of hepatic inflow correlated with HVPG in a small study of 12 patients [48]; however, the hepatic artery flow was not measured directly. An indirect measure was obtained by subtracting the portal vein flow from total hepatic blood flow (the difference between infra- and suprahepatic vena cava.

14.3.2 MR Markers of Hepatic Architecture and Splanchnic Haemodynamics

In a prospective study of patients undergoing HVPG measurements, liver T_1 relaxation time and splenic artery velocity were shown to correlate with HVPG [47]. These MR markers directly reflect the pathophysiological changes in the development and progression of portal hypertension. As discussed earlier, the liver T_1 relaxation time is associated with degree of fibrosis and inflammation in the liver. The T_1 measurement was respiratory triggered and multi-slice, and therefore a large volume of the liver could be sampled in a reasonable time. Interestingly the distribution of the liver T_1 values was shown to increase with the worsening portal hypertension, reflecting the increasing heterogeneity of T_1 values across the liver volume. This emphasises the sampling variability associated with liver biopsy and potentially transient elastography. The increased splenic artery velocity measured using PC-MR is likely to represent the hyperdynamic state in portal hypertension. In this study, 'within session' coefficient of variation of the splenic artery velocity was less than 10% in agreement with a previous study from the same group [49].

It was an interesting observation that HVPG can potentially be assessed noninvasively using a simple linear model of MRI parameters of liver T_1 relaxation time and SA velocity. Figure 14.1 highlights that this linear model provides good

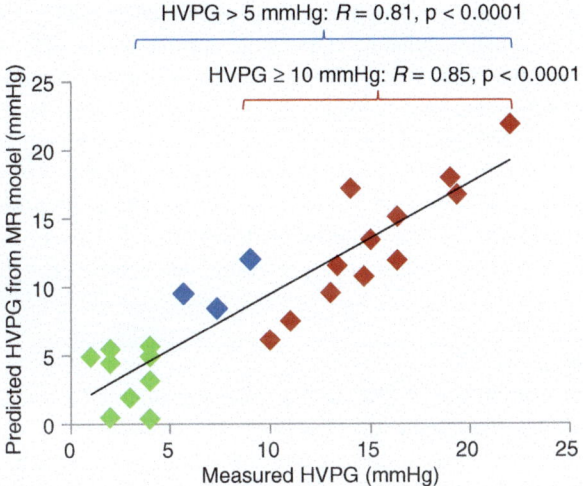

Fig. 14.4 The correlation between HVPG with MR model of liver T_1 relaxation time and splenic artery velocity

prediction of HVPG across the span of HVPG values from normal to clinically significant portal hypertension, better than SE-EPI liver T_1 relaxation time or SA velocity alone. The scan time required to collect the data for this model (Liver T_1 and triplicate SA data) was 5–10 min, dependent on breathing rate of the patient, with PC-MR data being planned whilst the respiratory triggered T_1 sequence is acquired (Fig. 14.4).

14.3.3 Potential Application and Future Directions

Various non-invasive markers of HVPG, including liver stiffness measurements, have been reported as being accurate as a binary predictor of the presence or absence of clinically significant portal hypertension (CSPH) (HVPG ≥10 mmHg) [50]. The Baveno VI consensus recommended that screening endoscopy can be avoided in patients with liver stiffness of <20 kPa and platelet count of >150,000 as the risk of having gastro-oesophageal varices requiring treatment is low [51]. However, we believe that the MR measures of hepatic architecture and splanchnic haemodynamics do have the advantage of being able to accurately estimate HVPG values on a continuous scale. This provides us with a tool to detect the development of portal hypertension as well as to monitor its progression beyond the threshold of CSPH (HVPG ≥10 mmHg) in patients with cirrhosis [52, 53].

We could potentially utilise this MR model to assess the treatment response in portal hypertensive patients by monitoring the change in portal pressure in response to therapy. Haemodynamic response (HVPG reduction of 20% from baseline or to <12 mmHg or) to non-selective beta blockers (NSBBs) has been associated with a significant reduction in the risk of variceal bleeding and decompensation [54].

However, carvedilol, a preferred NSBB with an additional alpha-1 receptor blockade effect, only achieves haemodynamic response in approximately 60% of the patients [55]. The non-responders can potentially be identified using the MR model, and alternative treatment can be initiated to reduce the risk of bleeding and decompensation.

Furthermore, the MR model can be used to aid the development of novel treatments in portal hypertension by investigating treatment efficacy as well as underlying mechanisms. This certainly would be an attractive proposition for the pharmaceutical industry as the experimental design with non-invasive and less expensive MR models would be preferable compared to direct HVPG measurements.

Conclusions

Although the current use of MRI in hepatology is mainly focused on investigation of focal abnormalities within the liver, the advances in the technology has allowed assessment of liver fibrosis and portal pressure. Currently, these measures are limited to experimental medicine studies. However, undoubtedly in the next decade, the multimodal quantitative MR methodology will be incorporated into the design of clinical trials and eventually the clinical algorithms in the diagnosis and management of patients with cirrhosis and portal hypertension.

References

1. Venkatesh SK, Yin M, Takahashi N, Glockner JF, Talwalkar JA, Ehman RL. Non-invasive detection of liver fibrosis: MR imaging features vs. MR elastography. Abdom Imaging. 2015;40(4):766–75.
2. Awaya H, Mitchell DG, Kamishima T, Holland G, Ito K, Matsumoto T. Cirrhosis: modified caudate-right lobe ratio. Radiology. 2002;224(3):769–74.
3. Ferrucci JT, Stark DD. Iron oxide-enhanced MR imaging of the liver and spleen: review of the first 5 years. AJR Am J Roentgenol. 1990;155(5):943–50.
4. Lucidarme O, Baleston F, Cadi M, Bellin MF, Charlotte F, Ratziu V, Grenier PA. Non-invasive detection of liver fibrosis: is superparamagnetic iron oxide particle-enhanced MR imaging a contributive technique? Eur Radiol. 2003;13(3):467–74.
5. Aguirre DA, Behling CA, Alpert E, Hassanein TI, Sirlin CB. Liver fibrosis: noninvasive diagnosis with double contrast material-enhanced MR imaging. Radiology. 2006;239(2):425–37.
6. Faria SC, Ganesan K, Mwangi I, Shiehmorteza M, Viamonte B, Mazhar S, Peterson M, Kono Y, Santillan C, Casola G, Sirlin CB. MR imaging of liver fibrosis: current state of the art. Radiographics. 2009;29(6):1615–36.
7. Pandharipande PV, Krinsky GA, Rusinek H, Lee VS. Perfusion imaging of the liver: current challenges and future goals. Radiology. 2005;234(3):661–73.
8. Materne R, Smith AM, Peeters F, Dehoux JP, Keyeux A, Horsmans Y, Van Beers BE. Assessment of hepatic perfusion parameters with dynamic MRI. Magn Reson Med. 2002;47(1):135–42.
9. Van Beers BE, Materne R, Annet L, Hermoye L, Sempoux C, Peeters F, Smith AM, Jamart J, Horsmans Y. Capillarization of the sinusoids in liver fibrosis: noninvasive assessment with contrast-enhanced MRI in the rabbit. Magn Reson Med. 2003;49(4):692–9.
10. Annet L, Materne R, Danse E, Jamart J, Horsmans Y, Van Beers BE. Hepatic flow parameters measured with MR imaging and Doppler US: correlations with degree of cirrhosis and portal hypertension. Radiology. 2003;229(2):409–14.

11. Hagiwara M, Rusinek H, Lee VS, Losada M, Bannan MA, Krinsky GA, Taouli B. Advanced liver fibrosis: diagnosis with 3D whole-liver perfusion MR imaging – initial experience. Radiology. 2008;246(3):926–34.

12. Thomsen HS, Marckmann P, Logager VB. Update on nephrogenic systemic fibrosis. Magn Reson Imaging Clin N Am. 2008;16(4):551–60. vii

13. Lewin M, Poujol-Robert A, Boelle PY, Wendum D, Lasnier E, Viallon M, Guechot J, Hoeffel C, Arrive L, Tubiana JM, Poupon R. Diffusion-weighted magnetic resonance imaging for the assessment of fibrosis in chronic hepatitis C. Hepatology. 2007;46(3):658–65.

14. Taouli B, Ehman RL, Reeder SB. Advanced MRI methods for assessment of chronic liver disease. AJR Am J Roentgenol. 2009;193(1):14–27.

15. Klasen J, Lanzman RS, Wittsack HJ, Kircheis G, Schek J, Quentin M, Antoch G, Haussinger D, Blondin D. Diffusion-weighted imaging (DWI) of the spleen in patients with liver cirrhosis and portal hypertension. Magn Reson Imaging. 2013;31(7):1092–6.

16. Aube C. Imaging modalities for the diagnosis of hepatic fibrosis and cirrhosis. Clin Res Hepatol Gastroenterol. 2015;39(1):38–44.

17. Zhang B, Liang L, Dong Y, Lian Z, Chen W, Liang C, Zhang S. Intravoxel incoherent motion MR imaging for staging of hepatic fibrosis. PLoS One. 2016;11(1):e0147789.

18. Lee Y, Lee SS, Kim N, Kim E, Kim YJ, Yun SC, Kuhn B, Kim IS, Park SH, Kim SY, Lee MG. Intravoxel incoherent motion diffusion-weighted MR imaging of the liver: effect of triggering methods on regional variability and measurement repeatability of quantitative parameters. Radiology. 2015;274(2):405–15.

19. Moon JC, Messroghli DR, Kellman P, Piechnik SK, Robson MD, Ugander M, Gatehouse PD, Arai AE, Friedrich MG, Neubauer S, Schulz-Menger J, Schelbert EB. Myocardial T1 mapping and extracellular volume quantification: a Society for Cardiovascular Magnetic Resonance (SCMR) and CMR Working Group of the European Society of Cardiology consensus statement. J Cardiovasc Magn Reson. 2013;15:92.

20. Thomsen C, Christoffersen P, Henriksen O, Juhl E. Prolonged T1 in patients with liver-cirrhosis – an invivo MRI study. Magn Reson Imaging. 1990;8(5):599–604.

21. Heye T, Yang SR, Bock M, Brost S, Weigand K, Longerich T, Kauczor HU, Hosch W. MR relaxometry of the liver: significant elevation of T1 relaxation time in patients with liver cirrhosis. Eur Radiol. 2012;22(6):1224–32.

22. Banerjee R, Pavlides M, Tunnicliffe EM, Piechnik SK, Sarania N, Philips R, Collier JD, Booth JC, Schneider JE, Wang LM, Delaney DW, Fleming KA, Robson MD, Barnes E, Neubauer S. Multiparametric magnetic resonance for the non-invasive diagnosis of liver disease. J Hepatol. 2014;60(1):69–77.

23. Mozes FE, Tunnicliffe EM, Pavlides M, Robson MD. Influence of fat on liver T1 measurements using modified Look-Locker inversion recovery (MOLLI) methods at 3T. J Magn Reson Imaging. 2016;44(1):105–11.

24. Pavlides M, Banerjee R, Sellwood J, Kelly CJ, Robson MD, Booth JC, Collier J, Neubauer S, Barnes E. Multiparametric magnetic resonance imaging predicts clinical outcomes in patients with chronic liver disease. J Hepatol. 2016;64(2):308–15.

25. Hoad CL, Palaniyappan N, Kaye P, Chernova Y, James MW, Costigan C, Austin A, Marciani L, Gowland PA, Guha IN, Francis ST, Aithal GP. A study of T1 relaxation time as a measure of liver fibrosis and the influence of confounding histological factors. NMR Biomed. 2015;28(6):706–14.

26. Agrawal S, Hoad CL, Francis ST, Guha IN, Kaye P, Aithal GP. Visual morphometry and three non-invasive markers in the evaluation of liver fibrosis in chronic liver disease. Scand J Gastroenterol. 2017;52(1):107–15.

27. Reynaert H, Thompson MG, Thomas T, Geerts A. Hepatic stellate cells: role in microcirculation and pathophysiology of portal hypertension. Gut. 2002;50(4):571–81.

28. Burkart DJ, Johnson CD, Morton MJ, Wolf RL, Ehman RL. Volumetric flow-rates in the portal venous system – measurement with cine phase-contrast MR imaging. Am J Roentgenol. 1993;160(5):1113–8.

29. Gouya H, Vignaux O, Sogni P, Mallet V, Oudjit A, Pol S, Legmann P. Chronic liver disease: systemic and splanchnic venous flow mapping with optimized cine phase-contrast MR imaging validated in a phantom model and prospectively evaluated in patients. Radiology. 2011;261(1):144–55.
30. Pelc LR, Pelc NJ, Rayhill SC, Castro LJ, Glover GH, Herfkens RJ, Miller DC, Jeffrey RB. Arterial and venous-blood flow – noninvasive quantitation with MR imaging. Radiology. 1992;185(3):809–12.
31. Hara AK, Burkart DJ, Johnson CD, Felmlee JP, Ehman RL, Ilstrup DM, Harmsen WS. Variability of consecutive in vivo MR flow measurements in the main portal vein. Am J Roentgenol. 1996;166(6):1311–5.
32. Wilson DJ, Ridgway JP, Evans JA, Robinson P. Measurement of hepatic arterial flow using phase contrast magnetic resonance imaging. Phys Med Biol. 2009;54(19):N439–49.
33. Bax L, Bakker CJG, Klein WM, Blanken N, Beutler JJ, Mali WPTRM. Renal blood flow measurements with use of phase-contrast magnetic resonance imaging: normal values and reproducibility. J Vasc Interv Radiol. 2005;16(6):807–14.
34. de Haan MW, Kouwenhoven M, Kessels AGH, van Engelshoven JMA. Renal artery blood flow: quantification with breath-hold or respiratory triggered phase-contrast MR imaging. Eur Radiol. 2000;10(7):1133–7.
35. de Haan MW, van Engelshoven JMA, Houben AJHM, Kaandorp DW, Kessels AGH, Kroon AA, de Leeuw PW. Phase-contrast magnetic resonance flow quantification in renal arteries – comparison with (133)Xenon washout measurements. Hypertension. 2003;41(1):114–8.
36. Burkart DJ, Johnson CD, Reading CC, Ehman RL. MR measurements of mesenteric venous flow – prospective evaluation in healthy-volunteers and patients with suspected chronic mesenteric ischemia. Radiology. 1995;194(3):801–6.
37. Li KCP, Whitney WS, Mcdonnell CH, Fredrickson JO, Pelc NJ, Dalman RL, Jeffrey RB. Chronic mesenteric ischemia – evaluation with phase-contrast cine MR-imaging. Radiology. 1994;190(1):175–9.
38. Yzet T, Bouzerar R, Baledent O, Renard C, Lumbala DM, Nguyen-Khac E, Regimbeau JM, Deramond H, Meyer ME. Dynamic measurements of total hepatic blood flow with Phase Contrast MRI. Eur J Radiol. 2010;73(1):119–24.
39. Yzet T, Bouzerar R, Allart JD, Demuynck F, Legallais C, Robert B, Deramond H, Meyer ME, Baledent O. Hepatic vascular flow measurements by phase contrast MRI and Doppler echography: a comparative and reproducibility study. J Magn Reson Imaging. 2010;31(3):579–88.
40. Bosch J, Groszmann RJ. Measurement of azygos venous blood flow by a continuous thermal dilution technique: an index of blood flow through gastroesophageal collaterals in cirrhosis. Hepatology. 1984;4(3):424–9.
41. Bosch J, Mastai R, Kravetz D, Bruix J, Rigau J, Rodes J. Measurement of azygos venous blood flow in the evaluation of portal hypertension in patients with cirrhosis. Clinical and haemodynamic correlations in 100 patients. J Hepatol. 1985;1(2):125–39.
42. Salama ZA, Kassem AM, Giovannini M, Hunter MS. Endoscopic ultrasonographic study of the azygos vein in patients with varices. Endoscopy. 1997;29(8):748–50.
43. Faigel DO, Rosen HR, Sasaki A, Flora K, Benner K. EUS in cirrhotic patients with and without prior variceal hemorrhage in comparison with noncirrhotic control subjects. Gastrointest Endosc. 2000;52(4):455–62.
44. Lomas DJ, Hayball MP, Jones DP, Sims C, Allison MED, Alexander GJM. Noninvasive measurement of Azygos venous-blood flow using magnetic-resonance. J Hepatol. 1995;22(4):399–403.
45. Debatin JF, Zahner B, Meyenberger C, Romanowski B, Schopke W, Marincek B, Fuchs WA. Azygos blood flow: phase contrast quantitation in volunteers and patients with portal hypertension pre- and postintrahepatic shunt placement. Hepatology. 1996;24(5):1109–15.
46. Gouya H, Grabar S, Vignaux O, Saade A, Pol S, Legmann P, Sogni P. Portal hypertension in patients with cirrhosis: indirect assessment of hepatic venous pressure gradient by measuring azygos flow with 2D-cine phase-contrast magnetic resonance imaging. Eur Radiol. 2016;26(7):1981–90.

47. Palaniyappan N, Cox E, Bradley C, Scott R, Austin A, O'Neill R, Ramjas G, Travis S, White H, Singh R, Thurley P, Guha IN, Francis S, Aithal GP. Non-invasive assessment of portal hypertension using quantitative magnetic resonance imaging. J Hepatol. 2016;65(6):1131–9.
48. Chouhan MD, Mookerjee RP, Bainbridge A, Punwani S, Jones H, Davies N, Walker-Samuel S, Patch D, Jalan R, Halligan S, Lythgoe MF, Taylor SA. Caval subtraction 2D phase-contrast MRI to measure total liver and hepatic arterial blood flow: proof-of-principle, correlation with portal hypertension severity and validation in patients with chronic liver disease. Investig Radiol. 2017;52(3):170–6.
49. Cox EF, Smith JK, Chowdhury AH, Lobo DN, Francis ST, Simpson J. Temporal assessment of pancreatic blood flow and perfusion following secretin stimulation using noninvasive MRI. J Magn Reson Imaging. 2015;42(5):1233–40.
50. Berzigotti A, Seijo S, Arena U, Abraldes JG, Vizzutti F, Garcia-Pagan JC, Pinzani M, Bosch J. Elastography, spleen size, and platelet count identify portal hypertension in patients with compensated cirrhosis. Gastroenterology. 2013;144(1):102–111.e1.
51. de Franchis R, Fac BV. Expanding consensus in portal hypertension report of the Baveno VI consensus workshop: stratifying risk and individualizing care for portal hypertension. J Hepatol. 2015;63(3):743–52.
52. Moitinho E, Escorsell N, Bandi JC, Salmeron JM, Garcia-Pagan JC, Rodis J, Bosch J. Prognostic value of early measurements of portal pressure in acute variceal bleeding. Gastroenterology. 1999;117(3):626–31.
53. Merkel C, Bolognesi M, Bellon S, Zuin R, Noventa F, Finucci G, Sacerdoti D, Angeli P, Gatta A. Prognostic usefulness of hepatic vein catheterization in patients with cirrhosis and esophageal-varices. Gastroenterology. 1992;102(3):973–9.
54. Garcia-Tsao G, Bosch J. Current concepts: management of varices and variceal hemorrhage in cirrhosis. N Engl J Med. 2010;362(9):823–32.
55. Sinagra E, Perricone G, D'Amico M, Tine F, D'Amico G. Systematic review with meta-analysis: the haemodynamic effects of carvedilol compared with propranolol for portal hypertension in cirrhosis. Aliment Pharmacol Ther. 2014;39(6):557–68.

Magnetic Resonance Elastography of the Liver

15

Sumeet K. Asrani and Jayant A. Talwalkar

15.1 Introduction

In the United States alone, an estimated 150,000 persons are diagnosed with chronic liver disease (CLD) annually with nearly 30,000 (20%) individuals having cirrhosis at initial presentation. Furthermore, over 75% of individuals are asymptomatic from their liver disease at evaluation [1]. In addition, the prevalence of non-alcoholic fatty liver disease (NAFLD) is between 8–45% with 9% of patients with nonalcoholic steatohepatitis (NASH) progressing to cirrhosis annually [2–4]. The global burden of CLD is expected to increase given the aging of the CLD population, especially the HCV infected birth cohort and in context of the obesity epidemic [5, 6]. In this setting, early identification of patients with cirrhosis or those highest at risk of progression of their liver disease at the population level is important.

Diagnosis of cirrhosis often relies on a combination of clinical history and examination, radiologic imaging as well as blood work to assess liver function. Assessment of fibrosis traditionally relies on obtaining a liver biopsy. Although liver biopsy is considered the gold standard for detecting hepatic fibrosis (see the specific chapter in this book), its use in clinical practice appears to be declining over time. Additionally, the ability to perform liver biopsy in large populations is limited by the risk for procedure-related complications, patient acceptance, cost, and inaccuracies associated with sampling error [7–9]. In turn, there remains a great need to introduce novel, effective methods to diagnose and risk stratify individuals with CLD.

S.K. Asrani, M.D., M.Sc.
Department of Medicine, Hepatology, Bylor University Medical Center, Dallas, Texas, USA
e-mail: Sumeet.asrani@bswhealth.org

J.A. Talwalkar, M.D., M.P.H. (✉)
Department of Medicine, Mayo Clinic College of Medicine, Rochester, MN, USA
e-mail: talwalkar.jayant@mayo.edu

© Springer International Publishing AG, part of Springer Nature 2018
A. Berzigotti, J. Bosch (eds.), *Diagnostic Methods for Cirrhosis and Portal Hypertension*, https://doi.org/10.1007/978-3-319-72628-1_15

225

15.2   Elastography

Given the practical limitations of using liver biopsy among the growing number of individuals with CLD, a number of noninvasive methods to detect liver fibrosis have been developed over the past decade to characterize the biologic properties and physical properties of liver disease. In general, these methods have been characterized as (1) serum tests containing panels of markers reflecting the biology of hepatic fibrogenesis and (2) functional imaging tests which measure unique physical characteristics associated with the development of fibrosis. More details regarding these methods are given in other chapters of this book, Among the imaging studies to date, the most widely studied and used are elastography techniques with ultrasound or magnetic resonance (MR) based examinations.

Elastography evaluates the intrinsic mechanical viscoelastic properties of liver parenchyma and allow for estimation of liver stiffness (LS), whereby elevated stiffness is associated with presence of advanced fibrosis. SWE captures the propagation of shear waves in tissues. Shear waves propagate faster in stiff tissue (e.g. cirrhosis) as compared to softer tissue. Shear waves can either be generated by controlled external vibration (e.g. vibration controlled transient elastography, VCTE), by acoustic radiation force impulse (either point SWE or 2DSWE) or by a continuous vibrating source (e.g. active driver in magnetic resonance elastography).

15.3   Magnetic Resonance Elastography

Magnetic resonance elastography (MRE) uses a modified phase-contrast imaging sequence to detect propagating shear waves within the tissue of interest (Fig. 15.1). A patient in an MRI scanner has a passive pneumatic drum driver placed over the right lobe of the liver. The passive driver is connected to the active driver with a plastic tube. The active driver (placed outside the room) generates dynamic low

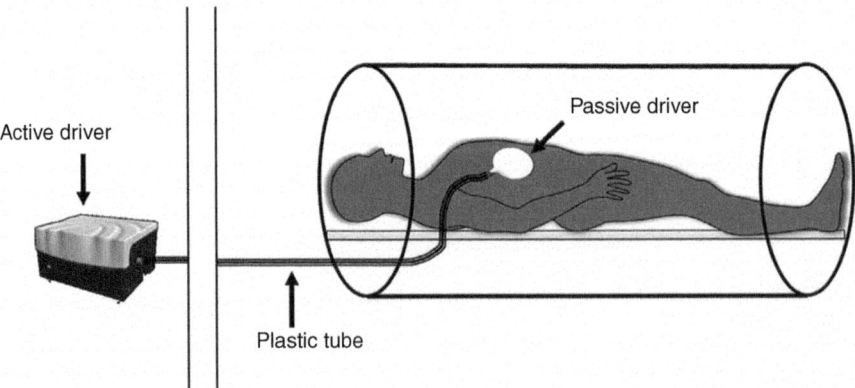

Fig. 15.1 Representative image of set up for Magnetic resonance Elastography. With permission from Venkatesh et al., 2015 MRE and the Liver

frequency mechanical waves (e.g. 60 Hz) which are transmitted to the passive driver. The flexible membrane of the passive driver creates vibrations. Subsequently, acoustic shear waves are generated by the driver for propagation into liver tissue. The sequences require four breath holds (11–16 s) and are completed within 1–2 min without the need for intravenous contrast administration. Subsequently, the LS values are calculated from wave displacement patterns and displayed as color-encoded images (elastograms). Region of interest analysis throughout 4–10 mm cross-sectional slices of liver (avoiding vascular structures) is then performed to calculate mean liver stiffness (LS) in kilo pascals, kPa [10, 11]. Elasticity quantification by MRE is based on the formula representing shear modulus, which is equivalent to one third of the Young's modulus which is used with VCTE [12].

15.4   Clinical Applications

15.4.1   Assessment of Fibrosis (Fig. 15.2)

Elevated LS quantified by MRE is associated with increasing liver fibrosis with a value below 2.9 kPa generally implying normal liver and a value above 5.2 kPa

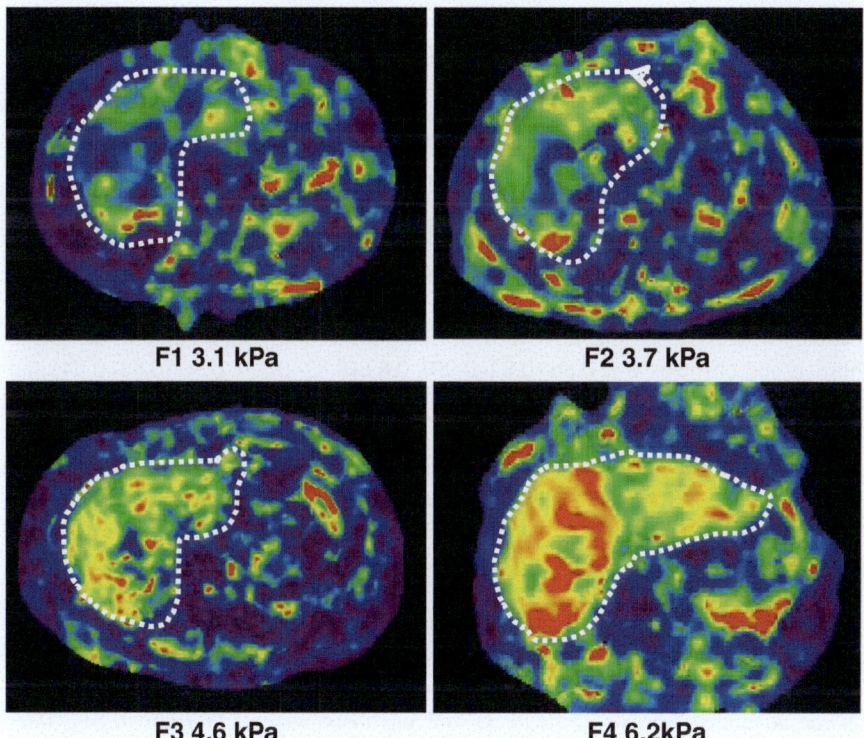

F1 3.1 kPa   **F2 3.7 kPa**

F3 4.6 kPa   **F4 6.2kPa**

Fig. 15.2 Representative images of Magnetic resonance elastography

implying the presence of cirrhosis [13–19]. Values of LS are approximately 1/3 that reported by US based techniques. LS as measured by MRE is highly reproducible with high interobserver agreement [20, 21]. LS among healthy controls is not influenced by age, gender, liver fat content or body mass index [22, 23]. The role of MRE has been examined across a spectrum of CLD etiologies including viral hepatitis, NAFLD, alpha 1 antitrypsin deficiency and in the post-transplant setting [24, 25]. Further it is feasible and highly accurate among the pediatric population, including those with obesity [26, 27]. A LS value ≥2.9 kPa separates *any* degree of liver fibrosis from normal liver with a sensitivity and specificity of 98% and 99%, respectively. Furthermore, MRE can discriminate between patients with *clinically significant hepatic fibrosis (F2-F4)* as compared to individuals with no to mild fibrosis (F0–F1) with sensitivity and specificity values in the 80–85% range, respectively [11, 15]. 10% of the cases are misclassified. MRE is highly accurate for the detection of *cirrhosis* with sensitivity and specificity values exceeding 90%, respectively [14, 15, 28].

In a recent meta-analysis, MRE at a cutoff of 4.96 had superior diagnostic accuracy for detecting presence of cirrhosis with the sensitivity, specificity, and area under the receiver-operating curve (AUROC) of 0.91, 0.92, and 0.98, respectively. In a meta-analysis of individual participant data, the mean AUROC for the diagnosis of any (≥stage 1), significant (≥stage 2), advanced fibrosis (≥stage 3), and cirrhosis was 0.84 (0.76–0.92), 0.88 (0.84–0.91), 0.93 (0.90–0.95), and 0.92 (0.90–0.94), respectively. Failure rate was 4.3%. In addition, results were similar regardless of etiology of liver disease or body mass index [29].

NAFLD: Given the influence of obesity and body habitus, increased skin to capsule distance, and incomplete examinations with US based non-invasive assessment of fibrosis (see below), MRE may serve as an important tool to diagnose presence of fibrosis in patients with NAFLD. In a prospective study, mean AUROC discriminating advanced fibrosis (stage 3–4) from stage 0–2 fibrosis was 0.92. A threshold of >3.63 kPa had a sensitivity of 0.86 (0.65–0.97), specificity of 0.91 (0.83–0.96), positive predictive value of 0.68 (0.48–0.84), and negative predictive value of 0.97 (0.91–0.99) for presence of advanced fibrosis [30]. In a meta-analysis of MRE in patients with NAFLD, mean AUROC for diagnosis of any, significant or advanced fibrosis and cirrhosis was 0.86 (0.82–0.90), 0.87 (0.82–0.93), 0.90 (0.84–0.94) and 0.91 (0.76–0.95), respectively. Diagnostic performance was similar regardless of BMI or degree of inflammation [31].

Primary Sclerosing Cholangitis: Among patients with PSC, a LS cutoff of 4.93 kPa has superior performance to detect cirrhosis [32]. MRE may be suitable for patients with small rib spaces, can be combined with MRCP and potentially pick up a patchy distribution of fibrosis that may be seen in PSC. Further, biliary obstruction which may falsely elevated stiffness with alternate techniques may not be an issue with MRE, though this is debated [33–35].

Post-transplant: In a meta-analysis of MRE among patients after liver transplantation the mean AUROC values for diagnosis of any (≥stage 1), significant (≥stage 2), or advanced fibrosis (≥stage 3) and cirrhosis were 0.73 (0.66–0.81), 0.69 (0.62–0.74), 0.83 (0.61–0.88) and 0.96 (0.93–0.98), respectively [36].

15.4.1.1   MRE Versus Other Modalities

MRE versus serum markers: Overall, diagnostic accuracy for assessment of fibrosis is better with radiologic markers (US or MR) as compared to serum marks [28, 37]. In comparing MRE versus other non-invasive markers, MRE had higher AUROC (0.96) than other clinical prediction rules such as ast to platelet ratio index (APRI), BARD, NAFLD fibrosis score and FIB-4 (0.81–0.86). MRE had lower rates of misclassification and correctly classified 75% of patients with intermediate FIB-4 score [38]. In a study of patients with chronic hepatitis C and B, MRE had a significantly greater area under the ROC curve than APRI score for discriminating among fibrosis stages F2–F4 [39].

MRE versus vibration controlled transient elastography (VCTE): It is unclear whether MRE is globally superior to US based techniques for diagnosis of advanced fibrosis. Studies comparing MRE and VCTE have conflicting reports on the superiority of one test of the other especially for intermediate stages [40, 41]. However, MRE may be more accurate for diagnosing fibrosis in patients with NAFLD as compared to VCTE.

In a prospective study of 141 patients with CLD (any etiology), MRE had a higher technical success rate vs. VCTE (94% vs. 84%). The diagnostic accuracy of MRE was also superior to both VCTE and APRI [15]. While comparable accuracy rates for detecting *cirrhosis* were observed for MRE and VCTE, the accuracy of MRE was significantly higher than VCTE for detecting *clinically significant* hepatic fibrosis (F2–F4) [42].

For viral hepatitis, MRE and VCTE accuracy were comparable for $\geq$F2 (AUROC 0.91 vs. 0.91) and $\geq$F3 (AUROC 0.93 vs. 0.90). Cutoff values of <5.2 and $\geq$8.9 kPa (VCTE) and <1.66 and $\geq$2.18 kPa (MRE) diagnosed 64% and 66% of patients correctly as F0–F1 or F2–F4, respectively [43].

MRE may be more accurate than VCTE at diagnosing fibrosis in patients with fatty liver disease. In a prospective, cross-sectional study, MRE detected any fibrosis (stage 1 or more) with an AUROC 0f 0.82 as compared to VCTE (0.67). MRE (as compared to VCTE) was better at detecting stage F2 (0.89 vs. 0.86), stage F3 (0.87 vs. 0.80) and F4 (0.87 vs. 0.69), respectively [44]. In another study from Japan, AUROC for $\geq$F2 was higher for MRE as compared to VCTE (0.91 vs. 0.82, $p < 0.01$) [45].

In a recent meta-analysis among patients with NAFLD, 2D SWE (0.95) and MRE (0.96) had the highest diagnostic accuracy in staging fibrosis as compared to VCTE (AUROC 0.88 with M probe and 0.85 with XL probe for VCTE). Diagnostic accuracy was better than serum based markers. Amongst serum markers, NAFLD fibrosis score (0.84) and FIB-4 (0.84) offered the best diagnostic performance [46].

MRE versus 2D-SWE: In a recent study, the technical success rates of MR elastography and 2D SWE were 96% and 92%, respectively. However, MRE provided significantly more reliable LS measurements than did 2D SWE (100% vs. 86.9%).There was moderate correlation in the LS measurements between the examination modalities ($r = 0.67$) [47].

MRE versus point SWE: MRE was more accurate than point SWE for diagnosing any fibrosis in NAFLD patients, especially those who are obese [48]. For diagnosing any fibrosis ($\geq$stage 1), the MRE AUROC was 0.8 versus 0.66 (point SWE). MRE was superior to point SWE for diagnosing any fibrosis in obese patients ($p < 0.01$) but not in nonobese patients ($p = 0.7$). The MRE AUROCs for diagnosing $\geq$stages 2, 3, and 4 fibrosis were 0.89, 0.93 and 0.88 as compared to 0.85, 0.90 and 0.86, respectively.

In a recently published clinical guideline technical review, it was suggested that MRE does not increase diagnostic accuracy in identifying cirrhosis in patients who truly have cirrhosis over VCTE in patients with HCV or NAFLD. However, in adults with NAFLD, MRE has higher diagnostic accuracy in ruling out cirrhosis in patients who do not have cirrhosis [19].

15.4.1.2 Strengths and Limitations

MRE may offer certain advantages over US based techniques. First, there are lower incomplete examinations with MRE. While the reproducibility of VCTE is excellent in experienced centers, its accuracy is diminished by the presence of inexperienced operators and patient factors including obesity and narrow rib interspaces [49, 50]. This is partly driven by limited wave penetration beyond a distance of 6–7 cm which can represent the width of subcutaneous tissues in some obese patients [50, 51]. Hence, MRE may play an increasingly important role in patients with NAFLD given that BMI and distribution of obesity (e.g. skin to capsule distance) does not appear to influence LS measurements by MRE. The reproducibility of MRE is excellent [52]. In a recent study comparing MRE and 2D SWE in the same individual, the rates of unreliable exam were higher with 2D SWE as compared to MRE (19% versus 0%) [47] Second, a larger region of interest is examined with MRE. While VCTE is designed to measure LS in a cylindrical-shaped area 1 cm wide and 4 cm long in the right lobe, MRE calculates LS over the entire cross-sectional areas of hepatic parenchyma from multiple slices.

There are however several limitations. For both US and MR based techniques, pathophysiological processes including acute inflammation, cholestasis, portal pressure, and hepatic congestion may independently contribute to increased LS [53–57]. Generalizability and accessibility may also be a concern. Though the use of MRE is increasing, it is not readily available and may need specialized training [58, 59]. Serum markers or US based examinations are more widely available and easier to incorporate into daily clinical practice. MRE requires a dedicated facility and involvement of a radiologist. However, MRE can be incorporated into care of CLD patients that routinely undergo MRI, such as those with PSC, but additional time and costs are required. Individuals with typical contraindications to MRI, such as claustrophobia and pacemaker, are unable to undergo MRE [12, 50]. Though wave propagation is not affected, the signal from the liver is poor [35]. Further, the standard MRE sequence is susceptible to presence of iron in the liver; newer MRE sequences not susceptible to iron presence are being developed, but are not validated yet. Further motion artifact is possible from the inability to hold breath.

15.4.2 Detection of Portal Hypertension

Complications associated with portal hypertension account for a significant proportion of morbidity and mortality among individuals with cirrhosis. As explained in a separate chapter in this book, the gold standard test for detecting portal hypertension involves measurement of the hepatic venous pressure gradient (HVPG). However, the measurement of HVPG in clinical practice has limitations [60, 61].

LS by VCTE correlates with HVPG, and accurately detects CSPH [62–64]. Despite the correlation between LS and HVPG is less precise beyond an HVPG value of 12 mmHg [65, 66], LS is currently the best non-invasive parameter to rule-out the presence of varices needing treatment (data are described in detail elsewhere in this book). Not surprisingly, LS measurement by MRE correlates independently with increasing HVPG [67]. In a single center study, a cutoff of 5.8 kPa had good sensitivity (96%) and negative predictive value (98%) for prediction of large varices though the specificity (60%) and positive predictive value (36%) was poor [68].

Spleen stiffness as a noninvasive predictor of portal hypertension was recently measured using MRE [69]. In addition to demonstrating that spleen stiffness was significantly higher among patients with liver fibrosis compared to healthy controls, the spleen stiffness was increased further among patients with cirrhosis and portosystemic collaterals versus patients with cirrhosis alone. Notably, a mean spleen stiffness ≥10.5 kPa was 100% sensitive in identifying all 17 patients with esophageal varices and cirrhosis in the study cohort. Therefore, spleen stiffness may provide additional information about the hemodynamic alterations within splenic and splanchnic circulations not captured by LS.

15.4.3 Predicting Progression (or Regression) of Liver Disease

As compared to the general population, individuals with compensated cirrhosis have a fivefold increase, whereas patients with decompensated disease have a tenfold increase in mortality [70]. Given that a majority of deaths in patients with compensated cirrhosis are due to progression to a decompensated state and the development of its ensuing complications, the ability to predict decompensation is important. If patients with compensated liver disease at the highest risk of decompensation can be identified, it may be possible to institute enhanced surveillance and prophylactic measures for this patient subset. The role of elastography in identifying this risk of transition has been reported. In a recent meta-analysis, elevated LS at baseline (either by US or MRE based techniques) was associated with a significant risk of hepatic decompensation (RR, 1.07; 95% CI, 1.03–1.11), hepatocellular cancer (RR, 1.11; 95% CI, 1.05–1.18), and death (RR, 1.22; 95% CI, 1.05–1.43) [71]. Specifically, in a single center study, subjects with decompensated cirrhosis had a higher mean LS (6.8 kPa versus 5.2 kPa). MRE was independently associated with decompensation after adjusting for relevant patient characteristics. Further among persons with compensated cirrhosis, the hazard for hepatic decompensation was 1.42 (95% CI 1.16–1.75) per unit increase in liver stiffness over time. The hazard of hepatic decompensation was 4.96 (95% CI 1.4–17.0, p = 0.019) for a subject with compensated disease and mean LSS value ⩾ 5.8 kPa as compared to an individual with compensated disease and lower mean LS values [72]. In patients with PSC, elevated LS was associated with development of decompensation. (HR, 1.55; 95% CI, 1.41–1.70) with the highest risk observed amongst patients with stiffness >6.0 kPa [32]. In another study elevated stiffness was associated with progression from Child A to Child B cirrhosis in patients with HCV. The 1-year risk (0.7%, 95% CI, 0.1–4.2%) of cirrhosis progression was negligible in patients with LS of <3.3 kPa or response to anti-viral treatment [73]. In a novel study, MRE of the kidney in patients with cirrhosis was associated with development of hepatorenal syndrome, whereby MRE-measured renal stiffness was significantly lower in patients with HRS (median stiffness 2.62 kPa at 60 Hz) compared with patients with normal renal function (median stiffness 3.41 kPa at 60 Hz) (p ≤ 0.01) [74]. Further, MRE may play a role in prediction of decompensation after liver resection. In a recent prospective study, LS was the only independent predictor of blood loss as well as major complications after hepatectomy. At a cutoff of 5.3 kPa the AUROC was 0.81 for prediction of major complications [75]. LS measurement may also offer prognostic information in prediction of decompensated disease after liver transplantation especially among persons with hepatitis C [76–78].

Improvement in stiffness may be a surrogate for improved outcomes. MRE may be used to monitor response to therapy. Among patients with NAFLD with at least a 5% reduction in BMI, there was a significant decrease in MRE-estimated LS [79]. MRE-estimated LS decreased from 2.79 kPa (±0.74) to 2.35 kPa (±0.39). It is unclear whether similar pattern would be seen in cirrhotics.

However, questions however remain about whether improvement in LS reflects actual regression or fibrosis or simply amelioration of dynamic component of liver disease and portal hypertension. Addressing this is very important for patients with cirrhosis. Achievement of LS below strict cutoffs for cirrhosis pretreatment may not reflect "regression of cirrhosis" and patients would still be at risk of complications of cirrhosis. Therefore it is still unclear whether surveillance strategies can be tailored for patients with marked reduction in LS [80].

15.4.4 Evaluation of Hepatic Mass

Recently, the role of MRE was applied to characterize LS among a variety of benign and malignant lesions [81]. Among 64 patients with 44 hepatic mass lesions, the mean stiffness of benign masses (nine hemangiomas, three focal nodular hyperplasias, and one hepatic adenoma) was 2.7 kPa, which is consistent with the LS of normal liver parenchyma. The mean stiffness of malignant tumors was 10.1 kPa. In this series, a cutoff value of 5 kPa completely separated all benign focal liver masses from malignant lesions. In a case control study, LS as quantified by MRE was an independent risk factor for HCC (odds ratio 1.4, 1.05–1.8) [82] However, other studies have failed to show this association [83].

MRE may improve the characterization of benign lesions which are atypical in presentation, especially when the distinction between atypical cavernous hemangioma, focal nodular hyperplasia or hepatic adenoma from malignant disease is not clear from conventional imaging techniques [84]. However, the use of contrast-enhanced techniques has been highly accurate for the diagnosis of hepatocellular carcinoma in patients with cirrhosis when lesions are at least 2 cm in size, contain arterial hypervascularity, and have a delayed venous washout pattern [85]. While the application of MRE for hepatocellular carcinoma does not seem to provide obvious incremental diagnostic value, it remains to be seen whether tumor stiffness can predict responses to non-surgical therapies including ablative procedures and pharmacological therapies. Furthermore, the measurement of LS after chemotherapy for colorectal hepatic metastases may help to identify individuals who may be at risk for hepatic sinusoidal injury.

Conclusion

The role of non-invasive methods in the management of patients with CLD continues to evolve. MRE offers staging of liver disease in a variety of patients especially among those with NAFLD. Beyond diagnosis, non-invasive measures may have a prognostic role. Measurement of LS may serve as a complementary tool to monitor progression of disease. Further studies are needed to evaluate whether a change in liver stiffness (improvement or deterioration) amongst patients followed serially is associated with development of relevant clinical outcomes. In addition, MRI based technology continues to evolve. For example in a recent study, 3 D-MRE (shear wave frequency 40 Hz) had even greater diagnostic accuracy than the commercially available 2D-MRE (shear wave frequency 60 Hz) in diagnosing advanced fibrosis (area under the receiver operator curve, AUROC 0.98 vs. 0.92, $p < 0.05$) using liver biopsy as reference standard. Finally, clinical algorithms are needed whereby non-invasive markers can seamlessly be incorporated in care of patients with CLD, keeping in mind the cost, accessibility and incremental clinical utility offered above and beyond that which may be gained by simple bedside clinical assessment.

References

1. Bell BP, Manos MM, Zaman A, Terrault N, Thomas A, Navarro VJ, et al. The epidemiology of newly diagnosed chronic liver disease in gastroenterology practices in the United States: results from population-based surveillance. Am J Gastroenterol. 2008;103(11):2727–36. quiz 37
2. Browning JD, Szczepaniak LS, Dobbins R, Nuremberg P, Horton JD, Cohen JC, et al. Prevalence of hepatic steatosis in an urban population in the United States: impact of ethnicity. Hepatology. 2004;40(6):1387–95.
3. Kanwal F, Kramer JR, Duan Z, Yu X, White D, El-Serag HB. Trends in the burden of nonalcoholic fatty liver disease in a United States Cohort of Veterans. Clin Gastroenterol Hepatol. 2016;14(2):301–8.e1–2.
4. Younossi ZM, Koenig AB, Abdelatif D, Fazel Y, Henry L, Wymer M. Global epidemiology of nonalcoholic fatty liver disease-meta-analytic assessment of prevalence, incidence, and outcomes. Hepatology. 2016;64(1):73–84.

5. Liu B, Balkwill A, Reeves G, Beral V. Body mass index and risk of liver cirrhosis in middle aged UK women: prospective study. BMJ. 2010;340:c912.
6. Kim WR, Brown RS Jr, Terrault NA, El-Serag H. Burden of liver disease in the United States: summary of a workshop. Hepatology. 2002;36(1):227–42.
7. Muir AJ, Trotter JF. A survey of current liver biopsy practice patterns. J Clin Gastroenterol. 2002;35(1):86–8.
8. Standish RA, Cholongitas E, Dhillon A, Burroughs AK, Dhillon AP. An appraisal of the histopathological assessment of liver fibrosis. Gut. 2006;55(4):569–78.
9. Everhart JE, Wright EC, Goodman ZD, Dienstag JL, Hoefs JC, Kleiner DE, et al. Prognostic value of Ishak fibrosis stage: findings from the hepatitis C antiviral long-term treatment against cirrhosis trial. Hepatology. 2010;51(2):585–94.
10. Muthupillai R, Lomas DJ, Rossman PJ, Greenleaf JF, Manduca A, Ehman RL. Magnetic resonance elastography by direct visualization of propagating acoustic strain waves. Science. 1995;269(5232):1854–7.
11. Yin M, Chen J, Glaser KJ, Talwalkar JA, Ehman RL. Abdominal magnetic resonance elastography. Top Magn Reson Imaging. 2009;20(2):79–87.
12. Talwalkar JA, Yin M, Fidler JL, Sanderson SO, Kamath PS, Ehman RL. Magnetic resonance imaging of hepatic fibrosis: emerging clinical applications. Hepatology. 2008;47(1):332–42.
13. Rouviere O, Yin M, Dresner MA, Rossman PJ, Burgart LJ, Fidler JL, et al. MR elastography of the liver: preliminary results. Radiology. 2006;240(2):440–8.
14. Yin M, Talwalkar JA, Glaser KJ, Manduca A, Grimm RC, Rossman PJ, et al. Assessment of hepatic fibrosis with magnetic resonance elastography. Clin Gastroenterol Hepatol. 2007;5(10):1207–13.e2.
15. Huwart L, Sempoux C, Salameh N, Jamart J, Annet L, Sinkus R, et al. Liver fibrosis: noninvasive assessment with MR elastography versus aspartate aminotransferase-to-platelet ratio index. Radiology. 2007;245(2):458–66.
16. Asbach P, Klatt D, Hamhaber U, Braun J, Somasundaram R, Hamm B, et al. Assessment of liver viscoelasticity using multifrequency MR elastography. Magn Reson Med. 2008;60(2):373–9.
17. Crespo S, Bridges M, Nakhleh R, McPhail A, Pungpapong S, Keaveny AP. Non-invasive assessment of liver fibrosis using magnetic resonance elastography in liver transplant recipients with hepatitis C. Clin Transpl. 2013;27(5):652–8.
18. Hennedige TP, Wang G, Leung FP, Alsaif HS, Teo LL, Lim SG, et al. Magnetic resonance elastography and diffusion weighted imaging in the evaluation of hepatic fibrosis in chronic hepatitis B. Gut Liver. 2017;11(3):401–8.
19. Singh S, Muir AJ, Dieterich DT, Falck-Ytter YT. American Gastroenterological Association Institute Technical Review on the role of elastography in chronic liver diseases. Gastroenterology. 2017;152(6):1544–77.
20. Lee YJ, Lee JM, Lee JE, Lee KB, Lee ES, Yoon JH, et al. MR elastography for noninvasive assessment of hepatic fibrosis: reproducibility of the examination and reproducibility and repeatability of the liver stiffness value measurement. J Magn Reson Imaging. 2014;39(2):326–31.
21. Runge JH, Bohte AE, Verheij J, Terpstra V, Nederveen AJ, van Nieuwkerk KM, et al. Comparison of interobserver agreement of magnetic resonance elastography with histopathological staging of liver fibrosis. Abdom Imaging. 2014;39(2):283–90.
22. Venkatesh SK, Wang G, Teo LL, Ang BW. Magnetic resonance elastography of liver in healthy asians: normal liver stiffness quantification and reproducibility assessment. J Magn Reson Imaging. 2014;39(1):1–8.
23. Lee DH, Lee JM, Han JK, Choi BI. MR elastography of healthy liver parenchyma: normal value and reliability of the liver stiffness value measurement. J Magn Reson Imaging. 2013;38(5):1215–23.
24. Kim RG, Nguyen P, Bettencourt R, Dulai PS, Haufe W, Hooker J, et al. Magnetic resonance elastography identifies fibrosis in adults with alpha-1 antitrypsin deficiency liver disease: a prospective study. Aliment Pharmacol Ther. 2016;44(3):287–99.

25. Ichikawa S, Motosugi U, Ichikawa T, Sano K, Morisaka H, Enomoto N, et al. Magnetic resonance elastography for staging liver fibrosis in chronic hepatitis C. Magn Reson Med Sci. 2012;11(4):291–7.
26. Xanthakos SA, Podberesky DJ, Serai SD, Miles L, King EC, Balistreri WF, et al. Use of magnetic resonance elastography to assess hepatic fibrosis in children with chronic liver disease. J Pediatr. 2014;164(1):186–8.
27. Schwimmer JB, Behling C, Angeles JE, Paiz M, Durelle J, Africa J, et al. Magnetic resonance elastography measured shear stiffness as a biomarker of fibrosis in pediatric nonalcoholic fatty liver disease. Hepatology. 2017;66(5):1474–85.
28. Venkatesh SK, Wang G, Lim SG, Wee A. Magnetic resonance elastography for the detection and staging of liver fibrosis in chronic hepatitis B. Eur Radiol. 2014;24(1):70–8.
29. Singh S, Venkatesh SK, Wang Z, Miller FH, Motosugi U, Low RN, et al. Diagnostic performance of magnetic resonance elastography in staging liver fibrosis: a systematic review and meta-analysis of individual participant data. Clin Gastroenterol Hepatol. 2015;13(3):440–51.e6.
30. Loomba R, Wolfson T, Ang B, Hooker J, Behling C, Peterson M, et al. Magnetic resonance elastography predicts advanced fibrosis in patients with nonalcoholic fatty liver disease: a prospective study. Hepatology. 2014;60(6):1920–8.
31. Singh S, Venkatesh SK, Loomba R, Wang Z, Sirlin C, Chen J, et al. Magnetic resonance elastography for staging liver fibrosis in non-alcoholic fatty liver disease: a diagnostic accuracy systematic review and individual participant data pooled analysis. Eur Radiol. 2016;26(5):1431–40.
32. Eaton JE, Dzyubak B, Venkatesh SK, Smyrk TC, Gores GJ, Ehman RL, et al. Performance of magnetic resonance elastography in primary sclerosing cholangitis. J Gastroenterol Hepatol. 2016;31(6):1184–90.
33. Schramm C, Eaton J, Ringe KI, Venkatesh S, Yamamura J, MRIwgot IPSCSG. Recommendations on the use of MRI in PSC-A position statement from the International PSC Study Group. Hepatology. 2017;66(5):1675–88.
34. Tan CH, Venkatesh SK. Magnetic resonance elastography and other magnetic resonance imaging techniques in chronic liver disease: current status and future directions. Gut Liver. 2016;10(5):672–86.
35. Venkatesh SK, Ehman RL. Magnetic resonance elastography of liver. Magn Reson Imaging Clin N Am. 2014;22(3):433–46.
36. Singh S, Venkatesh SK, Keaveny A, Adam S, Miller FH, Asbach P, et al. Diagnostic accuracy of magnetic resonance elastography in liver transplant recipients: a pooled analysis. Ann Hepatol. 2016;15(3):363–76.
37. Yoneda M, Thomas E, Sclair SN, Grant TT, Schiff ER. Supersonic shear imaging and transient elastography with the XL probe accurately detect fibrosis in overweight or obese patients with chronic liver disease. Clin Gastroenterol Hepatol. 2015;13(8):1502–9.e5.
38. Cui J, Ang B, Haufe W, Hernandez C, Verna EC, Sirlin CB, et al. Comparative diagnostic accuracy of magnetic resonance elastography vs. eight clinical prediction rules for non-invasive diagnosis of advanced fibrosis in biopsy-proven non-alcoholic fatty liver disease: a prospective study. Aliment Pharmacol Ther. 2015;41(12):1271–80.
39. Wu WP, Chou CT, Chen RC, Lee CW, Lee KW, Wu HK. Non-invasive evaluation of hepatic fibrosis: the diagnostic performance of magnetic resonance elastography in patients with viral hepatitis B or C. PLoS One. 2015;10(10):e0140068.
40. Talwalkar JA, Kurtz DM, Schoenleber SJ, West CP, Montori VM. Ultrasound-based transient elastography for the detection of hepatic fibrosis: systematic review and meta-analysis. Clin Gastroenterol Hepatol. 2007;5(10):1214–20.
41. Friedrich-Rust M, Ong MF, Martens S, Sarrazin C, Bojunga J, Zeuzem S, et al. Performance of transient elastography for the staging of liver fibrosis: a meta-analysis. Gastroenterology. 2008;134(4):960–74.
42. Huwart L, Sempoux C, Vicaut E, Salameh N, Annet L, Danse E, et al. Magnetic resonance elastography for the noninvasive staging of liver fibrosis. Gastroenterology. 2008;135(1):32–40.

43. Bohte AE, de Niet A, Jansen L, Bipat S, Nederveen AJ, Verheij J, et al. Non-invasive evaluation of liver fibrosis: a comparison of ultrasound-based transient elastography and MR elastography in patients with viral hepatitis B and C. Eur Radiol. 2014;24(3):638–48.
44. Park CC, Nguyen P, Hernandez C, Bettencourt R, Ramirez K, Fortney L, et al. Magnetic resonance elastography vs transient elastography in detection of fibrosis and noninvasive measurement of steatosis in patients with biopsy-proven nonalcoholic fatty liver disease. Gastroenterology. 2017;152(3):598–607.e2.
45. Imajo K, Kessoku T, Honda Y, Tomeno W, Ogawa Y, Mawatari H, et al. Magnetic resonance imaging more accurately classifies steatosis and fibrosis in patients with nonalcoholic fatty liver disease than transient elastography. Gastroenterology. 2016;150(3):626–37.e7.
46. Xiao G, Zhu S, Xiao X, Yan L, Yang J, Wu G. Comparison of laboratory tests, ultrasound, or MRE to detect fibrosis in patients with non-alcoholic fatty liver disease: a meta-analysis. Hepatology. 2017;66(5):1486–501.
47. Yoon JH, Lee JM, Woo HS, Yu MH, Joo I, Lee ES, et al. Staging of hepatic fibrosis: comparison of magnetic resonance elastography and shear wave elastography in the same individuals. Korean J Radiol. 2013;14(2):202–12.
48. Cui J, Heba E, Hernandez C, Haufe W, Hooker J, Andre MP, et al. Magnetic resonance elastography is superior to acoustic radiation force impulse for the diagnosis of fibrosis in patients with biopsy-proven nonalcoholic fatty liver disease: a prospective study. Hepatology. 2016;63(2):453–61.
49. Castera L, Bedossa P. How to assess liver fibrosis in chronic hepatitis C: serum markers or transient elastography vs. liver biopsy? Liver Int. 2011;31(Suppl 1):13–7.
50. Talwalkar JA. Elastography for detecting hepatic fibrosis: options and considerations. Gastroenterology. 2008;135(1):299–302.
51. Castera L, Foucher J, Bernard PH, Carvalho F, Allaix D, Merrouche W, et al. Pitfalls of liver stiffness measurement: a 5-year prospective study of 13,369 examinations. Hepatology. 2010;51(3):828–35.
52. Hines CD, Bley TA, Lindstrom MJ, Reeder SB. Repeatability of magnetic resonance elastography for quantification of hepatic stiffness. J Magn Reson Imaging. 2010;31(3):725–31.
53. Arena U, Vizzutti F, Corti G, Ambu S, Stasi C, Bresci S, et al. Acute viral hepatitis increases liver stiffness values measured by transient elastography. Hepatology. 2008;47(2):380–4.
54. Sagir A, Erhardt A, Schmitt M, Haussinger D. Transient elastography is unreliable for detection of cirrhosis in patients with acute liver damage. Hepatology. 2008;47(2):592–5.
55. Millonig G, Reimann FM, Friedrich S, Fonouni H, Mehrabi A, Buchler MW, et al. Extrahepatic cholestasis increases liver stiffness (FibroScan) irrespective of fibrosis. Hepatology. 2008;48(5):1718–23.
56. Millonig G, Friedrich S, Adolf S, Fonouni H, Golriz M, Mehrabi A, et al. Liver stiffness is directly influenced by central venous pressure. J Hepatol. 2010;52(2):206–10.
57. Chang PE, Miquel R, Blanco JL, Laguno M, Bruguera M, Abraldes JG, et al. Idiopathic portal hypertension in patients with HIV infection treated with highly active antiretroviral therapy. Am J Gastroenterol. 2009;104(7):1707–14.
58. Kayadibi H, Sertoglu E, Uyanik M. Biochemical markers, liver biopsy, or magnetic resonance elastography to detect or exclude advanced fibrosis in patients with nonalcoholic fatty liver disease. Hepatology. 2015;62(1):324–5.
59. Crossan C, Tsochatzis EA, Longworth L, Gurusamy K, Davidson B, Rodriguez-Peralvarez M, et al. Cost-effectiveness of non-invasive methods for assessment and monitoring of liver fibrosis and cirrhosis in patients with chronic liver disease: systematic review and economic evaluation. Health Technol Assess. 2015;19(9):1–409. v–vi
60. Bureau C, Metivier S, Peron JM, Selves J, Robic MA, Gourraud PA, et al. Transient elastography accurately predicts presence of significant portal hypertension in patients with chronic liver disease. Aliment Pharmacol Ther. 2008;27(12):1261–8.
61. Burroughs AK, Thalheimer U. Hepatic venous pressure gradient in 2010: optimal measurement is key. Hepatology. 2010;51(6):1894–6.

62. Groszmann RJ, Wongcharatrawee S. The hepatic venous pressure gradient: anything worth doing should be done right. Hepatology. 2004;39(2):280–2.
63. Lemoine M, Katsahian S, Ziol M, Nahon P, Ganne-Carrie N, Kazemi F, et al. Liver stiffness measurement as a predictive tool of clinically significant portal hypertension in patients with compensated hepatitis C virus or alcohol-related cirrhosis. Aliment Pharmacol Ther. 2008;28(9):1102–10.
64. Vizzutti F, Arena U, Romanelli RG, Rega L, Foschi M, Colagrande S, et al. Liver stiffness measurement predicts severe portal hypertension in patients with HCV-related cirrhosis. Hepatology. 2007;45(5):1290–7.
65. Lim JK, Groszmann RJ. Transient elastography for diagnosis of portal hypertension in liver cirrhosis: is there still a role for hepatic venous pressure gradient measurement? Hepatology. 2007;45(5):1087–90.
66. Castera L, Le Bail B, Roudot-Thoraval F, Bernard PH, Foucher J, Merrouche W, et al. Early detection in routine clinical practice of cirrhosis and oesophageal varices in chronic hepatitis C: comparison of transient elastography (FibroScan) with standard laboratory tests and non-invasive scores. J Hepatol. 2009;50(1):59–68.
67. Gharib AM, Han MAT, Meissner EG, Kleiner DE, Zhao X, McLaughlin M, et al. Magnetic resonance elastography shear wave velocity correlates with liver fibrosis and hepatic venous pressure gradient in adults with advanced liver disease. Biomed Res Int. 2017;2017:2067479.
68. Sun HY, Lee JM, Han JK, Choi BI. Usefulness of MR elastography for predicting esophageal varices in cirrhotic patients. J Magn Reson Imaging. 2014;39(3):559–66.
69. Talwalkar JA, Yin M, Venkatesh S, Rossman PJ, Grimm RC, Manduca A, et al. Feasibility of in vivo MR elastographic splenic stiffness measurements in the assessment of portal hypertension. AJR Am J Roentgenol. 2009;193(1):122–7.
70. Fleming KM, Aithal GP, Card TR, West J. All-cause mortality in people with cirrhosis compared with the general population: a population-based cohort study. Liver Int. 2012;32(1):79–84.
71. Singh S, Fujii LL, Murad MH, Wang Z, Asrani S, Ehman R, et al. Liver stiffness measurement predicts risk of decompensation, hepatocellular cancer and mortality in patients with chronic liver diseases: a systematic review and meta-analysis. Hepatology. 2013;58:956A.
72. Asrani SK, Talwalkar JA, Kamath PS, Shah VH, Saracino G, Jennings L, et al. Role of magnetic resonance elastography in compensated and decompensated liver disease. J Hepatol. 2014;60(5):934–9.
73. Takamura T, Motosugi U, Ichikawa S, Sano K, Morisaka H, Ichikawa T, et al. Usefulness of MR elastography for detecting clinical progression of cirrhosis from child-pugh class a to B in patients with type C viral hepatitis. J Magn Reson Imaging. 2016;44(3):715–22.
74. Low G, Owen NE, Joubert I, Patterson AJ, Graves MJ, Alexander GJ, et al. Magnetic resonance elastography in the detection of hepatorenal syndrome in patients with cirrhosis and ascites. Eur Radiol. 2015;25(10):2851–8.
75. Abe H, Midorikawa Y, Mitsuka Y, Aramaki O, Higaki T, Matsumoto N, et al. Predicting postoperative outcomes of liver resection by magnetic resonance elastography. Surgery. 2017;162(2):248–55.
76. Crespo G, Lens S, Gambato M, Carrion JA, Marino Z, Londono MC, et al. Liver stiffness 1 year after transplantation predicts clinical outcomes in patients with recurrent hepatitis C. Am J Transplant. 2014;14(2):375–83.
77. Kamphues C, Klatt D, Bova R, Yahyazadeh A, Bahra M, Braun J, et al. Viscoelasticity-based magnetic resonance elastography for the assessment of liver fibrosis in hepatitis C patients after liver transplantation. RoFo. 2012;184(11):1013–9.
78. Lee VS, Miller FH, Omary RA, Wang Y, Ganger DR, Wang E, et al. Magnetic resonance elastography and biomarkers to assess fibrosis from recurrent hepatitis C in liver transplant recipients. Transplantation. 2011;92(5):581–6.
79. Patel NS, Hooker J, Gonzalez M, Bhatt A, Nguyen P, Ramirez K, et al. Weight loss decreases magnetic resonance elastography estimated liver stiffness in nonalcoholic fatty liver disease. Clin Gastroenterol Hepatol. 2017;15(3):463–4.

80. D'Ambrosio R, Aghemo A, Fraquelli M, Rumi MG, Donato MF, Paradis V, et al. The diagnostic accuracy of Fibroscan for cirrhosis is influenced by liver morphometry in HCV patients with a sustained virological response. J Hepatol. 2013;59(2):251–6.

81. Venkatesh SK, Yin M, Glockner JF, Takahashi N, Araoz PA, Talwalkar JA, et al. MR elastography of liver tumors: preliminary results. AJR Am J Roentgenol. 2008;190(6):1534–40.

82. Motosugi U, Ichikawa T, Koshiishi T, Sano K, Morisaka H, Ichikawa S, et al. Liver stiffness measured by magnetic resonance elastography as a risk factor for hepatocellular carcinoma: a preliminary case-control study. Eur Radiol. 2013;23(1):156–62.

83. Anaparthy R, Talwalkar JA, Yin M, Roberts LR, Fidler JL, Ehman RL. Liver stiffness measurement by magnetic resonance elastography is not associated with developing hepatocellular carcinoma in subjects with compensated cirrhosis. Aliment Pharmacol Ther. 2011;34(1):83–91.

84. Garteiser P, Doblas S, Daire JL, Wagner M, Leitao H, Vilgrain V, et al. MR elastography of liver tumours: value of viscoelastic properties for tumour characterisation. Eur Radiol. 2012;22(10):2169–77.

85. Oki E, Kakeji Y, Taketomi A, Yamashita Y, Ohgaki K, Harada N, et al. Transient elastography for the prediction of oxaliplatin-associated liver injury in colon cancer patients: a preliminary analysis. J Gastrointest Cancer. 2008;39(1–4):82–5.

Part III

Invasive and Non-Invasive Diagnostic Methods in Special Conditions

Budd-Chiari Syndrome: The Western Perspective

16

Aurélie Plessier, Audrey Payancé, and Dominique Valla

Abbreviations

APLS	Antiphospholipid syndrome
BCS	BUDD Chiari Syndrome
BMB	Bone marrow biopsy
BMI	Body mass index
HCC	Hepatocellular carcinoma
HV	Hepatic vein
IVC	Inferior vena cava
MPN	Myeloproliferative neoplasm
OLT	Orthotopic liver transplantation
OP	Oestro-progestative
PH	Portal hypertension
PMI	Per million inhabitants
PNH	Paroxysomal noctural haemoglobinuria
TIPS	Transjugular porto systemic shunt

A. Plessier (✉) • A. Payancé • D. Valla
DHU Unity, Pole des Maladies de l'Appareil Digestif, Service d'Hépatologie,
Centre de Référence des Maladies Vasculaires du Foie, HUPNVS, APHP, Clichy, France
e-mail: aurelie.plessier@aphp.fr; dominique.valla@aphp.fr, dominique.valla@bjn.aphp.fr

© Springer International Publishing AG, part of Springer Nature 2018
A. Berzigotti, J. Bosch (eds.), *Diagnostic Methods for Cirrhosis and Portal Hypertension*, https://doi.org/10.1007/978-3-319-72628-1_16

16.1 Definition and Epidemiology

Budd-Chiari syndrome (BCS) is characterized by obstruction of the hepatic venous outflow tract at any level, from the small hepatic veins to the IVC at the entrance of the right atrium, whatever the cause [1, 2]. Primary BCS is related to thrombosis. Secondary BCS is related to enclosement or invasion of the veins by malignant tumors (e.g. hepatocellular carcinoma, renal adenocarcinoma, adrenal adenocarcinoma, primary hepatic hemangiosarcoma, epithelioid hemangioendothelioma, sarcoma of the IVC, right atrial myxoma, etc.) or parasitic infection (alveolar hydatid disease).

Sinusoidal obstruction syndrome (previously called veno-occlusive disease) and cardiac and pericardial diseases are excluded from the definition.

BCS is a rare disease, and epidemiological data are scarce. Former studies suggested that the prevalence and incidence varied depending on the geographic origin and was more frequently encountered in Asian populations. Recent studies do not confirm this view (Table 16.1). A prospective survey in French hepatology units in 2010 reported that the incidence and prevalence rates of primary BCS were 0.68 per million inhabitants (pmi) and 4.1 pmi, respectively, while when the incidence was estimated according to population-based analyses of hospital discharge diagnoses, the incidence in France during the same period (2010) was 2.36 pmi [3]. A recent publication from South Korea shows similar rates [4] (Table 16.1). In China, a metaanalysis of Chinese publications from 2000 to 2013 reported an incidence rate of 0.88 pmi per year and a prevalence of 7.69 pmi [5]. These results show that the different epidemiological approaches make it difficult to interpret the similarities and differences of European/American (Western) and Asian (Eastern) countries. Further studies are clearly needed.

The causes, site of obstruction and symptoms have also been shown to differ in Western and Eastern studies. The Western perspective will be discussed in this chapter.

Table 16.1 Incidence and prevalence of BCS throughout the world

	Japan [62]	Denmark [63]	France [3]	Sweden [64]	S Korea [4]	France [3]	China [5]	Italy [65]
Study period	1989	1981–85	2010	1990–01	2009–13	2012	2000–13	2000–12
Population based	No	Yes	No	Yes	Yes	Yes	No	Yes
Study population—10^6	123	5	44	1.3	424	51	1300	13
Incident cases—n	21	13	30	12	43	120	1150	287
Incidence—pmi per yr	0.17	0.5	0.68	0.8	0.87	2.36	0.88	2
Prevalence pmi	2.4	NA	4.24	1.4	5.29	NA	7.69	NA

16.2   Causes

16.2.1 Myeloproliferative Neoplasms (Table 16.2)

In the West, routine investigation of patients shows the presence of systemic prothombotic factors in 90%, with multiple factors in 20%. Myeloproliferative neoplasms (MPNs) account for most of these factors. MPNs include polycythemia vera, essential thrombocytemia and myelofibrosis. A non-invasive diagnostic investigation of MPN is performed in most patients with suspected BCS by testing for the V617F mutation in the Janus kinase 2 gene (*JAK2*). In a recent meta-analysis [6] the mean prevalence of *JAK2*V617F in BCS was 41.1% (95% CI, 32.3–50.6%). Indeed, in a group of 104 BCS patients, JAK2V617F was found in 47 (45%). When the diagnosis of MPN was first stratified according to the detection of *JAK2*V617F, a bone marrow biopsy (BMB) could be avoided in 40% [7].

Table 16.2 Associated causes to BCS and non-invasive or invasive diagnosis tools

	Europe [18]	China [66]	Noninvasive diagnosis	Invasive diagnosis
Risk factor frequency (%)				
Thrombophilia				
Inherited	21	0/0/No data on PC/PS/AT/ plasminogen	Factor V Leiden/Factor II mutation Protein C/Protein S/ Antithrombin/ Plasminogen deficiency	
Acquired	44	4	Antiphospholipid Ab Anti beta2 GP1 Ab Lupus anticoagulant	
Myeloproliferative neoplasm	49	4.1	*JAK2*V617F mutation Cal R mutation Spleen 16 cm and platelet >200 × 10⁹/L	BMB
Hyperhomocysteinemia	22	50		
Hormonal factors	38	NA		
Oral contraceptives	33	NA		
Pregnancy	6	NA		
PNH	19	0.6	Flow- cytometry for CD55 and CD59 deficient cells	BMB
Systemic factors Coeliac disease Behcet disease	23	0.9	Anti transglutaminase Ab Cerebral and thoraco abdominal contrast imaging/HLA typing	Duodenal biopsy
Local factors	6	NA	Contrast imaging	

JAK2V617F is absent in 10–20% of BCS/MPN patients, while a bone marrow biopsy or assessment of endogenous erythroid colony formation provides evidence of MPN. Mutations across *JAK2* exon 12 or the *MPL* gene are rarely identified in BCS/MPN patients (fewer than 1%). CALR mutations, the second most prevalent acquired genetic alteration in essential thrombocythemia and primary myelofibrosis, has only been found in 0–4% of patients with *JAK2*V617F negative BCS. In a recent study of 322 patients with splanchnic vein thrombosis (SVT), including 99 with BCS, only 1/99 had the CALR mutation. CALR mutations were almost exclusively found in patients with SVT without *JAK2*V617F when the height of the spleen was ≥16 cm and the platelet count >200 × 10^9/L. This suggests that when the spleen is enlarged and the platelet count is normal or increased, patients should first be screened for CALR mutations and only undergo invasive diagnostic BMB if the CALR mutation is negative [8]. Finally, compared to non BCS MPNs, BCS MPNs are strongly associated with a high prevalence of the *JAK2*V617F mutation.

MPN appears to negatively influence the outcome of BCS, with significantly poorer baseline prognostic features, earlier hepatic decompression procedures, a higher risk of TIPS obstruction, risk factors for post-transplant thrombotic complications in BCS patients who have undergone OLT and recurrent thrombosis after SVT [6–8].

Treatment of MPN is complex in these patients and further studies evaluating the influence of treatment on the outcome of BCS are needed [11]. Expert hematological management is required. In the East, the frequency of associated JAK 2 V617F + MPN to BCS is very low: 0–2% in Indian, Korean or Chinese BCS patients [12]. The CAL R mutation was negative in 100% of BCS Chinese patients [13].

The prevalence of overt *JAK2* V617F-positive MPN in splanchnic vein thrombosis (BCS and portal vein thrombosis) is significantly higher than the prevalence of the *JAK2* mutation in MPN patients with other deep vein thromboses [14]. The *JAK2* mutation itself may have local effects on the splanchnic venous system. A recent study showed that a subset of patients with *JAK2*V617F + MPN have endothelial cells (ECs) that harbor the JAK2 V617F mutation [15]. Similar results have been shown with *JAK2*V617F MPN-neg, as 80% of patients harbor the *JAK2*V617F mutation in bone marrow-derived endothelial cells [16]. These results suggest that the presence of *JAK2*V617F in endothelial cells may be a risk factor for the development of thrombosis.

16.2.2 Other Causes

As shown in Table 16.2, large European cohorts report a high prevalence of MPN, APLS, and factor V Leiden mutation, a significant number of patients with paroxysmal nocturnal hemoglobinuria (PNH), and most (46%) with more than one disorder [17, 18]. Thirty-eight percent of 40 patients with SVTs had a risk factor in addition to MPN, including a hypercoagulable disorder, PNH, an autoimmune disorder (such as a connective tissue disease), or ulcerative colitis [19]. In a case control study of 43 BCS patients, the relative risk of BCS was 11.3 (95% CI 4.8–26.5) for individuals with the factor V Leiden mutation, 2.1(95% CI 0.4–9.6) for those with a prothrombin gene mutation, and 6.8 (95% CI 1.9–24.4) for those with a protein C deficiency [12]. These results were similar to those in other surveys from the Mediterranean area, showing a higher prevalence of celiac and Behcet's disease [19–22]. In a case control study from the 1980s, pregnancy seemed to be a trigger for Budd-Chiari syndrome in patients with an underlying prothrombotic disorder [23]. The relative risk of hepatic-vein thrombosis in women who use oral contraceptives was 2.37 [24].

Therefore, screening for other causes is routinely recommended in the Western literature in patients with one identified cause, mainly by noninvasive techniques (Table 16.2).

16.3   Manifestations

Manifestations are diverse and range from an absence of symptoms to fulminant hepatic failure depending on the site of obstruction, the number of hepatic veins obstructed, and the presence of hepatic venous collaterals. In a recent multicenter European survey, ascites, present in 83% of patients, hepatomegaly in 67% and abdominal pain in 61%, were the main clinical features. In approximately 15% of cases, BCS and PVT occurred simultaneously. Table 16.3 shows the different features at presentation in Eastern/Western studies and the invasive/non-invasive

Table 16.3 Manifestations West vs East

Country	Europe [17, 18]	China [67, 68]	
Number of patients	157	169	Diagnosis tools
Venous obstruction IVC/IVC + HV/ HV %	Mostly HV 2/49/49	Mostly IVC 12/56/31	Doppler US/ Contrast imaging
Median age	38 (16–83)	38	
Sex F %	57	49	
Ascites (%)	81	82	Imaging
Abdominal pain (%)	62	NA	
Hepatomegaly (%)	67	NA	Imaging
Hepatic encephalopathy (%)	9	0.5	
Varices/GI bleed (%)	58/5	63/14	Upper GI endoscopy
Dilated veins body, trunk (%)	NA	30	
Leg edema (%)	28	51	
Platelet count ($10^3/mm^3$)	265 (10–896)	108 ± 5	
Serum bilirubin (μmol/L)	31 (4–325	30 ± 2	
Serum albumin (g/L)	34 (17–55)	37 ± 0.5	
Serum creatinine (μmol/L)	79 (36–589)	71 ± 2	
INR	1.4 (1–10.9)	1.32 ± 0.03	
Child-Pugh score	8 (5–13)	NA	
Invasive procedure %	56	NA	Angioplasty/TIPS/ LT

procedures performed to identify them. In studies in Eastern countries, IVC obstruction is more frequent, there were no symptoms in more patients and leg edema, dilated veins on the body and trunk and HCC is more frequent. In recent Indian and Chinese studies, simultaneous caval and hepatic vein obstruction was the most prevalent feature. The high frequency of IVC in Asian countries but not in Europe or the United States must still be clarified, but the different prevalence of the causes in Eastern and Western countries may provide a partial explanation.

The cumulative incidence of HCC in BCS has been shown to be 4% after a median 5-year follow up. Diagnosis will be described in the following section.

Thus, BCS should be suspected when ascites, liver enlargement and upper abdominal pain are all present, or when intractable ascites is in contrast to moderate alteration of liver function tests; when liver disease occurs in a patient with known risk factors for thrombosis; or when liver disease remains unexplained after other common or uncommon causes have been excluded. The diagnosis of BCS must be assessed in all patients with acute/chronic, a/symptomatic liver disease.

16.4 Diagnosis

16.4.1 Non Invasive Imaging

Non invasive imaging can confirm a diagnosis of BCS when hepatic venous outflow obstruction is identified based on the visualization of obstructive lesions of the hepatic veins/inferior vena cava and/or of hepatic vein collaterals. Nonspecific signs of hepatic venous obstruction include extrahepatic portosystemic collateral circulation, perfusion abnormalities, dysmorphy and signs of PH.

Doppler ultrasound is highly sensitive in adults and children when the radiologist has been informed of the suspected diagnosis, [25, 26]. Venous obstruction may be total or partial, focal or extensive, and may involve one or several HVs or the supra hepatic inferior vena cava. Diagnosis is confirmed if it shows: (a) a hypoechoic and heterogeneous vein in association with expansion of the vessel lumen (corresponding to a recent thrombus) (b) large intrahepatic or subcapsular collaterals connecting the hepatic veins or the diaphragmatic or intercostal veins (c) a spider web appearance usually located near the hepatic vein ostia, associated with the absence of a normal hepatic vein in the area; (d) an absent or flat hepatic vein wave form without fluttering; (e) stenosis identified in the presence of a localized increase in flow velocity (= aliasing effect: a turbulent flow pattern, and loss of the normal triphasic cardiac modulation); or (f) a hyperechoic cord replacing a normal vein.

MRI and CT are used to confirm the diagnosis. On contrast-enhanced cross-sectional imaging, acute HV thrombosis is seen as a filling defect in the obstructed vein, which is hypoattenuating on CT and hypointense on T1-weighted MRI sequences. Obstructed veins are enlarged during the acute phase of BCS. With long-standing thrombosis, heterogeneity of the hepatic parenchyma is more prominent on CT and MRI and may make it difficult to visualize fibrous tracts. As a result, non-visible HV is the most common finding on contrast-enhanced imaging. Nonspecific signs are a hypoattenuating and heterogeneous liver on CT and a marked difference in signal intensity between central and peripheral zones on MRI. On T1-weighted sequences, the central zone is generally hyperintense while the peripheral zones are hypointense. On T2-weighted sequences, the central zone is hypointense and peripheral zones are hyperintense. Contrast enhancement varies. Hepatic dysmorphy is a characteristic, but nonspecific feather with atrophic areas that have been affected for a long period, contrast with hypertrophic areas that have a compensatory venous drainage. Marked segment I hypertrophy is suggestive of BCS and is due to preservation of the HV in this segment which drains directly into the retrohepatic IVC proximal to the ostia of the main HVs. However, segment I enlargement is not specific for BCS, because it is a common finding in cirrhosis.

Multiple regenerative nodules of various sizes are frequent in BCS, but they are frequently <3 cm in diameter. These nodules have been called "FNH-like" nodules [27]. They are hypo- or hyperechoic on ultrasound while on MRI they are more often iso- or slightly hyperintense on T1-weighted images, and iso- or slightly hypointense on T2-weighted images. Nodules are hypervascular and homogenous during the arterial phase on CT and MRI, without washout during the portal and late phases. The differential diagnosis between these nodules and HCC or adenomas may be difficult [28]. Although the sensitivity, specificity, positive predictive value (PPV) and negative predictive value (NPV) of contrast-enhanced ultrasound to differentiate malignant from benign thrombosis based on the enhancement of venous obstruction is excellent (95–100%) [29], there are no data on the efficacy of contrast-enchanced ultrasound to distinguish malignant from non malignant BCS nodules.

Measurement of liver stiffness (LS) by FibroScan transient elastography is an effective noninvasive tool to assess changes in stiffness before and shortly after an endovascular intervention, which may provide some information on changes in hepatic congestion [30]. Significant differences were found between mean LS measurements before and within 24 h after an endovascular procedure (Z-score = 4.372) and between mean LS values before and 3 months after treatment (Z-score = 3.408). These results provide indirect insight into the technical outcome and therapeutic benefits of endovascular procedures in patients with BCS.

16.4.2 Invasive Diagnostic Tools

Venography is only recommended when the diagnosis is uncertain or to characterize the liver anatomy before treatment. Liver biopsy is rarely needed because it is only recommended for the identification of small hepatic vein thrombosis when imaging has failed to demonstrate obstruction of the large veins or to diagnose HCC. HCC is strongly suggested:

- in patients with three nodules or less,
- when a nodule is larger than 3 cm in diameter,
- when a nodule is heterogeneous or washout occurs during the venous phase,

- when significant changes occur in two consecutive imaging techniques,
- if diffusion is restricted on MRI,
- or when AFP levels increases [1, 31, 32]. When a nodule is sampled, it is important to simultaneously perform a biopsy of the adjacent liver for comparison as
  well as hepatocellular adenoma (HCA) immunohistochemical analysis. Indeed
  in a recent study, 6/32 BCS patients had HCA immunostaining nodules, with one
  positive beta catenin and one HCC [33].

16.5   Therapy

A minimally invasive therapeutic strategy is proposed to Western BCS patients
[9, 34, 35] and presented in Fig. 16.1. First, medical therapy is begun, including
anticoagulation therapy, treatment of PH, and treatment of the cause. If the
patient has accessible stenosis of the HV or of the vena cava and a recanalization
procedure is feasible, angioplasty/and or stenting of the vein is performed. In
patients who do not respond to treatment, TIPS is proposed, and finally, orthotopic liver transplantation (OLT). Nevertheless, several aspects of the management strategy need be clarified. First, criteria of response to treatment must be
validated, and the delay of response must be confirmed. Also, a small group of
patients with severe BCS has been identified with a poor prognosis despite TIPS,
and these patients might benefit from early OLT. However, even though the BCS-
TIPS prognostic index (PI) score (based on international normalized ratio, bilirubin, and age) has been strongly associated with survival and was discriminative
[17, 34], it is difficult to identify these patients on an individual basis. On multivariate analysis, ascites, male sex, and higher creatinine levels were significantly
associated with invasive interventions (angioplasty/stent, TIPS or OLT) [18].
Several prognostic scores exist (Clichy, Rotterdam, Meld, and Barcelona) and

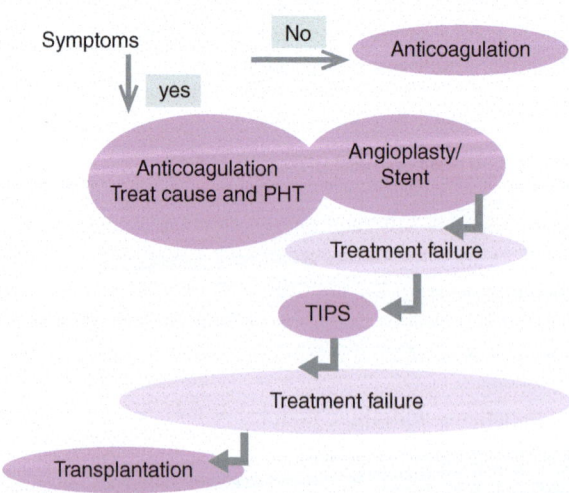

Fig. 16.1 Therapeutic strategy according to response to therapy

are currently used for stratification in clinical studies, although none of them seems to be reliable on an individual basis [17, 34, 36–39]. The levels and initial course of serum alanine aminotransferase seem to be a good predictor of 3-year survival: patients with initially high transaminases and a limited decrease within the first 48 h had a 3 year-survival rate of 30% compared to 70% in patients who were initially diagnosed with low transaminases. Finally, a recent Indian study measuring liver stiffness (transient elastography) with FibroScan used as a surveillance tool to assess the continued benefits of an endovascular intervention. Significant differences were found between mean LS measurements before and within 24 h after the intervention (Z-score = 4.372) and between mean values before and 3 months after treatment (Z-score = 3.408) in 15 patients who underwent periodic measurements. These data must be correlated with long-term outcome, further validation is needed, and the influence of "congestion" probably requires clarification [30].

16.5.1 Efficacy and Complications of Medical Therapy

There are no randomized studies to confirm the efficacy of anticoagulation therapy in BCS. The benefits of this treatment include an improved outcome in non-transplant as well as transplant patients since the implementation of systematic anticoagulation [40, 41], a high risk of thrombosis due to a high association rate to prothombotic diseases; case studies describing improvement following oral anticoagulant treatment, worsening when treatment is stopped and a noticeable improvement when it is reintroduced [42], as well as recanalization in rare cases of thrombosed hepatic veins and in half of patients with acute portal vein thrombosis [43]. In most centers, low molecular heparin has been used followed by long-term administration of coumarine derivatives, whatever the underlying thrombotic risk factor. Bleeding rates and heparin-induced thrombopenia seem to be more frequent and more severe in BCS anticoagulated patients than in those receiving anticoagulation for deep venous thromboembolism (VTE) [44, 45]. In a study of 94 consecutive patients, 47 had 92 major bleeding episodes (22.8 per 100 patient-years), with 40 episodes related to invasive therapy for BCS. In another more recent European study of 139 patients (88.5%) receiving long-term anticoagulation, 28 bleeding complications occurred in 24 patients (17%). The main causes of bleeding were related to PH (n = 14; 2 deaths) and intracranial hemorrhage (n = 3; 1 death) [17]. Invasive procedures and PH are major causes of bleeding, while excess anticoagulation probably plays a secondary role [17, 46]. Ascites paracentesis is an invasive procedure with a high risk of peritoneal bleeding, thus short interruption of anticoagulation for paracentesis should probably be considered to prevent heamoperitoneum. Treatment for the complications of PH is similar to that for cirrhosis. There are no data on the risk of bleeding during esophageal banding due to anticoagulation in BCS.

Although only preliminary data are available, treatment of the cause seems to improve the outcome for the liver [10, 47, 48].

16.5.2 Efficacy and Complications of Angioplasty/Stenting

The rate of patients who undergo angioplasty/stenting with the goal of restoring physiological sinusoidal flow and reducing morbidity and mortality, is low in Western countries [17, 49]. This treatment is only indicated in 5–30% of Western BCS patients because accessible stenosis is only encountered in 25% of patients (partial or segmental stenosis is present in 60% of patients with IVC obstruction and 25–30% of those with HV obstruction), and post angioplasty re-stenosis is frequent (although it is reduced when combined with a stent). In the EN vie study, 22/157 (14%) of patients had angioplasty/stent/or thrombolysis; only 5% did not require an alternative therapy, the procedure was completely effective in 32% and mortality due to liver failure occurred in 4% [17]. A recent retrospective study of 32 angioplasties and 31 stents in 155 BCS patients with a 27-year follow-up, reported technical success in 100% and symptom resolution in 73%. Secondary patency at 10 years was 79% and 64% in the stenting and venoplasty groups, respectively, with a low rate of procedural complications (9.5%) and no hepatic encephalopathy. Ten patients required TIPS, and eight surgery [49].

These results are in contrast to numerous Chinese and Indian studies reporting excellent results [50–57]. In a recent Indian study, interventional endovascular therapy was performed in 233/334 (70%) of patients, with a technical success rate of 90%. A complete clinical response was obtained in 166 patients (71.2%) [57]. Similar results were obtained in China [53, 54]. Future studies must take into account potential biases. In particular, when specialized healthcare is not available, the diagnosis of BCS related to an obstructed inferior vena cava is more probable due to the presence of a prominent cavo-caval subcutaneous circulation, while BCS due to hepatic venous obstruction with a patent IVC is more apt to obtain a non-specific diagnosis of cirrhosis. This type of bias could confound the outcome (which will be spontaneously better in patients with IVC obstruction).

16.5.3 Efficacy and Complications of TIPS

The one, 3 and 5-year actuarial survival rate following TIPS was 88%, 83% and 72%, respectively, while the OLT-free survival rate was 85%, 78 and 72%, respectively, in a European study [17]. Two other recent studies have reported excellent long-term 10-year survival (72–76%) [9, 58]. Early (27–34%) and late complications include bleeding, thrombosis, hepatic encephalopathy (20–25%) and TIPS dysfunction (30%) [9, 17, 34, 58]. Results suggest that there is a learning curve for TIPS for the management of BCS because of the specific technical and perioperative management associated with the etiology of disease [35].

16.5.4 Efficacy and Complications of OLT

When a "minimally invasive" strategy was applied in the Envie study, 20/157 (13%) of the patients underwent OLT. Four of these patients died. In another large European retrospective questionnaire survey, the 1-, 5-, and 10-year survival rate of 248 patients from 51 centers was 76%, 71% and 68%, respectively. Most of these patients were managed before radiological interventions were extensively used for BCS. Therefore, some of the patients who were transplanted would probably have been candidates for TIPS. Most early deaths (<3 months) were due to infection and multiple organ failure with graft failure or hepatic artery thrombosis in 18%. Late death (>1 year) occurred in 9/248 patients due to recurrent BCS in four [59]. Two recent studies evaluated the impact of MPN: 29/41 patients (71%) with MPN survived ≥3 years [mean age 36 ± 11 years old; women n = 27 (93%)]. Five- and 10-year survival rates were not significantly different in patients with and without MPN (P = 0.81 and P = 0.66 respectively) [60]. Thrombosis and bleeding occurred in 24–33% of patients [60, 61] and retransplantation in 30%. The *JAK2* mutation was strongly associated with the development of thrombotic complications following LT (P = 0.005) [62]. There was no evidence of progression to overt myelofibrosis or acute myeloid leukemia in the long-term follow-up [60]. Therefore, MPN does not seem to influence survival following OLT, while it strongly influences bleeding and thrombotic complications. Close perioperative and long-term hematological follow-up is needed in these patients.

Conclusion

Management of BCS has significantly changed in the past 30 years with a strategy of providing minimally invasive diagnosis and treatment. Imaging tools are highly sensitive and specific when performed by trained, informed radiologists. Further studies are needed to identify the prognostic value of liver stiffness measurements with an assessment of congestion. Individual prognostic tools are needed. The treatment strategy involves expertise in anticoagulation management, TIPS and OLT to find a balance between the risk of thrombosis and the risk of bleeding. Treatment of the cause is always difficult because the normal criteria are often affected by the presence of PH, liver failure, and shunts.

References

1. European Association for the Study of the Liver. Electronic address: easloffice@easloffice. eu. EASL clinical practice guidelines: vascular diseases of the liver. J Hepatol. 2016;64(1): 179–202.
2. DeLeve LD, Valla D-C, Garcia-Tsao G, American Association for the Study Liver Diseases. Vascular disorders of the liver. Hepatology. 2009;49(5):1729–64.
3. Allaire M, Ollivier-Hourmand I, Morello R, Chagneau-Derrode C, Dumortier J, Goria O, et al. P1288: Budd chiari syndrome (BCS) in France from a large national cohort. J Hepatol. 2015;62:S842.
4. Ki M, Choi HY, Kim K-A, Kim BH, Jang ES, Jeong S-H. Incidence, prevalence and complications of Budd-Chiari syndrome in South Korea: a nationwide, population-based study. Liver Int. 2016;36(7):1067–73.
5. Zhang W, Qi X, Zhang X, Su H, Zhong H, Shi J, et al. Budd-Chiari syndrome in China: a systematic analysis of epidemiological features based on the Chinese literature survey. Gastroenterol Res Pract. 2015;2015:738548.

6. Smalberg JH, Arends LR, Valla DC, Kiladjian J-J, Janssen HLA, Leebeek FWG. Myeloproliferative neoplasms in Budd-Chiari syndrome and portal vein thrombosis: a meta-analysis. Blood. 2012;120(25):4921–8.

7. Kiladjian J-J, Cervantes F, Leebeek FWG, Marzac C, Cassinat B, Chevret S, et al. The impact of JAK2 and MPL mutations on diagnosis and prognosis of splanchnic vein thrombosis: a report on 241 cases. Blood. 2008;111(10):4922–9.

8. Poisson J, Plessier A, Kiladjian J-J, Turon F, Cassinat B, Andreoli A, et al. Selective testing for calreticulin gene mutations in patients with splanchnic vein thrombosis: a prospective cohort study. J Hepatol. Epub 2017 May 5

9. Hayek G, Ronot M, Plessier A, Sibert A, Abdel-Rehim M, Zappa M, et al. Long-term outcome and analysis of dysfunction of transjugular intrahepatic portosystemic shunt placement in chronic primary Budd-Chiari syndrome. Radiology. 2017;283(1):280–92. Epub 2016 Oct 31

10. De Stefano V, Qi X, Betti S, Rossi E. Splanchnic vein thrombosis and myeloproliferative neoplasms: molecular-driven diagnosis and long-term treatment. Thromb Haemost. 2016;115(2):240–9.

11. Pieri L, Paoli C, Arena U, Marra F, Mori F, Zucchini M, et al. Safety and efficacy of ruxolitinib in splanchnic vein thrombosis associated with myeloproliferative neoplasms. Am J Hematol. 2017;92(2):187–95.

12. Janssen HL, Meinardi JR, Vleggaar FP, van Uum SH, Haagsma EB, van Der Meer FJ, et al. Factor V Leiden mutation, prothrombin gene mutation, and deficiencies in coagulation inhibitors associated with Budd-Chiari syndrome and portal vein thrombosis: results of a case-control study. Blood. 2000;96(7):2364–8.

13. Zhang P, Ma H, Min Q, Zu M, Lu Z. CALR mutations in Chinese Budd-Chiari syndrome patients. Eur J Gastroenterol Hepatol. 2016;28(3):361–2.

14. Austin SK, Lambert JR. The JAK2 V617F mutation and thrombosis. Br J Haematol. 2008;143(3):307–20.

15. Teofili L, Martini M, Iachininoto MG, Capodimonti S, Nuzzolo ER, Torti L, et al. Endothelial progenitor cells are clonal and exhibit the JAK2(V617F) mutation in a subset of thrombotic patients with Ph-negative myeloproliferative neoplasms. Blood. 2011;117(9):2700–7.

16. Helman R, Pereira W de O, Marti LC, Campregher PV, Puga RD, Hamerschlak N, et al. Granulocyte whole exome sequencing and endothelial JAK2V617F in patients with JAK2V617F positive Budd-Chiari syndrome without myeloproliferative neoplasm. Br J Haematol. Epub 2016 Sep 21.

17. Seijo S, Plessier A, Hoekstra J, Dell'era A, Mandair D, Rifai K, et al. Good long-term outcome of Budd-Chiari syndrome with a step-wise management. Hepatology. 2013;57(5): 1962–8.

18. Darwish Murad S, Plessier A, Hernandez-Guerra M, Fabris F, Eapen CE, Bahr MJ, et al. Etiology, management, and outcome of the Budd-Chiari syndrome. Ann Intern Med. 2009;151(3):167–75.

19. De Stefano V, Za T, Ciminello A, Betti S, Rossi E. Causes of adult splanchnic vein thrombosis in the mediterranean area. Mediterr J Hematol Infect Dis. 2011;3(1):e2011063.

20. Jadallah KA, Sarsak EW, Khazaleh YM, Barakat RMK. Budd-Chiari syndrome associated with coeliac disease: case report and literature review. Gastroenterol Rep. Epub 2016 Sep 7.

21. Ben Ghorbel I, Ennaifer R, Lamloum M, Khanfir M, Miled M, Houman MH. Budd-Chiari syndrome associated with Behçet's disease. Gastroenterol Clin Biol. 2008;32(3):316–20.

22. Seyahi E, Caglar E, Ugurlu S, Kantarci F, Hamuryudan V, Sonsuz A, et al. An outcome survey of 43 patients with Budd-Chiari syndrome due to Behçet's syndrome followed up at a single, dedicated center. Semin Arthritis Rheum. 2015;44(5):602–9.

23. Bissonnette J, Durand F, de Raucourt E, Ceccaldi P-F, Plessier A, Valla D, et al. Pregnancy and vascular liver disease. J Clin Exp Hepatol. 2015;5(1):41–50.

24. Valla D, Le MG, Poynard T, Zucman N, Rueff B, Benhamou JP. Risk of hepatic vein thrombosis in relation to recent use of oral contraceptives. A case-control study. Gastroenterology. 1986;90(4):807–11.

25. Faraoun SA, Boudjella MEA, Debzi N, Benidir N, Afredj N, Guerrache Y, et al. Budd-Chiari syndrome: an update on imaging features. Clin Imaging. 2016;40(4):637–46.

26. Pariente D, Franchi-Abella S. Paediatric chronic liver diseases: how to investigate and follow up? Role of imaging in the diagnosis of fibrosis. Pediatr Radiol. 2010;40(6):906–19.

27. Cazals-Hatem D, Vilgrain V, Genin P, Denninger M-H, Durand F, Belghiti J, et al. Arterial and portal circulation and parenchymal changes in Budd-Chiari syndrome: a study in 17 explanted livers. Hepatology. 2003;37(3):510–9.

28. Moucari R, Rautou P-E, Cazals-Hatem D, Geara A, Bureau C, Consigny Y, et al. Hepatocellular carcinoma in Budd-Chiari syndrome: characteristics and risk factors. Gut. 2008;57(6):828–35.

29. Raza SA, Jang H-J, Kim TK. Differentiating malignant from benign thrombosis in hepatocellular carcinoma: contrast-enhanced ultrasound. Abdom Imaging. 2014;39(1):153–61.

30. Mukund A, Pargewar SS, Desai SN, Rajesh S, Sarin SK. Changes in liver congestion in patients with Budd-Chiari syndrome following endovascular interventions: assessment with transient elastography. J Vasc Interv Radiol. Epub 2017 Jan 30.

31. Faraoun SA, Boudjella MEA, Debzi N, Afredj N, Guerrache Y, Benidir N, et al. Budd-Chiari syndrome: a prospective analysis of hepatic vein obstruction on ultrasonography, multidetector-row computed tomography and MR imaging. Abdom Imaging. 2015;40(6):1500–9.

32. Martens P, Maleux GA, Devos T, Monbaliu D, Heye S, Verslype C, et al. Budd-Chiari syndrome: reassessment of a step-wise treatment strategy. Acta Gastro-Enterol Belg. 2015;78(3):299–305.

33. Sempoux C, Paradis V, Komuta M, Wee A, Calderaro J, Balabaud C, et al. Hepatocellular nodules expressing markers of hepatocellular adenomas in Budd-Chiari syndrome and other rare hepatic vascular disorders. J Hepatol. 2015;63(5):1173–80.

34. Garcia-Pagán JC, Heydtmann M, Raffa S, Plessier A, Murad S, Fabris F, et al. TIPS for Budd-Chiari syndrome: long-term results and prognostics factors in 124 patients. Gastroenterology. 2008;135(3):808–15.

35. Plessier A, Sibert A, Consigny Y, Hakime A, Zappa M, Denninger M-H, et al. Aiming at minimal invasiveness as a therapeutic strategy for Budd-Chiari syndrome. Hepatology. 2006;44(5):1308–16.

36. Langlet P, Escolano S, Valla D, Coste-Zeitoun D, Denie C, Mallet A, et al. Clinicopathological forms and prognostic index in Budd-Chiari syndrome. J Hepatol. 2003;39(4):496–501.

37. Rautou P-E, Moucari R, Cazals-Hatem D, Escolano S, Denié C, Douarin L, et al. Levels and initial course of serum alanine aminotransferase can predict outcome of patients with Budd-Chiari syndrome. Clin Gastroenterol Hepatol. 2009;7(11):1230–5.

38. Rautou P-E, Moucari R, Escolano S, Cazals-Hatem D, Denié C, Chagneau-Derrode C, et al. Prognostic indices for Budd-Chiari syndrome: valid for clinical studies but insufficient for individual management. Am J Gastroenterol. 2009;104(5):1140–6.

39. Darwish Murad S, Kim WR, de Groen PC, Kamath PS, Malinchoc M, Valla D-C, et al. Can the model for end-stage liver disease be used to predict the prognosis in patients with Budd-Chiari syndrome? Liver Transpl. 2007;13(6):867–74.

40. Min AD, Atillasoy EO, Schwartz ME, Thiim M, Miller CM, Bodenheimer HC. Reassessing the role of medical therapy in the management of hepatic vein thrombosis. Liver Transpl Surg. 1997;3(4):423–9.

41. Zeitoun G, Escolano S, Hadengue A, Azar N, El Younsi M, Mallet A, et al. Outcome of Budd-Chiari syndrome: a multivariate analysis of factors related to survival including surgical porto-systemic shunting. Hepatology. 1999;30(1):84–9.

42. Ouwendijk RJ, Koster JC, Wilson JH, Stibbe J, Lameris JS, Visser W, et al. Budd-Chiari syndrome in a young patient with anticardiolipin antibodies: need for prolonged anticoagulant treatment. Gut. 1994;35(7):1004–6.

43. Plessier A, Darwish-Murad S, Hernandez-Guerra M, Consigny Y, Fabris F, Trebicka J, et al. Acute portal vein thrombosis unrelated to cirrhosis: a prospective multicenter follow-up study. Hepatology. 2010;51(1):210–8.

44. Plessier A, Rautou P-E, Valla D-C. Management of hepatic vascular diseases. J Hepatol. 2012;56(Suppl 1):S25–38.

45. Zaman S, Wiebe S, Bernal W, Wendon J, Czuprynska J, Auzinger G. Increased prevalence of heparin-induced thrombocytopenia in patients with Budd-Chiari syndrome: a retrospective analysis. Eur J Gastroenterol Hepatol. 2016;28(8):967–71.

46. Rautou P-E, Douarin L, Denninger M-H, Escolano S, Lebrec D, Moreau R, et al. Bleeding in patients with Budd-Chiari syndrome. J Hepatol. 2011;54(1):56–63.
47. Chagneau-Derrode C, Roy L, Guilhot J, Gloria O, Ollivier-Hourmand I, Bureau C, et al. Impact of cytoreductive therapy on the outcome of patients with myeloproliferative neoplasms and hepatosplanchnic vein thrombosis. 58th ed; 2013. p. 857A.
48. Desbois AC, Rautou PE, Biard L, Belmatoug N, Wechsler B, Resche-Rigon M, et al. Behcet's disease in Budd-Chiari syndrome. Orphanet J Rare Dis. 2014;9:104.
49. Tripathi D, Sunderraj L, Vemala V, Mehrzad H, Zia Z, Mangat K, et al. Long-term outcomes following percutaneous hepatic vein recanalization for Budd-Chiari syndrome. Liver Int. 2017;37(1):111–20.
50. Zhang QQ, Xu H, Zu MH, Gu YM, Shen B, Wei N, et al. Strategy and long-term outcomes of endovascular treatment for Budd-Chiari syndrome complicated by inferior vena caval thrombosis. Eur J Vasc Endovasc Surg. 2014;47(5):550–7.
51. Huang Q, Shen B, Zhang Q, Xu H, Zu M, Gu Y, et al. Comparison of long-term outcomes of endovascular management for membranous and segmental inferior vena cava obstruction in patients with primary Budd-Chiari syndrome. Circ Cardiovasc Interv. 2016;9(3):e003104.
52. Qi X, Guo X, Fan D. Difference in Budd-Chiari syndrome between the West and China. Hepatology. 2015;62(2):656.
53. Fu Y-F, Li Y, Cui Y-F, Wei N, Li D-C, Xu H. Percutaneous recanalization for combined-type Budd-Chiari syndrome: strategy and long-term outcome. Abdom Imaging. 2015;40(8):3240–7.
54. Ding P-X, Zhang S-J, Li Z, Fu M-T, Hua Z-H, Zhang W-G. Long-term safety and outcome of percutaneous transhepatic venous balloon angioplasty for Budd-Chiari syndrome. J Gastroenterol Hepatol. 2016;31(1):222–8.
55. Fan X, Liu K, Che Y, Wang S, Wu X, Cao J, et al. Good clinical outcomes in Budd-Chiari syndrome with hepatic vein occlusion. Dig Dis Sci. 2016;61(10):3054–60.
56. Sharma VK, Ranade PR, Marar S, Nabi F, Nagral A. Long-term clinical outcome of Budd-Chiari syndrome in children after radiological intervention. Eur J Gastroenterol Hepatol. 2016;28(5):567–75.
57. Shalimar, Kumar A, Kedia S, Sharma H, Gamanagatti SR, Gulati GS, et al. Hepatic venous outflow tract obstruction: treatment outcomes and development of a new prognostic score. Aliment Pharmacol Ther. 2016;43(11):1154–67.
58. Tripathi D, Macnicholas R, Kothari C, Sunderraj L, Al-Hilou H, Rangarajan B, et al. Good clinical outcomes following transjugular intrahepatic portosystemic stent-shunts in Budd-Chiari syndrome. Aliment Pharmacol Ther. 2014;39(8):864–72.
59. Mentha G, Giostra E, Majno PE, Bechstein WO, Neuhaus P, O'Grady J, et al. Liver transplantation for Budd-Chiari syndrome: a European study on 248 patients from 51 centres. J Hepatol. 2006;44(3):520–8.
60. Potthoff A, Attia D, Pischke S, Mederacke I, Beutel G, Rifai K, et al. Long-term outcome of liver transplant patients with Budd-Chiari syndrome secondary to myeloproliferative neoplasms. Liver Int. 2015;35(8):2042–9.
61. Westbrook RH, Lea NC, Mohamedali AM, Smith AE, Orr DW, Roberts LN, et al. Prevalence and clinical outcomes of the 46/1 haplotype, Janus kinase 2 mutations, and ten-eleven translocation 2 mutations in Budd-Chiari syndrome and their impact on thrombotic complications post liver transplantation. Liver Transpl. 2012;18(7):819–27.
62. Okuda H, Yamagata H, Obata H, Iwata H, Sasaki R, Imai F, et al. Epidemiological and clinical features of Budd-Chiari syndrome in Japan. J Hepatol. 1995;22(1):1–9.
63. Almdal TP, Sørensen TI. Incidence of parenchymal liver diseases in Denmark, 1981 to 1985: analysis of hospitalization registry data. The Danish Association for the Study of the Liver. Hepatology. 1991;13(4):650–5.
64. Rajani R, Melin T, Björnsson E, Broomé U, Sangfelt P, Danielsson A, et al. Budd-Chiari syndrome in Sweden: epidemiology, clinical characteristics and survival – an 18-year experience. Liver Int. 2009;29(2):253–9.

65. Ageno W, Dentali F, Pomero F, Fenoglio L, Squizzato A, Pagani G, et al. Incidence rates and case fatality rates of portal vein thrombosis and Budd-Chiari syndrome. Thromb Haemost. Epub 2017 Feb 9.
66. Cheng D, Xu H, Lu Z-J, Hua R, Qiu H, Du H, et al. Clinical features and etiology of Budd-Chiari syndrome in Chinese patients: a single-center study. J Gastroenterol Hepatol. 2013;28(6):1061–7.
67. Han G, Qi X, Zhang W, He C, Yin Z, Wang J, et al. Percutaneous recanalization for Budd-Chiari syndrome: an 11-year retrospective study on patency and survival in 177 Chinese patients from a single center. Radiology. 2013;266(2):657–67.
68. Qi X, Wu F, Fan D, Han G. Prevalence of thrombotic risk factors in Chinese Budd-Chiari syndrome patients: results of a prospective validation study. Eur J Gastroenterol Hepatol. 2014;26(5):576–7.

Budd-Chiari Syndrome and Inferior Vena Cava Obstruction: The Asian Perspective

17

Qiuhe Wang and Guohong Han

17.1 Introduction

Budd-Chiari syndrome (BCS) includes a group of liver vascular diseases scarcely seen in western countries but that has a relatively higher incidence in Asian countries [1, 2]. BCS is characterized by vascular obstruction of the hepatic outflow, occurring at any level from hepatic venules to right atrium [3], and obstruction of inferior vena cava (IVC) is thus incorporated in this category. Unrecognized BCS has a potential to develop recurrent ascites, portal hypertension with complications, liver cirrhosis and hepatocellular carcinoma [4], whereas well-diagnosed BCS patients receiving adequate treatment can achieve a 5-year survival of around 75% [5]. The diagnostic workout of BCS, therefore, is of great significance and expertise to avoid missed diagnosis and misdiagnosis is required. The current review aims at summarizing the updated knowledge on non-invasiveness diagnosis of BCS particularly from the Asian perspective.

17.2 Who Should Be Suspected of BCS?

Due to the heterogeneity of the disease, clinical manifestation of BCS can be diverse, ranging from asymptomatic to fulminant liver failure [6]. Although the classical triad, abdominal pain, ascites, and hepatomegaly can be seen frequently in BCS patients [7], up to 20% patients are asymptomatic at diagnosis [8]. Asymptomatic BCS are usually diagnosed in routine medical examination, e.g. finding of direct signs of hepatic vein obstruction in abdominal ultrasound. For symptomatic patients, the most frequent clinical features of BCS recorded in recent

Q. Wang • G. Han (✉)
Department of Liver Disease and Digestive Interventional Radiology, National Clinical
Research Center for Digestive Diseases and Xijing Hospital of Digestive Diseases,
Fourth Military Medical University, Xi'an, China
e-mail: hangh@fmmu.edu.cn

© Springer International Publishing AG, part of Springer Nature 2018
A. Berzigotti, J. Bosch (eds.), *Diagnostic Methods for Cirrhosis and Portal Hypertension*, https://doi.org/10.1007/978-3-319-72628-1_17

published articles from Asian countries are listed in Table 17.1 [9–17]. The most frequently seen clinical manifestations are ascites, hepatomegaly, abdominal distension, and pedal edema, whereas variceal bleeding, hepatic encephalopathy, and jaundice are less common. It should be noted that, in countries with a relatively high incidence of IVC obstruction, such as China, lower limb fatigue and pigmentation are also common presentations [10, 11, 13, 14, 18, 19].

Generally, BCS should be suspected in a patient with following presentations: (1) simultaneous ascites, liver enlargement and upper abdominal pain; (2) intractable ascites with mildly altered liver function tests; (3) known underlying thrombophilia condition, either inherited or acquired; (4) fulminant hepatic failure associating with liver enlargement and ascites; (5) unexplained chronic liver disease after excluding alcoholism, chronic viral hepatitis B or C, autoimmunity, iron overload, Wilson's disease and alpha-1 antitrypsin deficiency [4]. It should be noted that these manifestations, although suggestive of BCS, are not specific, and its absence does not exclude the diagnosis since clinical manifestations are largely determined by the existence and patency of large intrahepatic or extrahepatic collaterals [6, 20]. For the same reason, the duration of symptoms is not indicative of prognosis.

17.3   How to Diagnose BCS?

When BCS is suspected, patients should receive a step-wise diagnostic work out for minimal invasiveness to diagnose or rule out BCS (Fig. 17.1).

17.3.1 Ultrasonography

Given the typical vascular disorder nature of BCS, abdominal Doppler ultrasonography is usually considered as a must for BCS since it meets the most important goal of identifying stenosis or obstruction with a relatively high sensitivity and specificity, of over 80% [21], with low cost, easy accessibility and most important, noninvasiveness. However, diagnosing BCS with ultrasound require expertise and experience, and the accuracy of diagnosis may partly be influenced by patient body size/composition [22].

Doppler-ultrasound is able to detect stenosis or obstruction occurring at levels from hepatic veins to inferior vena cava. Suggestive findings are: (1) no flow or flow in an abnormal direction in all or part of the hepatic veins; (2) stenosis of hepatic veins, aliasing at the hepatic ostium; (3) high flow velocity at the site of stenosis; (4) phasic to absent, reversed, turbulent or continuous flow in the IVC, hepatic veins, or both [23]; and (5) slow hepatofugal flow (<11 cm/s) at the level of portal vein [24].

Gray-scale ultrasonography, or B-mode ultrasonography, can also be useful in making the diagnosis by disclosing direct or indirect signs of BCS (Table 17.2) [23, 25–29].

Table 17.1 Summary of major symptoms at presentation in Asian BCS patients (% of patients)

First author	Year	Country	Ascites	Hepatomegaly	Abdominal distention	Pedal edema	Abdominal pain	Abdominal wall varices	Splenomegaly	Lower limb varices	Variceal bleeding	Jaundice	Encephalopathy
Amarapurka	2008	India	86	–	–	12	–	28	20	–	8	20	4
Han	2013	China	52	–	75	54	12	32	–	–	12	–	0.5
Cheng	2013	China	53	28	31	52	21	50	78	42	21	–	–
Nozari	2013	Iran	76	60	38	–	60	–	34	–	–	18	–
Qi	2014	China	94	–	6	55	22	29	–	–	43	–	6
Shalimar	2016	India	80	58	–	46	27	30	38	–	23	20	6
Kucukay	2016	Turkey	88	97	–	–	84	94	40	–	–	–	–
Ki	2016	Korea	21	–	–	–	–	–	–	–	10	–	–
Cui	2016	China	95	–	100	–	34	–	–	–	9	12	–

Fig. 17.1 Step-wise diagnostic work-up of BCS aiming at minimal invasiveness

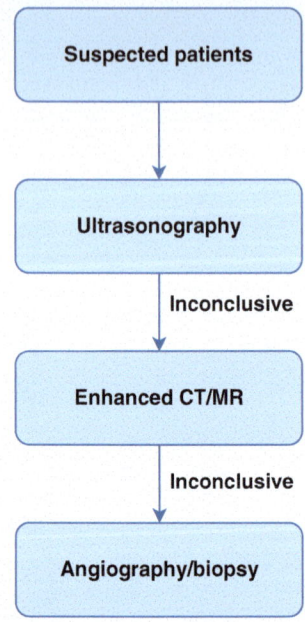

Table 17.2 Direct and indirect signs of BCS at gray-scale ultrasonography

Direct signs	Indirect signs
Hepatic veins • Non-visualized or tortuous hepatic veins • Replacement of the hepatic vein by a fibrous, echogenic cord • Stenosis with proximal dilatation, intraluminal echogenicity, thickened walls, and thrombosis • A smaller caliber of a hepatic vein than normal while the other being considerably large	**Liver** • Hepatomegaly • Caudate lobe enlargement • Hemorrhagic hepatic infarction
IVC • Localized, marked narrowing consistent with a web or a thrombus, uncommonly, aneurysm formation • Long segment narrowing without enlarged caudate lobe • Narrowing due to compression by the enlarged caudate lobe • A caudate vein ≥3 mm in diameter draining directly into IVC	**Collaterals** • Intrahepatic collaterals that communicate with systemic veins via collaterals from an occluded hepatic vein to a non-occluded hepatic vein or to the caudate lobe veins • Hepatic veins to the supra-hepatic IVC **Others** • Splenomegaly • Ascites

Abbreviations: *IVC* inferior vena cava

17.3.2 Computer Tomography (CT)

Contrast-enhanced CT is recommended as a second line diagnostic modality for BCS patients. Compared with ultrasonography, enhanced CT is advantageous in depicting not only the patency of hepatic veins and IVC, but also morphological changes and parenchymal abnormalities such as necrotic areas, liver perfusion, and intrahepatic/extrahepatic collaterals [30, 31], and thus is especially recommended whenever a transjugular intrahepatic portosystemic shunt (TIPS) is considered for a BCS patient [6, 26].

The two most characterized signs of BCS at an early stage under CT are obstruction in hepatic outflow tract or lack of visualization of hepatic veins and heterogeneously enhanced liver parenchymal [4, 32]. In terms of hepatic outflow obstruction, although non-visualized or thrombosis in hepatic veins can be observed with CT, false-positive or indeterminate rates may be as high as 50%, whereas membranous "web" obstruction in IVC, frequently seen type of obstruction in eastern Asia [11, 15, 18, 33–35], can hardly be detected [36]. These limitations makes CT a second choice modality to accurately identify type and site of obstruction [37]. Heterogenous enhancement of liver parenchyma is also described as patchy enhancement or mottled appearance [32], and is a result of the blood flow stasis within the sinusoids and portal vein with increased enhancement of the central part of the liver parenchyma and decreased enhancement in the periphery [27, 28, 38, 39]. An enlarged caudate lobe with increased enhancement is usually present [40].

As the disease progresses and move towards chronic stage, intrahepatic and extrahepatic collateral veins develop and sometimes may even be the only suggestive clue when other evidence of BCS are absent [24]. Another important morphological abnormality in patients with protracted BCS is the development of multiple regenerative nodules as a probable response to a localized portal perfusion loss and compensatory arterialization in areas with remnant hepatic venous outflow [41–44]. These regenerative nodules can be considerably enhanced and thus some patients may be misdiagnosed as hepatocellular carcinoma (HCC). However, the benign nodules are characterized by homogeneous hyper-enhancement on arterial phase images and remain slightly hyper-enhanced on portal venous phase images, whereas HCC nodules usually demonstrate heterogeneous hyper-enhancement on arterial phase and hypo-enhanced at portal phase [24]. In long-lasting BCS, radiological appearance similar to liver cirrhosis with spontaneous portosytemic shunts may be seen [30].

17.3.3 Magnetic Resonance Imaging (MRI)

MRI is an alternative to CT in patients with inconclusive ultrasonography results [45]. More importantly, MRI can be used in patients with impaired renal function that cannot receive radiologic contrast media. It is also advantageous for better anatomic orientation of the vessels (for example, visualizing the entire length of the IVC) and may differentiate acute from subacute and chronic BCS [45, 46].

MRI can show hepatic vein or IVC obstruction, hepatomegaly, heterogeneous signal intensity of the parenchyma, caudate lobe enlargement, and regenerative nodules.

Enhanced MR images acquired with T1-weighted sequences can clearly delineate the occlusion of hepatic outflow tract. Notably, Enhanced MRI is particularly useful in differentiating regenerative nodules from HCC nodules [47, 48]. Regenerative nodules are bright on T1-weighted MR images and strongly hyper-vascular and are mainly isointense or hypo-intense compared to the liver parenchymal on T2-weighted images [24, 41–44]. In contrast, the HCC nodules are usually hypo-intense compared to the liver on T1-weighted images and hyper-intense on T2-weighted images [24].

MR angiography, especially 3D MR angiography, can be helpful in providing the vascular anatomy and collaterals in multiple projections. Findings of aberrantly shaped arterial and portal vessels are indirect signs of severe structural changes in parenchyma [27], and differentiating fresh thrombus from organized or tumor thrombus are facilitated [31, 44].

17.3.4 Angiography/Venography

Angiography (venography) is currently considered as the golden standard for diagnosing BCS [2, 6, 49] to demonstrate not only the level, but also the extent and morphology of obstruction, allowing identification of membranes, webs, and segmental stenoses or obstructions. Furthermore, at angiography a transjugular liver biopsy and measurement of the hepatic venous pressure gradient can be performed [50], which may help in diagnosis and in evaluating treatment success [30, 51] and may help in clinical decision-making. In patients who in which a transvenous approach fails, transhepatic angiography may be considered [11, 13, 28].

At venography, the BCS is characterized by demonstrating the "spider web pattern", which is considered to be formed by collaterals between small hepatic vein branches [52]. Fine collaterals at an early stage give rise to a "fine spider web", while long-standing collaterals are thicker, giving rise to a "coarse spider web". In some patients, retro-hepatic portion of IVC demonstrates a compressed shape due to hypertrophy of the caudate lobe [32].

17.3.5 Liver Biopsy

In BCS liver biopsy is usually performed to exclude other causes of liver disease rather than to confirm the diagnosis, owing to the sampling error caused by the patchy liver involvement [53]. Typical findings are centrilobular congestion and necrosis, along with sinusoidal dilatation, yet the specificity of these findings is limited.

17.4 What Should Be Further Investigated?

Classification of BCS according to the type and site of obstruction [1, 7, 20, 26, 47, 54, 55], should be made at diagnosis in order to select the appropriate treatment modality. Classification criteria are listed in Table 17.3 [21, 56–59].

Table 17.3 Classification of BCS according to site and type of obstruction

Site of obstruction	Type of obstruction
Hepatic veins	**Webs and membranes**
• Terminal hepatic veins (central veins), intercalated veins	**Short-length stenosis**
	Smooth tapering less than 4 cm in length of
• Interlobular veins (collecting veins)	venous lumen
• Segmental hepatic vein branches	
IVC	**Intraluminal thrombus**
• Hepatic segment	**Fibrous cord**
• Suprahepatic segment	
Combined	**Nonspecific changes**
• IVC combined with one or more hepatic veins	Diffuse reduction in caliber, tortuous or irregular appearance

Abbreviations: *IVC* inferior vena cava

Table 17.4 Thrombophilic disorders that should be included in the diagnostic work-up of BCS

Inherited thrombophilia	Acquired thrombophilia
Factor V Leiden mutation	Myeloproliferative neoplasm
Factor II G20210A mutation	Antiphospholipid syndrome
Protein C deficiency	Hyperhomocysteinemia
Protein S deficiency	Paroxysmal nocturnal hemoglobinuria
Antithrombin III deficiency	Oral contraceptive use
MTHFR C677T mutation	Behcet's disease

Abbreviations: *MTHFR* methylenetetrahydrofolate reductase

Additional investigations include:

17.4.1 Etiological Factors

Most western BCS patients have underlying thrombophilia as etiology. The three most frequent etiology in these countries, i.e. myeloproliferative neoplasms (MPN), factor V Leyden mutation and antiphospholipid syndrome, are scarcely seen in Asian patients [9, 15, 17, 60–63]. Moreover, despite that Chinese patients have a high prevalence of methylenetetrahydrofolate reductase C677T gene mutation [62], the association between this mutation and occurrence of thrombosis in hepatic veins and IVC remains uncertain, thus the major cause of BCS in eastern countries is still unclear and most cases are considered idiopathic [63–65]. However, screening for thrombophilic disorders (Table 17.4) is still recommended in order to initiate specific treatment as soon as possible, especially for MPN patients [2]. The latest guidelines recommended testing calreticulin (CALR) mutation in all suspected MPN patients without JAK2 V617F mutation. However, according to a recent study, spleen size >16 cm and platelet count ≤200 × 10^9 have a specificity of 100%, suggesting that such patients do not require CALR mutation tests [66] (Fig. 17.2). This finding is especially significant for Asian patients, since the incidence of both JAK2 and CALR mutations are rather low in these countries [62, 67].

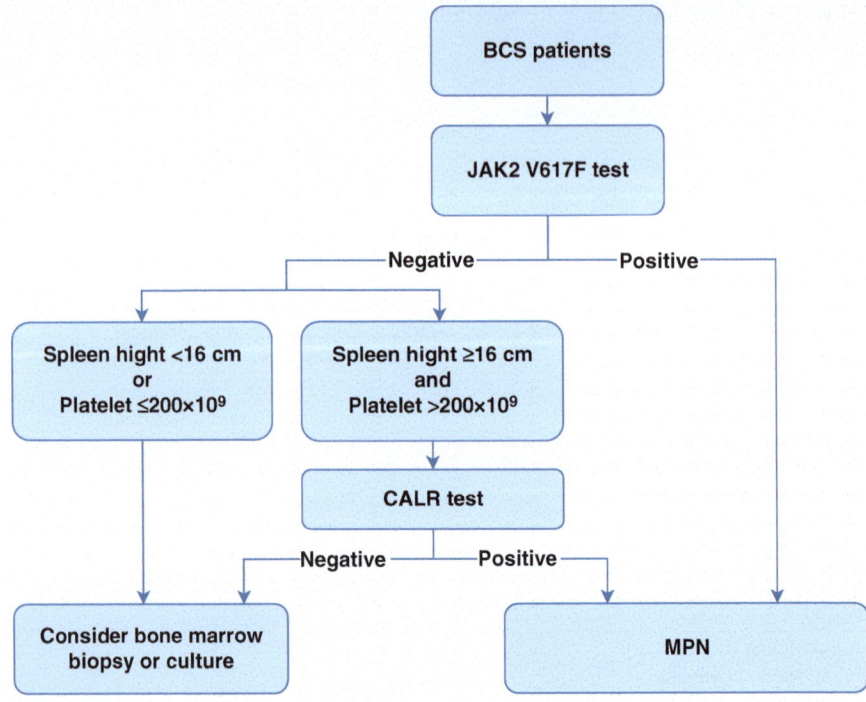

Fig. 17.2 Selective CALR test in BCS patients with suspected MPN

It should be noted that BCS patients may have more than one etiological factor [5], thus one positive finding in the etiology work-up should not prevent further investigations.

17.4.2 Liver Function Tests

Liver function tests offer little help in the diagnosis of BCS but reflects the severity of liver injury and is crucial for evaluating prognosis [22]. Specifically, alanine aminotransferase (ALT) elevated to five times the upper limit of normal values as well as a slow decline 3 days after ALT peak were reported to be associated with poor prognosis in BCS patients [68]. This has not been validated in Asian patients. Child-Pugh score and MELD score are also predictive of patient outcome in BCS [69]. Although other prognostic scores have been suggested [17, 70–72], predictive ability require further validation for their generalization [69].

17.4.3 Existence of Associated Portal Vein Thrombosis (PVT)

Occluded hepatic outflow tract lead to increased sinusoidal pressure and decreased portal flow velocity, which may contribute to portal vein thrombosis [1]. The possible existence of underlying thrombophilic disorder may further increase the risk of PVT. PVT is seen in about 15–20% in BCS patients in western countries, but there is no data from Asian countries. BCS patients with concomitant PVT tend to have a worse prognosis [73–75], and TIPS might be the better option for these patients [75].

Screening for PVT in BCS with Doppler is done first with ultrasonography and confirmed with CT or NMR [76].

17.4.4 HCC Surveillance

The prevalence of HCC among BCS patients is relatively high in Asian countries ranging from 2.8 % to 41 % [35, 77–80]. Some studies have suggested that IVC involvement, a common type of obstruction in many Asian countries, is related to a higher incidence of HCC [81–83], which might be accountable for the high HCC prevalence in these regions [80, 84]. These significant problems indicate that HCC surveillance is crucial.

As is mentioned above, the difficulties in differentiating HCC nodules and benign regenerative nodules is the most prominent issue in HCC surveillance. Moucari et al. reported that α fetoprotein (AFP) above 15 ng/ml is highly suggestive of HCC, and in patients with AFP ≤15 ng/ml, heterogenous or large (≥3 cm) nodules is strongly associated with HCC [82]. Biopsy of the largest nodule is recommended in these patients. Thereafter, close surveillance at 3-month intervals was suggested for the first year, and every 6-month thereafter [82]. Still, specific data in Asian patients is lacking.

Conclusion

An evidence-based diagnostic work-up specifically designed for Asian patients is lacking. We recommend a step-wise approach including ultrasonography as first line modality, CT/MR as second line modality, and angiography as confirmatory gold-standard. After diagnosis, screening for thrombophilic disorders is suggested, despite most Asian patients are considered idiopathic. Other investigations including liver function, assessment of concomitant portal vein thrombosis, and especially HCC surveillance should be performed.

Acknowledgement *Conflict of Interest*: The authors declare that they have no conflict of interest.

References

1. Menon KV, Shah V, Kamath PS. The Budd-Chiari syndrome. N Engl J Med. 2004;350:578–85.
2. EASL Clinical Practice Guidelines. Vascular diseases of the liver. J Hepatol. 2016;64:179–202.
3. Valla DC. Budd-Chiari syndrome and veno-occlusive disease/sinusoidal obstruction syndrome. Gut. 2008;57:1469–78.
4. Janssen HL, Garcia-Pagan JC, Elias E, Mentha G, Hadengue A, Valla DC. Budd-Chiari syndrome: a review by an expert panel. J Hepatol. 2003;38:364–71.

5. Darwish Murad S, Plessier A, Hernandez-Guerra M, Fabris F, Eapen CE, Bahr MJ, et al. Etiology, management, and outcome of the Budd-Chiari syndrome. Ann Intern Med. 2009;151:167–75.
6. DeLeve LD, Valla DC, Garcia-Tsao G. Vascular disorders of the liver. Hepatology. 2009;49:1729–64.
7. Martens P, Nevens F. Budd-Chiari syndrome. United European Gastroenterol J. 2015;3: 489–500.
8. Hadengue A, Poliquin M, Vilgrain V, Belghiti J, Degott C, Erlinger S, et al. The changing scene of hepatic vein thrombosis: recognition of asymptomatic cases. Gastroenterology. 1994;106:1042–7.
9. Amarapurkar DN, Punamiya SJ, Patel ND. Changing spectrum of Budd-Chiari syndrome in India with special reference to non-surgical treatment. World J Gastroenterol. 2008;14:278–85.
10. Cheng D, Xu H, Lu ZJ, Hua R, Qiu H, Du H, et al. Clinical features and etiology of Budd-Chiari syndrome in Chinese patients: a single-center study. J Gastroenterol Hepatol. 2013;28:1061–7.
11. Han G, Qi X, Zhang W, He C, Yin Z, Wang J, et al. Percutaneous recanalization for Budd-Chiari syndrome: an 11-year retrospective study on patency and survival in 177 Chinese patients from a single center. Radiology. 2013;266:657–67.
12. Nozari N, Vossoghinia H, Malekzadeh F, Kafami L, Mirheidari M, Malekzadeh R. Long-term outcome of Budd-Chiari syndrome: a single center experience. Middle East J Dig Dis. 2013;5:146–50.
13. Qi X, Guo W, He C, Zhang W, Wu F, Yin Z, et al. Transjugular intrahepatic portosystemic shunt for Budd-Chiari syndrome: techniques, indications and results on 51 Chinese patients from a single centre. Liver Int. 2014;34:1164–75.
14. Cui YF, Fu YF, Li DC, Xu H. Percutaneous recanalization for hepatic vein-type Budd-Chiari syndrome: long-term patency and survival. Hepatol Int. 2016;10:363–9.
15. Ki M, Choi HY, Kim KA, Kim BH, Jang ES, Jeong SH. Incidence, prevalence and complications of Budd-Chiari syndrome in South Korea: a nationwide, population-based study. Liver Int. 2016;36:1067–73.
16. Kucukay F, Akdogan M, Bostanci EB, Ulus AT, Kucukay MB. Percutaneous transluminal angioplasty for complete membranous obstruction of suprahepatic inferior vena cava: long-term results. Cardiovasc Intervent Radiol. 2016;39:1392–9.
17. Shalimar, Kumar A, Kedia S, Sharma H, Gamanagatti SR, Gulati GS, et al. Hepatic venous outflow tract obstruction: treatment outcomes and development of a new prognostic score. Aliment Pharmacol Ther. 2016;43:1154–67.
18. Zhang CQ, Fu LN, Xu L, Zhang GQ, Jia T, Liu JY, et al. Long-term effect of stent placement in 115 patients with Budd-Chiari syndrome. World J Gastroenterol. 2003;9:2587–91.
19. Li WD, Yu HY, Qian AM, Rong JJ, Zhang YQ, Li XQ. Risk factors for and causes and treatment of recurrence of inferior vena cava type of Budd-Chiari syndrome after stenting in China: a retrospective analysis of a large cohort. Eur Radiol. 2017;27:1227–37.
20. Valla DC. Primary Budd-Chiari syndrome. J Hepatol. 2009;50:195–203.
21. Bolondi L, Gaiani S, Li Bassi S, Zironi G, Bonino F, Brunetto M, et al. Diagnosis of Budd-Chiari syndrome by pulsed Doppler ultrasound. Gastroenterology. 1991;100:1324–31.
22. Goel RM, Johnston EL, Patel KV, Wong T. Budd-Chiari syndrome: investigation, treatment and outcomes. Postgrad Med J. 2015;91:692–7.
23. Bargallo X, Gilabert R, Nicolau C, Garcia-Pagan JC, Ayuso JR, Bru C. Sonography of Budd-Chiari syndrome. AJR Am J Roentgenol. 2006;187:W33–41.
24. Brancatelli G, Vilgrain V, Federle MP, Hakime A, Lagalla R, Iannaccone R, et al. Budd-Chiari syndrome: spectrum of imaging findings. AJR Am J Roentgenol. 2007;188:W168–76.
25. Bargallo X, Gilabert R, Nicolau C, Garcia-Pagan JC, Bosch J, Bru C. Sonography of the caudate vein: value in diagnosing Budd-Chiari syndrome. AJR Am J Roentgenol. 2003;181:1641–5.
26. Aydinli M, Bayraktar Y. Budd-Chiari syndrome: etiology, pathogenesis and diagnosis. World J Gastroenterol. 2007;13:2693–6.
27. Erden A. Budd-Chiari syndrome: a review of imaging findings. Eur J Radiol. 2007;61:44–56.
28. Ferral H, Behrens G, Lopera J. Budd-Chiari syndrome. AJR Am J Roentgenol. 2012;199:737–45.

29. Trivedi CR, Thakkar H, Sannananja B, Shah HU. Ultrasound and Doppler features of Budd-Chiari syndrome in pediatric population. Ultrasound Q. 2015;31:45–54.
30. Kamath PS. Budd-Chiari syndrome: Radiologic findings. Liver Transpl. 2006;12:S21–2.
31. Zimmerman MA, Cameron AM, Ghobrial RM. Budd-Chiari syndrome. Clin Liver Dis. 2006;10:259–73. viii
32. Mathieu D, Vasile N, Menu Y, Van Beers B, Lorphelin JM, Pringot J. Budd-Chiari syndrome: dynamic CT. Radiology. 1987;165:409–13.
33. Yamada R, Sato M, Kawabata M, Nakatsuka H, Nakamura K, Kobayashi N. Segmental obstruction of the hepatic inferior vena cava treated by transluminal angioplasty. Radiology. 1983;149:91–6.
34. Yang XL, TO C, Chen CR. Successful treatment by percutaneous balloon angioplasty of Budd-Chiari syndrome caused by membranous obstruction of inferior vena cava: 8-year follow-up study. J Am Coll Cardiol. 1996;28:1720–4.
35. Park H, Yoon JY, Park KH, Kim DY, Ahn SH, Han KH, et al. Hepatocellular carcinoma in Budd-Chiari syndrome: a single center experience with long-term follow-up in South Korea. World J Gastroenterol. 2012;18:1946–52.
36. Lim JH, Park JH, Auh YH. Membranous obstruction of the inferior vena cava: comparison of findings at sonography, CT, and venography. AJR Am J Roentgenol. 1992;159:515–20.
37. Gupta S, Barter S, Phillips GW, Gibson RN, Hodgson HJ. Comparison of ultrasonography, computed tomography and 99mTc liver scan in diagnosis of Budd-Chiari syndrome. Gut. 1987;28:242–7.
38. Camera L, Mainenti PP, Di Giacomo A, Romano M, Rispo A, Alfinito F, et al. Triphasic helical CT in Budd-Chiari syndrome: patterns of enhancement in acute, subacute and chronic disease. Clin Radiol. 2006;61:331–7.
39. Mukund A, Gamanagatti S. Imaging and interventions in Budd-Chiari syndrome. World J Radiol. 2011;3:169–77.
40. Copelan A, Remer EM, Sands M, Nghiem H, Kapoor B. Diagnosis and management of Budd Chiari syndrome: an update. Cardiovasc Intervent Radiol. 2015;38:1–12.
41. Bas K, Yaprak O, Dayangac M, Ulusoy OL, Dogusoy GB, Yuzer Y, et al. Living-donor liver transplant in 3 patients with Budd-Chiari syndrome: case report. Exp Clin Transplant. 2012;10:172–5.
42. Heller MT, Hattoum A. Imaging of acute conditions affecting the hepatic vasculature. Emerg Radiol. 2012;19:329–39.
43. Jang HJ, Khalili K, Yu H, Kim TK. Perfusion and parenchymal changes related to vascular alterations of the liver. Abdom Imaging. 2012;37:404–21.
44. Patil P, Deshmukh H, Popat B, Rathod K. Spectrum of imaging in Budd Chiari syndrome. J Med Imaging Radiat Oncol. 2012;56:75–83.
45. Noone TC, Semelka RC, Siegelman ES, Balci NC, Hussain SM, Kim PN, et al. Budd-Chiari syndrome: spectrum of appearances of acute, subacute, and chronic disease with magnetic resonance imaging. J Magn Reson Imaging. 2000;11:44–50.
46. Brancatelli G, Federle MP, Grazioli L, Golfieri R, Lencioni R. Large regenerative nodules in Budd-Chiari syndrome and other vascular disorders of the liver: CT and MR imaging findings with clinicopathologic correlation. AJR Am J Roentgenol. 2002;178:877–83.
47. McKusick MA. Imaging findings in Budd-Chiari syndrome. Liver Transpl. 2001;7:743–4.
48. Maetani Y, Itoh K, Egawa H, Haga H, Sakurai T, Nishida N, et al. Benign hepatic nodules in Budd-Chiari syndrome: radiologic-pathologic correlation with emphasis on the central scar. AJR Am J Roentgenol. 2002;178:869–75.
49. de Franchis R. Expanding consensus in portal hypertension: Report of the Baveno VI Consensus Workshop: stratifying risk and individualizing care for portal hypertension. J Hepatol. 2015;63:743–52.
50. Klein AS, Molmenti EP. Surgical treatment of Budd-Chiari syndrome. Liver Transpl. 2003;9:891–6.
51. Plessier A, Sibert A, Consigny Y, Hakime A, Zappa M, Denninger MH, et al. Aiming at minimal invasiveness as a therapeutic strategy for Budd-Chiari syndrome. Hepatology. 2006;44:1308–16.

52. Plessier A, Valla DC. Budd-Chiari syndrome. Semin Liver Dis. 2008;28:259–69.
53. Tang TJ, Batts KP, de Groen PC, van Hoek B, Haagsma EB, Hop WC, et al. The prognostic value of histology in the assessment of patients with Budd-Chiari syndrome. J Hepatol. 2001;35:338–43.
54. Budd G. Diseases of the liver. Philadelphia: Lea & Blanchard; 1846.
55. Langlet P, Escolano S, Valla D, Coste-Zeitoun D, Denie C, Mallet A, et al. Clinicopathological forms and prognostic index in Budd-Chiari syndrome. J Hepatol. 2003;39:496–501.
56. Ludwig J, Hashimoto E, McGill DB, van Heerden JA. Classification of hepatic venous outflow obstruction: ambiguous terminology of the Budd-Chiari syndrome. Mayo Clin Proc. 1990;65:51–5.
57. Valla D, Hadengue A, el Younsi M, Azar N, Zeitoun G, Boudet MJ, et al. Hepatic venous outflow block caused by short-length hepatic vein stenoses. Hepatology. 1997;25:814–9.
58. Kreel L, Freston JW, Clain D. Vascular radiology in the Budd-Chiari syndrome. Br J Radiol. 1967;40:755–9.
59. Menu Y, Alison D, Lorphelin JM, Valla D, Belghiti J, Nahum H. Budd-Chiari syndrome: US evaluation. Radiology. 1985;157:761–4.
60. Qi X, Guo X, Fan D. Difference in Budd-Chiari syndrome between the West and China. Hepatology. 2015;62:656.
61. De Stefano V, Qi X, Betti S, Rossi E. Splanchnic vein thrombosis and myeloproliferative neoplasms: molecular-driven diagnosis and long-term treatment. Thromb Haemost. 2016;115:240–9.
62. Qi X, Wu F, Ren W, He C, Yin Z, Niu J, et al. Thrombotic risk factors in Chinese Budd-Chiari syndrome patients. An observational study with a systematic review of the literature. Thromb Haemost. 2013;109:878–84.
63. Augustin S, Pons M, Santos B, Ventura M, Genescà J. Portal hypertension VI: Proceedings of the sixth Baveno consensus workshop: stratifying risk and individualizing care. Switzerland: Springer International Publishing; 2016.
64. Bosy-Westphal A, Ruschmeyer M, Czech N, Oehler G, Hinrichsen H, Plauth M, et al. Determinants of hyperhomocysteinemia in patients with chronic liver disease and after orthotopic liver transplantation. Am J Clin Nutr. 2003;77:1269–77.
65. Frederiksen J, Juul K, Grande P, Jensen GB, Schroeder TV, Tybjaerg-Hansen A, et al. Methylenetetrahydrofolate reductase polymorphism (C677T), hyperhomocysteinemia, and risk of ischemic cardiovascular disease and venous thromboembolism: prospective and case-control studies from the Copenhagen City Heart Study. Blood. 2004;104:3046–51.
66. Poisson J, Plessier A, Kiladjian JJ, Turon F, Cassinat B, Andreoli A, et al. Selective testing for calreticulin gene mutations in patients with splanchnic vein thrombosis: a prospective cohort study. J Hepatol. 2017;67(3):501–7.
67. Zhang P, Ma H, Min Q, Zu M, Lu Z. CALR mutations in Chinese Budd-Chiari syndrome patients. Eur J Gastroenterol Hepatol. 2016;28:361–2.
68. Rautou PE, Moucari R, Cazals-Hatem D, Escolano S, Denie C, Douarin L, et al. Levels and initial course of serum alanine aminotransferase can predict outcome of patients with Budd-Chiari syndrome. Clin Gastroenterol Hepatol. 2009;7:1230–5.
69. Rautou PE, Moucari R, Escolano S, Cazals-Hatem D, Denie C, Chagneau-Derrode C, et al. Prognostic indices for Budd-Chiari syndrome: valid for clinical studies but insufficient for individual management. Am J Gastroenterol. 2009;104:1140–6.
70. Malinchoc M, Kamath PS, Gordon FD, Peine CJ, Rank J, ter Borg PC. A model to predict poor survival in patients undergoing transjugular intrahepatic portosystemic shunts. Hepatology. 2000;31:864–71.
71. Zeitoun G, Escolano S, Hadengue A, Azar N, El Younsi M, Mallet A, et al. Outcome of Budd-Chiari syndrome: a multivariate analysis of factors related to survival including surgical portosystemic shunting. Hepatology. 1999;30:84–9.
72. Darwish Murad S, Valla DC, de Groen PC, Zeitoun G, Hopmans JA, Haagsma EB, et al. Determinants of survival and the effect of portosystemic shunting in patients with Budd-Chiari syndrome. Hepatology. 2004;39:500–8.

73. Mahmoud AE, Helmy AS, Billingham L, Elias E. Poor prognosis and limited therapeutic options in patients with Budd-Chiari syndrome and portal venous system thrombosis. Eur J Gastroenterol Hepatol. 1997;9:485–9.
74. Watanabe H, Shinzawa H, Saito T, Ishibashi M, Shirahata N, Miyano S, et al. Successful emergency treatment with a transjugular intrahepatic portosystemic shunt for life-threatening Budd-Chiari syndrome with portal thrombotic obstruction. Hepato-Gastroenterology. 2000;47:839–41.
75. Darwish Murad S, Valla DC, de Groen PC, Zeitoun G, Haagsma EB, Kuipers EJ, et al. Pathogenesis and treatment of Budd-Chiari syndrome combined with portal vein thrombosis. Am J Gastroenterol. 2006;101:83–90.
76. Ganger DR, Klapman JB, McDonald V, Matalon TA, Kaur S, Rosenblate H, et al. Transjugular intrahepatic portosystemic shunt (TIPS) for Budd-Chiari syndrome or portal vein thrombosis: review of indications and problems. Am J Gastroenterol. 1999;94:603–8.
77. Dilawari JB, Bambery P, Chawla Y, Kaur U, Bhusnurmath SR, Malhotra HS, et al. Hepatic outflow obstruction (Budd-Chiari syndrome). Experience with 177 patients and a review of the literature. Medicine (Baltimore). 1994;73:21–36.
78. Paul SB, Shalimar, Sreenivas V, Gamanagatti SR, Sharma H, Dhamija E, et al. Incidence and risk factors of hepatocellular carcinoma in patients with hepatic venous outflow tract obstruction. Aliment Pharmacol Ther. 2015;41:961–71.
79. Franchis R. Portal hypertension VI: Proceedings of the sixth Baveno consensus workshop: stratifying risk and individualizing care. Switzerland: Springer International Publishing; 2016.
80. Ren W, Qi X, Yang Z, Han G, Fan D. Prevalence and risk factors of hepatocellular carcinoma in Budd-Chiari syndrome: a systematic review. Eur J Gastroenterol Hepatol. 2013;25:830–41.
81. Rector WG Jr, Xu YH, Goldstein L, Peters RL, Reynolds TB. Membranous obstruction of the inferior vena cava in the United States. Medicine (Baltimore). 1985;64:134–43.
82. Moucari R, Rautou PE, Cazals-Hatem D, Geara A, Bureau C, Consigny Y, et al. Hepatocellular carcinoma in Budd-Chiari syndrome: characteristics and risk factors. Gut. 2008;57:828–35.
83. Shrestha SM. Liver cirrhosis in hepatic vena cava syndrome (or membranous obstruction of inferior vena cava). World J Hepatol. 2015;7:874–84.
84. Seijo S, Plessier A, Hoekstra J, Dell'era A, Mandair D, Rifai K, et al. Good long-term outcome of Budd-Chiari syndrome with a step-wise management. Hepatology. 2013;57:1962–8.

Extrahepatic Portal Vein Obstruction: Asian and Global Perspective

18

Rakhi Maiwall and Shiv Kumar Sarin

18.1 Introduction

The first case of portal vein thrombosis was described by Stewart and Balfour in the late 1860s in a patient with splenomegaly, ascites and variceal dilatation [1]. The portal vein comprises of 75% of the total blood flow to the liver and forms the backbone of the portal venous system. It is 8 cm wide valveless conduit formed by the confluence of the superior mesenteric and splenic veins behind the neck of the pancreas. Thrombosis of the portal vein refers to the thrombotic and non-thrombotic occlusion of the portal vein as well as cavernoma formation. It refers to thrombosis of the trunk of the portal vein with or without extension into the right and left intrahepatic branches. The thrombotic process may even extend to the splenic or superior mesenteric veins. Portal vein thrombosis is known to exist in association with cirrhosis or malignancy or without any associated condition i.e. non-malignant and non-cirrhotic portal vein thrombosis. Portal cavernoma is a sequel of chronic portal vein thrombosis wherein the vein is replaced by numerous tortuous vascular channels. As these collateral channels are insufficient to bypass the entire blood flow from the spleno-mesenteric axis therefore the clinical signs of portal hypertension are frequently present [2].

18.2 Prevalence

Extra Hepatic Portal Venous Obstruction (EHPVO) is considered as a separate entity which refers to the development of portal cavernoma in the absence of associated liver disease and is the commonest cause of non-cirrhotic portal hypertension in Asia where EHPVO is the cause of portal hypertension in almost 80–85%

R. Maiwall, M.B.B.S., M.D., D.M. (✉) • S.K. Sarin
Department of Hepatology, Institute of Liver and Biliary Sciences, New Delhi, India
e-mail: rakhi_2011@yahoo.co.in

© Springer International Publishing AG, part of Springer Nature 2018
A. Berzigotti, J. Bosch (eds.), *Diagnostic Methods for Cirrhosis and Portal Hypertension*, https://doi.org/10.1007/978-3-319-72628-1_18

of children presenting with variceal bleeds and about 40% of adults presenting with portal hypertension [2]. The prevalence of PVT in compensated cirrhotics is around 0.6–16%, in advanced cirrhotics awaiting liver transplantation 8–25%, and about 36–70% in the explanted liver on histopathology [3–5]. In a systematic review the prevalence of PVT in patients with hepatocellular carcinoma was reported to be 36%, in patients with primary biliary cirrhosis 3.6%, in primary sclerosing cholangitis in 8%, and 16% in alcohol related and Hepatitis B related cirrhosis. In a recent autopsy study the lifetime risk of PVT in general population was reported to be 1% [6].

18.3   Etiology and Pathophysiological Basis of PVT

The main pathophysiological basis of portal venous thrombosis is based on the "*Virchow's triad*" which comprises of venous stasis, hypercoagulability and endo-thelial injury.

Rigorous search is required to diagnose an underlying thrombophilic condition in almost 80% of the patients and less than 20% of the cases of PVT are now con-sidered as idiopathic [7–11]. Indeed, two or more factors are seen in 40% of the patients [12–15].

In adults, abdominal malignancies are the cause of PVT in almost 50%, the com-monest being pancreatic and hepatocellular carcinoma [12, 15].

PVT may occur due to pylephlebitis or septic thrombosis of the portal vein in patients with intraabdominal infections or inflammation, such as pancreatitis, diver-ticulitis or appendicitis. In most of these patients, the thrombotic process is either due sluggish flow, hypercoagulability or constriction or invasion of the portal vein.

In Asian countries, the development of EHPVO in children is commonly related to sepsis or omphalitis in the neonatal period. Umbilical vein catheterization has been identified as important risk factor in neonates [16]. However, spontaneous recanalization (either complete or partial) of the umbilical vein has been reported by follow up ultrasonography in an Indian study [17]. Abdominal sepsis has also been identified as a risk factor in 11% of PVT in a large prospective study [18]. A strong association between Bacteroides fragilis infection and PVT has been suggested [19]. The transient development of anticardiolipin antibodies has been suggested as a pathophysiological link between this infection and PVT [20].

18.4   Inherited and Acquired Thrombophilias

In almost one-third of the patients primary myeloproliferative disorders, either occult (in 16.7%) or manifest (13.8%) are the cause of PVT (Tables 18.1 and 18.2). The identification of Janus-kinase (JAK2) V617F mutation, which is seen in 17–35% of the PVT patients, has led to an increase in the diagnosis of the myelo-proliferative disorders. In a recent meta-analysis comprising 23 studies, irrespective of the underlying etiological factors, the pooled prevalence of JAK2 was noted in

Table 18.1 Proposed classification of PVT in cirrhosis

Site of PVT (Type 1, 2a, 2b, 3)
  Type 1: Only trunk
  Type 2: Only branch: 2a, one branch; 2b, both branches
  Type 3: Trunk and branches

Degree of portal venous system occlusion (O, NO)
  O: Occlusive: No flow visible in PV lumen on imaging/Doppler study
  NO: Non-occlusive: Flow visible in PV lumen through imaging/Doppler study

Duration and Presentation (R, Ch)
  R: Recent (first time detected in previously patent PV, presence of hyperdense thrombus on
    imaging, absent or limited collateral circulation, dilated PV at the site of occlusion)
  Asymptomatic (As)
  Symptomatic: (S), Acute PVT features (with or without ABI)
  Ch: Chronic (no hyperdense thrombus; previously diagnosed PVT, portal cavernoma and
    clinical features of PHT)
  Asymptomatic
  Symptomatic: features of portal hypertension (with or without PHT)

Extent of PV system occlusion (S, M, SM)
  Splenic vein (S), mesenteric vein (M) or both (SM)

Type and presence of underlying liver disease
  Cirrhotic
  Non-cirrhotic Liver Disease
  Post-Liver Transplant
  HCC
  Local Malignancies and associated conditions

24% of patients with PVT which decreased to 19% after exclusion of known myelo-proliferative disorders (MPD) [21]. A more recent meta-analysis including 855 patients with PVT the mean prevalence of MPD and JAK2V617F mutation was 31.5% and 27.7% respectively. These results lead to the suggestion of including JAK2 in the routine work up of patients with PVT [22].

In Asians, in a Chinese study, the prevalence of JAK2 mutation was reported to be 24–26.6% in non-cirrhotic non-malignant PVT versus just 1.4% in cirrhosis with PVT [23]. Further, this study found that in non-malignant and non-cirrhotic patients with PVT, higher platelet counts and older age were independent predictors of the JAK2V617F mutation. In an Indian study, the prevalence of JAK2 mutation was reported in 14% in patients with abdominal vein thrombosis [24]. Other prothrombotic conditions that cause PVT include paroxysmal nocturnal hemoglobinuria (PNH), hyperhomocysteinemia, antiphospholipid syndrome, and inherited thrombophilic states, such as Protein C deficiency (in 0–9.1%), Protein S (0.9–30%) and antithrombin III deficiencies (0–4.5%) (Tables 18.1–18.6). Less frequent mutations include factor V Leiden (1.3–7.6%), factor II mutation (G20210A in 0–22%) and methylene-tetrahydrofolate-reductase (MTHFR) gene mutation [8–10]. An important caveat here is that the levels of these can be low in parenchymal liver disease, which calls for confirmation of the diagnosis by screening first degree family members [10, 25]. D'Amico and colleagues showed predominant role of PAI-14G-4G and MTHFR677TT in abdominal thrombosis in non-cirrhotic non-malignant splanchnic vein thrombosis in a cohort of 235 Caucasian patients, 54 with portal

Table 18.2 Risk Factors for the development of portal vein thrombosis

Systemic thrombophilia inherited:	Inflammatory diseases
• Factor V Leiden mutation	• Behcet's Disease
• Factor II-Prothrombin mutation-G20210A	• Pancreatitis
• Protein C deficiency	• Diverticulitis
• Protein S deficiency	• Appendicitis
• Antithrombin deficiency	• Cholecystitis
• Methylenetetrahydrofolate reductase mutationTT677	• Inflammatory Bowel Disease
	Hepatobiliary malignancy: • Hepatocellular carcinoma • Pancreatic Carcinoma • Cholangiocarcinoma
Acquired Thrombophilias: • Myeloproliferative disorder including polycythemia vera	Sluggish Portal Vein Flow
• Paroxysmal nocturnal hemoglobinuria	• Liver Cirrhosis
• Pregnancy or puerperium	• Budd-Chiari Syndrome
• Antiphospholipid syndrome	• Sinusoidal obstruction syndrome
• Oral contraceptives	• Nodular Regenerative Hyperplasia
• Hyperhomocysteinemia	
• Nephrotic Syndrome	Miscellaneous
• Sickle Cell Anemia	• Living at high altitude
• Increased factor VIII levels	• Choledochal cyst
• Thrombin activatable fibrinolysis inhibitor gene (TAFI)	• Bladder Cancer
Iatrogenic injury of the portal vein:	
• Umbilical vein catheterization	
• Splenectomy	
• Abdominal Surgery	
• Alcohol Injection	
• Colectomy	
• Endoscopic Sclerotherapy	
• Radiofrequency Ablation	
• Fundoplication	
• Peritoneal Dialysis	

vein thrombosis. In a recent meta-analysis which included nine studies, the pooled prevalence of inherited antithrombin, Protein C, and Protein S deficiencies were 3.9%, 5.6%, and 2.6%, respectively.

18.5   Cirrhosis Associated Hypercoagulability and Portal Vein Thrombosis

In the context of cirrhosis, PVT is attributed to the underlying hypercoagulable state that is present despite the fact that these patients have increased international normalized ratio [26, 27]. Cirrhosis is characterized by an imbalance between the pro (increased levels of factor VIII) and anticoagulation proteins (decreased levels of protein C due to impaired synthesis) [28]. Consequent to this, the balance is tilted either towards bleeding or thrombosis [28–31]. Long back, in a study by Amitrano and colleagues, wherein a cohort of 701 patients of cirrhosis were screened for presence or absence of PVT and inherited thrombophilias, it was seen that almost 11% of these patients had PVT, which was symptomatic in 57% and asymptomatic in the rest. Majority of these patients had advanced liver disease and were Child Pugh B or C. Further, it was seen that amongst all the thrombophilic risk factors studied, only the mutation G20210A of the prothrombin gene was independently associated with PVT and this risk was increased fivefold in patients who harboured this mutation [32]. Following this, Mangia and colleagues studied the frequencies of three common prothrombotic mutations (factor V Leiden, the G20210A mutation of the prothrombin gene, and homozygosity for C677T methylenetetrahydrofolate reductase) in 219 cirrhotic patients, 43 with PVT. They found a 29% prevalence of these mutations, which was not different in patients with or without PVT, suggesting a non-causative role of these mutations in the context of PVT associated with liver cirrhosis [33].

18.6   Venous Stasis and Reduced Portal Vein Blood Flow

Involvement of portal vein in intraabdominal malignancies is an important cause of PVT due to slow flow. In a study done in patients with cirrhosis, it was shown that even though the plasma levels of protein C, protein S and antithrombin were lower in patients with PVT, a reduced portal vein flow velocity was the only significant variable that was independently associated with PVT development [34]. Similar to this, in another study in which 150 patients with viral related cirrhosis were studied, the cumulative incidence of PVT was reported as 12.8%, 20%, and 38.7% at 1, 5, and 8-10 years, respectively. It was further shown that baseline flow volume in the largest collateral vessel was an independent risk factor for thrombosis [35].

18.7   Endothelial Injury

Various intraabdominal inflammatory conditions like pancreatitis, cholecystitis, appendicitis, diverticulitis and liver abscess predispose to PVT by causing direct injury to the portal vein or septic thrombosis of the portal vein. Plessier and colleagues evaluated 102 patients with acute PVT wherein they documented a local risk factor in 21% while almost 52% of these patients had underlying thrombophilic condition [36]. Other conditions like splenectomy, colectomy, abdominal trauma and other intraabdominal surgeries cause PVT via the same mechanism [5, 15, 26, 37–46]. Acute PVT has also been documented in patients undergoing radiofrequency ablation or transarterial chemoembolization for hepatocellular carcinoma [41, 42]. It is also an important complication after liver transplantation [5, 44]

18.8   Classification

Currently there is no formal classification of EHPVO/PVT. However, based on the Baveno V guidelines it has been suggested that PVT can be classifies based on the site, clinical presentation (acute or chronic), degree of occlusion i.e. (partial or complete) and extent (extension into the splenic or superior mesenteric veins) and type of underlying liver disease. Further, it is also important to consider whether it is symptomatic or asymptomatic, progressive or self-resolving and etiologically as malignant, cirrhotic or non-malignant and non-cirrhotic [26]. Recently, an expert group had suggested a new classification system for PVT in the context of patients with cirrhosis (Table 18.1) [47].

18.9   Natural History of Extrahepatic Portal Venous Obstruction

Variceal bleeding is the most frequent complication of EHPVO in children. In a study of 207 patients with EHPVO who were followed prospectively with a prior history of variceal bleeding, transient ascites was observed in 16%, hypersplenism in 22% (symptomatic in 6%). Further, 127 patients had more than one episode of bleeding, mean episodes was 0.94/year, the severity of bleeding being maximum in age group of 12–19 years [48]. In another cohort study of 198 EHPVO patients which were followed for 20 years after the eradication of esophageal varices, 34 (17.2%) had rebleeding after variceal eradication; rebleeding occurred at a mean of 5.4 years [49]. The causes of rebleeding were: recurrence of the esophageal varices in 21 patients, gastric fundal varices in eight patients, portal gastropathy in three, and ectopic varices in two patients.

Natural history studies of PVT in cirrhosis have shown a variable progression of PVT. Non-progressive or resolving PVT has been demonstrated in 33–75% of the patients [36]. The course of PVT is usually benign in the absence of cirrhosis and malignancy. In acute thrombosis recanalization occurs in one-third to one-half of patients. Presence of ascites and thrombosis of the splenic vein are important determinants of failure of recanalization [36]. In the context of cirrhosis, partial PVT has been shown to be of no clinical relevance. In patients with advanced cirrhosis awaiting liver transplantation, complete portal vein thrombosis was associated with a worse survival and patients who have either a complete or partial recanalization had a better outcome [50, 51]. Luca and colleagues followed up 42 patients with cirrhosis with untreated non-malignant partial PVT with multidetector CT scans. They found that at a mean follow-up of 27 months, partial PVT worsened in 20 (48%) patients, improved in 19 (45%), and was stable in three (7%). The probability of hepatic decompensation was 41% and 57% at 1 year and 2 years respectively. No association could be ascertained between progression or regression of partial PVT and clinical outcome [52]. In another multicentric (43 liver units), longitudinal study of 1243 cirrhotics done in France and Belgium over 6 years, Doppler ultrasound was done to assess development of portal vein thrombosis and its potential consequences on liver disease progression. Also, G20210A and factor V gene mutations were done in stored serum samples. It was noted that the development of PVT was independently associated with the severity of liver disease at baseline, but not with progression prior to its development, and that it does not cause worsening or progression of the liver disease. Further, no association was detected between PVT and genetic thrombophilic mutations [53].

18.10 Clinical Presentation

18.10.1 Acute PVT

Acute PVT may be asymptomatic or may be associated with symptoms of bowel ischemia, which depends upon the rapidity and extension of the thrombotic process. Acute obstruction of portal vein extending into the superior mesenteric vein and mesenteric arch can lead to mesenteric ischemia and intestinal infarction. This is secondary to complete obstruction of the venous outflow. Acute PVT may initially present with abdominal pain and fever. Transient ascites can be seen and is usually due to intestinal venous congestion.

Patients with liver cirrhosis rarely present with acute PVT. Usually liver function is well-preserved in these patients, possibly due to a compensatory increase in the hepatic arterial blood flow. Acute PVT in patients with cirrhosis can result in an acute increase in portal pressure which may further lead to gastrointestinal bleeding, ascites and deterioration of liver function. The thrombus in the portal vein may either resolve spontaneously or extend proximally to the intrahepatic branches or distally to the superior mesenteric veins [40, 54–57].

18.10.2 Chronic PVT

Chronic PVT is frequently recognised on the development of portal hypertension related complications i.e. variceal bleed, hypersplenism or portal biliopathy. Other complications include neurological abnormalities secondary to portalsystemic shunting (hepatic encephalopathy, usually mild or minimal) [18, 58] and intestinal ischemia.

Acute variceal bleed is the most common complication of portal cavernoma. Growth retardation is also frequently seen in childhood due to reduced portal blood flow, resistance to growth hormone and deficiency of insulin-like growth factor. Variceal bleed is also the most frequent complication in adults. The bleeds are usually well-tolerated because of the preserved liver functions and mortality due to bleeding is infrequent. These patients usually have large gastroesophageal varices, more frequently have gastric and ectopic varices than patients with cirrhosis; however portal hypertensive gastropathy is infrequent [27, 40, 58–64]. Splenomegaly and hypersplenism are almost universally present in these patients and symptomatic hypersplenism is a common indication for shunt surgery. Abnormal coagulation profile (low factor V, VIII, protein C and S and antithrombin-III) are commonly seen; restitution of portal vein patency may cause reversion of the coagulation parameters [19]. In a study of EHPVO and NCPF patients, a significantly prolonged international normalized ratio and a decrease in fibrinogen and platelet aggregation was documented. Moreover, patients with EHPVO had a significant prolongation in partial thromboplastin time and increased levels of fibrinogen degradation product levels which were normal in NCPF patients. Hypersplenism did not significantly influence the coagulation profile in either NCPF or EHPVO patients [65].

Portal biliopathy is defined as abnormalities of the intra or extrahepatic bile ducts which include indentations of the paracholedochal collaterals, strictures, angulation and displacement of ducts with formation of stones and clustering of the intrahepatic branches in the hepatic ducts. This is seen in almost 80–100% of the cases, however is infrequently symptomatic. Jaundice and cholangitis, gallstones, hemobilia and secondary biliary cirrhosis are known complications of portal biliopathy [20, 52].

Incidence of intestinal ischemia is not widely reported and intestinal infarction is very rarely seen [35, 52, 66]. Harki and colleagues evaluated the clinical presentation and characteristics in a cohort of 15 patients with PVT using visible light spectroscopy (VLS). These were compared to a reference population and patients with cirrhosis. Decreased mucosal oxygenation in at-least single location of the GI tract was found in 75%, VLS measurements were mostly decreased in the descending duodenum in patients with PVT and symptoms typical for GI ischemia were reported in 63% with PVT [29].

18.11 Diagnosis

18.11.1 Liver Function Tests

The tests of liver function are near-normal and may be abnormal in patients with cirrhosis. Mild and asymptomatic increase in alkaline phosphatase and gamma-glutamyl transpeptidase may be present in patients with portal biliopathy. Abnormal coagulation profile may be noted in EHPVO patients [65].

18.11.2 Ultrasound

The advantages of ultrasound is that it is easily available, reliable and an excellent non-invasive method to diagnose portal vein thrombosis in majority of patients. Acute PVT on sonography appears as a hyperechoic material in the vessel lumen with adequate distension of the portal vein and its tributaries. If the thrombus appears anechoic then a Doppler study is required for its demonstration [66, 67]. Presence of portal cavernoma establishes the diagnosis of chronic PVT. This appears as a distinctive tangle of tortous vessels in porta and is commonly associated with splenomegaly, splenoportal collaterals and portosystemic shunts [66]. Sonographic features of portal vein thrombosis include an echogenic thrombus within the lumen of the vein in 67%, presence of portal vein collateral circulation 48%, enlargement of the thrombosed segment of the vein in 38%, and cavernoma in 19% [68]. Further, echogenic endoluminal thrombi are observed in both malignant and benign disease. Sonography, is unable to characterize neoplastic thrombi and only a combination of an echogenic thrombus and an adjacent hepatic mass was strongly suggestive of malignancy [67]. The sensitivity and specificity of ultrasound colour Doppler is 89% and 92%, respectively for the diagnosis of PVT [69]. To diagnose the extension of thrombus, Doppler sonography is not a reliable test as it is difficult to visualise the mesenteric veins. Recently, endoscopic ultrasound can also be used for the diagnosis of PVT with a comparable sensitivity and specificity to colour Doppler and rather appears more accurate in assessment of portal vein infiltration or invasion in the context of intraabdominal malignancies [26, 69].

18.11.3   Contrast-Enhanced CT and Magnetic Resonance Imaging

These are more sensitive and specific tests when compared to Doppler ultrasound to diagnose thrombus extension, bowel ischemia, congestion and infarction as well as the status of the adjacent organs. The thrombus appears isodense to adjacent soft tissue in a noncontrast CT. It may show as hyper-attenuating material in the portal vein lumen in acute or recent PVT [70]. Using iodinated contrast injection, lack of luminal enhancement, increased and decreased hepatic enhancement respectively in the arterial and portal venous phases is demonstrated [71]. In contrast to a bland thrombus that is usually seen as a low density, non-enhancing defect within portal vein, a tumour thrombus demonstrates enhancement on contrast administration. Intestinal infarction is also accurately diagnosed with CT showing thickening of the intestinal wall following contrast administration or lack of mucosal enhancement. MRI compares to CT in the diagnosis, however, may be less reliable in the presence of ascites. At spin-echo MR, the thrombus appears isointense on T1-weighted images, hyperintense if recent, and usually more hyperintense on T2 images. Gradient-echo MR might help to better delineate images obtained on spin-echo MR image. Addition of MR angiography is very useful adjunct for demonstration of flow direction, patency and portal cavernoma. MR-portography can identify porto-splenic collaterals and portal venous vessels same as Doppler ultrasound but with a better accuracy [66, 72, 73]. Differentiation between bland versus tumor thrombus can be done reliably by contrast ultrasonography, diffusion-weighted MRI, 18F-FDG PET or dual-energy spectral CT [11, 47, 72, 74–77].

18.11.4   Endoscopy

Esophageal varices are seen in 20–55% of patients with chronic PVT. Gastric varices are more commonly seen in almost 40% of cases and ectopic varices in the antroduodenal location in a few [26, 59, 61, 78]. Ectopic varices in duodenum, gallbladder bed and anorectal region are significantly more frequent in patients with

PVT than in patients with cirrhosis [63, 64, 79]. Portal hypertensive gastropathy is seen as early as one month after an acute PVT. These patients might also develop varices on follow up.

18.11.5 Liver Biopsy

A liver biopsy will help to rule out a chronic liver disease associated with PVT in patients with altered liver biochemistry or ultrasound appearance of cirrhosis. The utility of liver biopsy was also demonstrated in a study of 45 children to assess their outcomes post Meso-Rex bypass. In this study, these children were followed for 3.65 years and clinical, histologic and morphometric features of the liver histology were correlated with surgical outcome after Meso-Rex bypass. Portal fibrosis, bridging, parenchymal nodules, portal inflammation, hepatocellular swelling, steatosis, dilatation of portal lymphatics, and periductal fibrosis did not show a significant difference between the two groups. The diameter of the portal vein and bile duct area index were significantly smaller in the unsuccessful group (P = 0.004 and 0.003, respectively). Further, they showed that a portal vein area index <0.08 had a lower chance of successful surgical outcome. The authors concluded that a low portal vein area index and intraoperative portal blood inflow may be important negative prognostic factors for MRB outcome in children with idiopathic EHPVT [80].

18.11.6 Hemodynamic Studies

In a study to evaluate alterations of systemic and pulmonary vascular systems in patients with EHPVO and prior history of variceal bleed as compared to patients with compensated cirrhosis matched for variceal status, and body surface area, the median (range) cardiac index in EHPVO was lower, 3.8 (2.3–7.7) l min^{-1} m^{-2} versus 4.4 (2.8–8.9) l min^{-1} m^{-2} (P = 0.468) however a similar systemic vascular resistance index and pulmonary vascular resistive index was documented in EHPVO patients i.e. 1835 (806–3400) dynes cm^{-5} m^{-2} as compared to cirrhotics (1800 [668–3022], P = 0.520) and (71 [42–332] vs 79 [18–428], P = 0.885) respectively. Therefore, patients with EHPVO manifest a hyperdynamic circulatory state similar to that of compensated cirrhotics with a similar grade of portal hypertension [81]. Further, the hepatic venous pressure gradient is usually normal in patients with EHPVO while it is high in patients with cirrhosis.

18.11.7 Elastography

Elastography seems to be an excellent non-invasive modality to rule out cirrhosis. It includes both ultrasound based elastography and magnetic resonance based elastography imaging. Ultrasound based elastography i.e. transient elastography (TE; FibroScan, Echosens, Paris, France) is a technique that uses both ultrasound (5 MHz) and low-frequency (50 Hz) shear waves caused by a vibrator, the propagation velocity of the later is directly related to tissue stiffness. In patients with cirrhosis the TE values are in majority above 13–17 kPa. Acoustic Radiation Force Imaging is another ultra-sound based non-invasive procedure that is similar to TE and is also used to assess liver fibrosis. MR elastography is another non-invasive technique for assessment of liver fibrosis that should be more accurate, but has the disadvantages over ultrasound based elastographic methods of its limited availability and high cost [71, 82, 83].

18.11.8 Assessment of Portal Biliopathy

The diagnosis of portal biliopathy is usually made by magnetic resonance angiography and cholangiography (MRA/MRC), that is the investigation of choice. Based on this, the portal cavernoma cholangiopathy (PCC) can be classified into different degrees of severity; i.e. no abnormalities, grade I (irregularities or angulations of the biliary tree), grade II (indentations or strictures without dilatation) and grade III (strictures with dilation). Chandra et al. had proposed a classification system for PCC based on direct chol-angiography. Type I which is associated with involvement of extrahepatic bile ducts, type II which indicates involvement of intrahepatic bile ducts, type III a is associated with involvement of both extrahepatic bile duct and unilateral intrahepatic bile duct involvement and type III b which indicates involvement of extrahepatic bile duct and bilateral intrahepatic bile duct involvement. Endoscopic retrograde cholangiography (ERCP) should be restricted to symptomatic cases requiring therapeutic intervention like those with symptomatic cholangitis or choledocholithiasis. Endoscopic ultrasonog-raphy may also show the characteristic lesions of portal biliopathy [68, 84, 85].

18.11.9 Work Up for Inherited or Acquired Thrombophilia

After the establishment of diagnosis of PVT, the underlying etiological diagnosis should be identified by doing a complete evaluation of all possible inherited and thrombophilic disorders (Table 18.2). This is important as it has its impact on the overall management and the decision regarding requirement and duration of antico-agulation [78, 86–88].

18.12 Management

18.12.1 Acute PVT

The goals of treatment of acute PVT are: (1) To reverse the thrombotic process; (2) To prevent extension of thrombosis; (3) Prevent recurrence; (4) Treatment of complications.

Anticoagulation remains the mainstay of therapy to enable early recanalization. It should be initiated with subcutaneous low molecular weight heparin (LMWH) which is as effective as intravenous unfractionated heparin and it does not require laboratory monitoring (i.e., heparin-induced thrombocytopenia). After 2–3 weeks, this can be switched to oral vitamin K antagonists with a target INR in the range of 2–3. The rates of recanalization decrease with delayed initiation, from 69% when anticoagulation was instituted within first week to 25% when instituted in second week [89]. Other predictive factors for lack of recanalization are severity and extent of the initial thrombus within the portal vasculature, the presence of ascites and presence of more than one prothrombotic disorder [57, 66, 90, 91]. Early initiation of anticoagulation also leads to a reduction in serious life-threatening complications like peritonitis due to bowel necrosis and development of significant portal hypertension. Anticoagulation should be maintained for at-least 6 months, although in patients with prothrombotic disorder(s), personal and family history of venous thromboembolism or those who have developed serious complications should be maintained lifelong [92].

18.12.2 Thrombolytic Therapy

Local thrombolytic therapy which incorporates introduction of a catheter introduced into the portal vein either transhepatically or through a transjugular approach may be curative in some patients with acute PVT [90, 91, 93, 94]. The thrombolytic drugs that are used include infusion of drugs like recombinant tissue plasminogen activator, urokinase and streptokinase. In a retrospective study by Hollingshead et al. three patients had complete resolution, 12 had partial resolution, and five had no resolution of thrombus. None of these patients required bowel resection after thrombolytic therapy. Therefore, transcatheter thrombolysis was beneficial in avoiding death, resolving thrombus, improving symptoms and avoiding bowel resection [93].

18.12.3 Thrombectomy

Surgical thrombectomy is associated with recurrence of thrombosis, surgical morbidity and mortality and hence not recommended [66]. Mechanical thrombectomy by percutaneous transhepatic route has the advantage of rapidly removing thrombus in a recently developed PVT (<30 days), although its drawbacks include intimal or vascular trauma to the portal vein, that may promote recurrent thrombosis. Aspiration thrombectomy, either percutaneously or during TIPS placement, have been tried successfully [94].

18.13 Management of Chronic Portal Vein Thrombosis

18.13.1 Primary Prevention

In a randomized controlled trial by Villa et al. enoxaparin was administered at 4000 IU daily for 48 weeks in 70 patients (34-active arm and 36 controls) with

Child B7 to C10 cirrhosis and no PVT. No patient in the treatment arm developed PVT while 27.7% developed PVTin the control arm. Furthermore, the development of ascites, hepatic encephalopathy, spontaneous bacterial peritonitis and portal hypertensive bleeding were significantly lower in the treatment arm as compared to the control arm. Moreover, the actuarial probability of survival was significantly higher in the treatment arm. The pathophysiological basis of this benefit was proposed to be due to a reduction in bacterial translocation. No major adverse effects or haemorrhagic complications were reported with the use of enoxaparin [95].

18.13.2 Secondary Prevention

Senzoloand colleagues [96] prospectively evaluated treatment with nadraparin (n = 35) given for 6 months as compared to standard medical treatment in subjects with cirrhosis with partial or complete PVT. Patients who received treatment achieved complete recanalization more often (60% versus 5%) with almost a similar incidence of stable or partial recanalization (20% versus 24%). The control group had a very high frequency of thrombus progression (71%). Other studies evaluating the utility of anticoagulation in patients with established PVT have reported recanalization rates varying from 39–75% and thrombus progression rates of 0–14% [78].

Therapy is generally not recommended in patients with chronic PVT or EHPVO unless there is presence of an underlying prothrombotic state.

In patients with advanced cirrhosis and PVT, anticoagulation may be associated with a high risk of gastrointestinal and other sites bleed as oesophageal varices or thrombocytopenia are frequently present in patients with end-stage liver disease. This makes mandatory to provide adequate prophylactic measures to prevent variceal bleeding before starting anticoagulation.

Francoz et al. [75] evaluated cirrhotics and found that survival was significantly lower in those with complete PVT at the time of transplantation. There was also a higher rate of recanalization in patients who received anticoagulation. Delgado et al. [97] reported that re-thrombosis after complete recanalization occurred in 38% of cirrhotics after the anticoagulation therapy was stopped. On the contrary, Thatipelli et al. [1] were against the routine and prolonged use of anticoagulation, considering a low rate of recurrent thrombosis and substantial risk of bleeding complications. Summary of key studies of non-cirrhotic, non-malignant portal vein thrombosis (Table 18.3) and in patients with cirrhosis with portal vein thrombosis (Table 18.4).

18.13.3 Thrombolysis

In a recent pilot study, thrombolytic treatment of recent PVT with intravenous r-tPA and LMWH in nine patients with cirrhosis was shown to be promising [98]. Complete or partial regression of thrombosis was achieved in 89%.

Table 18.3 Summary of key studies on management of non-cirrhotic, non-malignant portal vein thrombosis

Author/year (Reference)	Study design	No. of patients	PVT	Type of anticoagulation	Duration	Recanalization (Complete or partial)
Plessier et al. (2010) [57]	Prospective	95	Acute	LMWH-61 UF-23 OA-11		39%
Turnes et al. (2008) [143]	Retrospective	27	Acute	Either drug	6 months or lifelong	44%
Sogaard et al. (2007) [144]	Retrospective	17	Acute and chronic PVT	Not specified—16/17		62.5%
Amitrano et al. (2007) [61]	Prospective	21	Splanchnic vein thrombosis	IV heparin and OA	6 months or lifelong	45.5.%
Romano et al. (2006) [145]	Retrospective	12	Post-splenectomy PVT	IV Heparin and OA		58.3%
Condat et al. (2000) [146]	Retrospective	141	Recent splanchnic vein thrombosis or portal cavernoma	IV Heparin and OA	1–4 months	93%
Sheen et al. (2000) [139]	Retrospective	9	Acute PVT	IV Heparin and OA	3 months	55.5%

LMWH light molecular weight heparin, *OA* oral anticoagulation

18.13.4 New Oral Anti-Coagulants

The newer anticoagulants include dabigatran, rivoraxaban, edoxaban and apixaban. These are direct inhibitors of thrombin or activated factor Xa [98–115]. The advantages of these drugs include oral administration, non-requirement of continuous monitoring by any blood tests, and no effect on INR, which is a very important prognostic variable in patients with cirrhosis and a component of the MELD score. The most important disadvantage is the lack of any specific antidote in the case of significant bleeding (except for dabigatran) and drug-drug interactions with use of P-glycoprotein substrates [106]. Recently, the use of rivaroxaban has been described for management of acute PVT in patients with compensated cirrhosis, however, there is still no data on the safety and efficacy of these drugs in patients with advanced cirrhosis where bleeding is a major concern. Even though the published literature suggests for the use of anticoagulants in advanced cirrhotics on the transplant waiting list weighing their risk versus benefit, there are still no guidelines. The data regarding the duration, the type of anticoagulant and also data on the safety of newer drugs is still awaited. Other situations that merit initiation of early anticoagulation in the setting of cirrhosis include presence of intestinal ischemia heralding an infarction, and even asymptomatic patients with mesenteric venous occlusion or the presence of inherited thrombophilia.

Table 18.4 Summary of studies on management of portal vein thrombosis in patients with cirrhosis

Author/year	Study design	Study population	Anticoagulation	Follow up	Duration	Type	Recanalization (Complete/partial)
Francoz (2005) [75]	P	Listed for transplantation	19 treated 10 untreated	36 months	8.1 months	LMWX followed by oral anticoagulants	42% vs 0%
Garcovich (2011) [147]	R	Cirrhotic patients with non-malignant PVT	15 untreated 15 treated	6 months	3–6 months	LMWH	46.6% vs 33.3%
Senzolo (2012) [96]	P	Cirrhotic patients with non-malignant PVT	35 treated 21 untreated	24 months	6 months	LMWH	63.6% vs 4.7%
Cai (2013) [148]	R	Patients with hypersplenism caused by cirrhotic portal hypertension	5-treated	37 months	3 months	LMWH-2 patients 3-Warfarin	80%
Chung (2014) [149]	R	Cirrhotic patients with non-malignant portal hypertension	14 treated 14 untreated	4 months	3.7 months	Oral anticoagulants	78.5% vs 35.7%
Risso (2014) [150]	R	Cirrhotic patients with non-malignant portal hypertension awaiting liver transplantation	50 treated 20 untreated	–	–	–	70% vs 40%
Chen (2015) [151]	R	Cirrhotic patients with non-malignant portal hypertension	30-treated 36 untreated	33 months	7.6 months	Oral anticoagulants	68% vs 15.3%
Wang (2016) [152]	RCT	Cirrhotic patients with PVT who underwent TIPS	31 treated 33 untreated	12 months	12 months	Oral anticoagulants	100% vs 93.7%

R retrospective, *P* prospective, *RCT* randomized controlled trial

18.13.5 TIPS

TIPS could be an effective alternative to anticoagulation for management of portal vein thrombosis with a goal to re-canalize the portal vein and to prevent recurrent thrombosis (Table 18.5). It can be effectively used in patients who have other complications of portal hypertension and are awaiting liver transplantation [107–109]. Feasibility of TIPS has been reported to be close to 70–100%, mostly in patients

Table 18.5 Summary of case series on transjugular intrahepatic portosystemic shunt (TIPS) for portal vein thrombosis in cirrhosis

Author	Years	N	Type of stent	Child class N (%)	Indication of TIPS	PVT characteristics	Outcome
Luca et al. [110]	2003–2010	70	13 bare Wallstent, 57 covered Viatorr ePTFE covered	A17(24) B42(60) C11(16)	Bleeding 48 Ascites/ Hydrothorax18 Specific treatment for PVT4	Complete-24 Cavernoma-2	Complete recanalization40(57%), 38 maintained patency at follow up 20.7 months
Perarnau et al. [153]	1990–2004	34	Palmaz or Wallstent bare stents	A3(1?) B11(52) C7(3?)	Bleeding27 Ascites 5 Other2	Complete acute 15 Cavernoma19	26/34(72%) long term patency at 30 months
Senzolo et al. [113]	1994–2005	28	26 Memotherm bare stents, 3 Viatorr covered stents	–	Bleeding-15 Ascites-5 Portal Biliopathy-3 PVT-1	Complete 8 (3-cavernoma) Partial5	Stent thrombosis in 2 (both Budd-Chiari syndrome) Primary patency 18 months
Han et al. [107]	2001–2008	57	Uncovered stents	A25(?4) B26(46) C6(3C)	Bleeding-56 Ascites -1	Complete14 (Cavernoma30) Partial 35	Patency maintained in 26 /43 patients 17-required shunt revisions
Van Ha et al. [154]	1995–2003	15	12 bare Wallstent, 1 bare Zilver stent	B11(73) C4(27)	Bleeding-10 Ascites-5	Complete4 Complete with cavernoma4 Partial7	Mean follow up of 17 months , 1 stent occlusions
D'Avola et al. [109]	1995–2009	15	Bare and covered stents	Mean Child score8	Prevention of complete PVT pre-liver transplant 8 Bleeding-6 Ascites1	All partial PVT	3/15 TIPSS thrombosis, median follow up to LT 185 days 100% PV patency at transplant
Bauer et al. [155]	1999–2005	9	3 covered stents, 6 bare stents	–	Maintain PV patency for future liver transplant	Complete7 Partial2 Cavernoma4	1/9 re-thrombosed 2 patients transplanted with no PVT
Blum et al. [94]	Case series	7	All bare stents	–	Bleeding-7	–	All successful

with partial PVT. There are no randomized controlled trials comparing TIPS to anticoagulation and standard medical treatment, still the data suggests low rate of rethrombosis and recurrent bleeds. Systemic anticoagulation is therefore only indicated in the presence of an underlying prothrombotic state [110, 111]. In a study of 15 cirrhotics awaiting liver transplantation with partial PVT who underwent TIPS, no differences were documented in the post-transplant outcomes, transplant operating times or requirement of blood products. Similarly, Wang and colleagues compared a group of 25 patients with cirrhosis and PVT treated with TIPS as compared to controls who were managed conservatively [112]. Patients who underwent TIPS had successful portal vein recanalisation as well as reduction in the rates of variceal bleeding, without any benefit in survival [113].

18.14   Management of Complications

18.14.1   Portal Hypertensive Bleed

18.14.1.1   Endoscopic and Drug Therapy

According to the current guidelines, acute variceal bleed in patients with PVT is treated in the same way as for patients with cirrhosis.

There are no studies addressing the role of primary prophylaxis in PVT. The use of beta-blockers is associated with a concern of extension of thrombosis due to a reduction in the splanchnic blood flow [116]. Similar concerns have been associated with the use of vasopressors and endoscopic therapy [117]. Beta-blockers have been shown to reduce the risk of variceal rebleed and improve survival [118]. Endoscopic variceal ligation is both a safe and highly effective treatment [119, 120]. Patients with chronic PVT have an acceptable long term survival rate of 85.7% at 1 and 82% at 5 years. Presence of jaundice and ascites impact negatively and use of beta blockers and anticoagulation were associated with improved outcomes [121].

18.14.1.2   Shunt Surgery

Shunt surgery is a definitive treatment option in patients with portal cavernoma, symptomatic portal biliopathy, failed endotherapy for variceal or ectopic variceal bleed, and severe growth retardation. However, almost one-third of the patients with PVT also have other site thrombosis with extension to splenic and superior mesenteric veins that may limit the options for shunt surgery [47]. Surgical shunts may be selective or non-selective. Non-selective shunts are either end-to-side or side-to-side portacaval, proximal lieno-renal, meso-caval or large diameter interposition porta-caval or meso-caval shunts. Selective shunts include distal lieno-renal shunt and mesenteric-left portal vein bypass (Rex shunt). The Rex shunt is the most physiological shunt which returns the blood flow to the liver [122, 123]. It restores mesenteric blood flow to the liver and may improve the growth potential in children. Before attempting surgery, patency of the Rex recess should be demonstrated. The distal spleno-renal shunt (Warren shunt) has been shown to be effective in control of bleeding and long-term survival in patients with PVT [124–127].

18.14.1.3 Non-Shunt Surgery

Oesophageal transection with or without splenectomy can be done for refractory bleeding but has been abandoned because of the high-risk of late rebleeding and reappearance of varices [128].

18.14.1.4 Liver Transplantation in Portal Vein Thrombosis

Liver transplantation is indicated for life threatening complications of PVT which cannot be managed conservatively or by shunt surgery such as encephalopathy, hypoxia or pulmonary artery hypertension. Patients with cirrhosis and PVT for the same MELD have a worse outcome as compared with those without PVT (Table 18.6) [82, 129, 130]. PVT is considered to increase the complexity of the liver transplantation, with an increase in the operative time and transfusion requirements, as well as re-thrombosis. To improve outcomes, various surgical techniques like have been tried, including thrombectomy, thromboendovenectomy with venous reconstruction, portocaval liver, use of jump graft, use of interposition venous graft between the donor and the recipient portal vein, extra-anatomic reconstruction involving the autologous vessels and PV arterialization [82, 131–133]. Based on the Yerdel's classification patients with Grade 1–2 PVT can be adequately managed by end-to-end portal vein anastomosis with or without thrombectomy. Patients with Grade 3, if the distal segment of SMV is patent, can be treated with PV reconstruction. Further, the dilated branches of the portal venous system could be constructed as inflow vessels or alternatively anastomosis to the coronary vein can be done. In the absence of a suitable vein, an interposition graft of donor iliac vein can be used for anastomosis to the SMV. For patients with grade 4 Yerdel's porto-caval hemitransposition is the most common approach. Alternatively, reno-portal anastomosis or anastomosis to the coronary vein or to a collateral vein can be tried. Even with this approach, residual portal hypertension is still noted in 50% of cases [132], with a variceal bleeding risk of 20%, persistence of ascites in 58% and renal dysfunction in 26%. In patients where there is extensive porto-mesenteric thrombosis,

Table 18.6 Summary of key studies of portal vein thrombosis and liver transplantation

Author/year	Number of patients	PVT characteristics	Outcome
Englesbe et. al. (2010) [114]	2291 (2001–2007)	–	PVT not predictive of wait-list mortality
Sringeri et al. (2013) [115]	1491 (2000–2012)	–	PVT was predictive of post-transplant mortality Prolonged operative time and increased blood transfusion requirement
Ravaioli et al. (2011) [156]	889 (1998–2008)	Partial-56% Complete-44%	Significant improvement in survival for patients with complete PVT in the second era (2003–2008) (57% vs 89% at 1 year)
Yerdel et al. (2000) [157]	779 (1987–1996)	Grade 1-24 Grade 2-23 Grade 3-6 Grade 4-10	Reduced 5 year survival between PVT and non-PVT subjects (65.3% vs 76.3%) Improved 5-year survival from first and second era in all patients

combined liver and intestine transplantation is the most accepted approach [132]. The rate of re-thrombosis is 10% without the use of anticoagulation, which decreases to 6% with use of anticoagulants as prophylaxis. The use of intra portal pump has also been shown to have reduced rethrombosis rates (7% vs 30%) [132].

18.14.2 Symptomatic Hypersplenism

Shunt surgery with splenectomy is usually done for symptomatic hypersplenism. In a study from India in 22 children with symptomatic hypersplenism, partial spleen resection was performed by ligation of blood vessels to caudal two thirds of the spleen along with the creation of the Warren DSRS shunt. The platelets and leucocytes counts were normalized after surgery and patients remained asymptomatic during the entire period of follow up (1–9 years) with an improved quality of life and growth [47].

18.14.3 Growth Failure in Children

Growth retardation is quite common in children with EHPVO. In a study of 61 children from India with EHPVO, 51% of children were short for their age (height <90% of expected), compared with 16% in matched controls [134]. In another study [135] growth retardation (height less than fifth percentile for age) was documented in 54.5% of the 33 children with EHPVO versus 5.7% of 35 controls. A decreased growth velocity despite adequate nutrition was also seen [134]. Mehrotra et al. [136] found that children with EHPVO had significantly lower mid-arm circumference and triceps skin-fold thickness as compared to healthy controls. Menon et al. [136] reported surgical porto-systemic shunts resulted in improved growth in 76% of 30 children with EHPVO, which supports the idea that portal enteropathy and subsequent malabsorption are the most plausible reasons for growth impairment. In the second hypothesis, shunting of blood away from the liver with features of growth hormone resistance with increased levels of growth hormone and decreased levels of insulin-like growth factor-1 (IGF-1) and insulin-like growth factor binding protein-3 (IGFBP-3) have been documented. Growth parameters have shown to improve significantly at 12 and 24 months follow up, after restoration of blood flow to the liver and decrease in portal hypertension by mesenterico-left portal vein bypass (MLPVB) in children [137–139]. Growth retardation constitutes a relative indication for mesenterico-left portal bypass surgery or Rex shunt.

18.14.4 Minimal Hepatic Encephalopathy

Minimal hepatic encephalopathy (MHE) has recently been reported in patients with extrahepatic portal venous obstruction (EHPVO). In a study of 31 EHPVO patients, MHE was reported in 45%, blood ammonia levels were elevated in all, and were significantly higher in the MHE than no MHE group. Further, critical flicker frequency (CFF) was abnormal in 21% (3/14) with MHE and significantly increased mean diffusivity (MD) and decreased (MTR) were observed in the MHE group, suggesting presence of interstitial cerebral oedema. This correlated positively with blood ammonia level (r = 0.65, P = 0.003) and Glutamine (r = 0.60, P = 0.003) levels in these patients [139]. In yet another study from India, patients with extrahepatic portal vein obstruction were shown to have inflammation and hyperammonemia made evident by higher levels of proinflammatory cytokines in the blood (TNF-α, IL-6, ammonia, and brain glutamine levels). A significant correlation between hyperammonemia, pro-inflammatory cytokines, and cerebral edema was documented as the pathophysiological basis of MHE in EHPVO patients [140]. Further, studies have shown lactulose to be an effective treatment for MHE [141, 142].

18.14.5 Portal Biliopathy

Portal biliopathy even though very common is rarely symptomatic. Symptomatic patients are usually adults, which suggests that portal biliopathy is a slowly progressive disease and is related to the duration of portal hypertension. In symptomatic patients, stones need endoscopic treatment, patients with stricture or cholangitis require biliary stenting, while balloon dilatation, sphincterotomy and/or stone extraction can give symptomatic relief. For dominant biliary strictures and/or endoscopic failures or as a definitive management in patients with a patent mesenteric or splenic vein portosystemic shunting is usually considered, which may lead to amelioration of the biliary obstruction. In patients with persistent obstruction a second stage hepaticojejunostomy may also be needed if biliary strictures persist (Fig. 18.1).

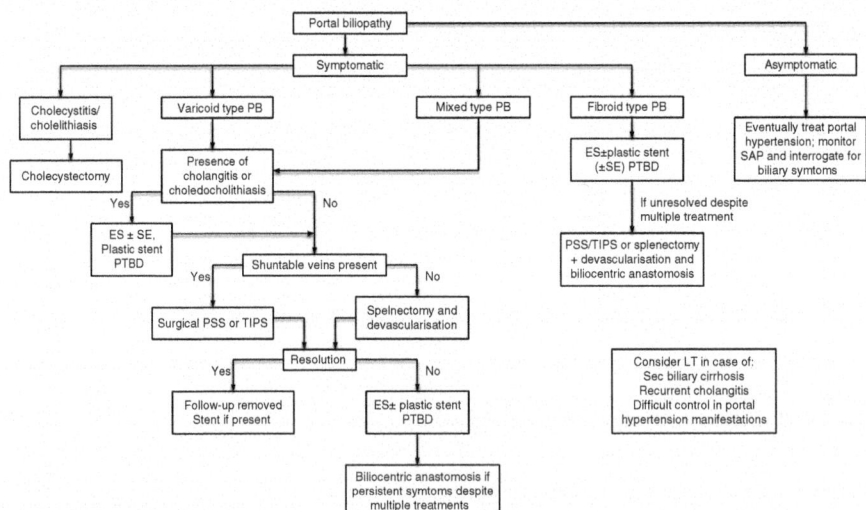

Fig. 18.1 An algorithmic approach to management of portal biliopathy in patients with portal vein thrombosis

Conclusion

Portal vein thrombosis (PVT) is a frequent complication in patients with cirrhosis associated with significant morbidity and mortality.

In Asia, PVT occurs frequently in non-cirrhotic subjects and is the most common cause of portal hypertension. Cirrhosis, intraabdominal inflammatory states and malignant conditions are important causes of PVT. The majority of patients have an underlying prothrombotic state which therefore should be rigorously looked for. The proposed new classification is a way forward to understand the pathophysiological basis, presentation and response to treatment for PVT. Doppler ultrasound is the most sensitive and easily available test for the diagnosis of PVT, although MRI angiography is preferable to assess extension of the thrombosis. Shunt surgery remains the definitive treatment option for cavernomatous PVT amongst which the Rex shunt should be offered whenever possible in children to prevent growth failure.

Use of anticoagulation in cirrhotics with acute PVT is promising with appreciable results and no added significant bleeding risk, and should be especially considered for patients awaiting liver transplantation after having treated any gastroesophageal varices. Liver transplantation, even though challenging, is feasible even in the presence of portal vein thrombosis. There is an unmet need in research on exact type and duration of anticoagulation, need of primary prophylaxis and safety and efficacy of newer anticoagulants in the context of PVT in cirrhosis, wherein there is a complete lack of consensus recommendations and the area still needs to be explored by well-designed randomized controlled trials.

Acknowledgements *Disclosures*: None to declare from authors.
Conflict of Interest: None to declare.
Writing assistance: None.

References

1. Franceschet I, Zanetto A, Ferrarese A, Burra P, Senzolo M. Therapeutic approaches for portal biliopathy: A systematic review. World J Gastroenterol. 2016;22(45):9909–20. https://doi.org/10.3748/wjg.v22.i45.9909. Review. PubMed PMID: 28018098; PubMed Central PMCID: PMC5143758
2. Pargewar SS, Desai SN, Rajesh S, Singh VP, Arora A, Mukund A. Imaging and radiological interventions in extra-hepatic portal vein obstruction. World J Radiol. 2016;8(6):556–70.
3. Al Khalloufi K, Laiyemo AO. Management of rectal varices in portal hypertension. World J Hepatol. 2015;7(30):2992–8. https://doi.org/10.4254/wjh.v7.i30.2992. Review. PubMed PMID: 26730278; PubMed Central PMCID: PMC4691702
4. Shneider BL, de Ville de Goyet J, Leung DH, Srivastava A, Ling SC, Duché M, McKiernan P, Superina R, Squires RH, Bosch J, Groszmann R, Sarin SK, de Franchis R, Mazariegos GV. Primary prophylaxis of variceal bleeding in children and the role of Meso-Rex Bypass: summary of the Baveno VI Pediatric Satellite Symposium. Hepatology. 2016;63(4):1368–80.
5. Trebicka J, Strassburg CP. Etiology and complications of portal vein thrombosis. Viszeralmedizin. 2014;30(6):375–80. https://doi.org/10.1159/000369987. Review. PubMed PMID: 26288604; PubMed Central PMCID: PMC4513836

6. Le Roy B, Gelli M, Serji B, Memeo R, Vibert E. Portal biliopathy as a complication of extrahepatic portal hypertension: etiology, presentation and management. J Visc Surg. 2015;152(3):161–6. https://doi.org/10.1016/j.jviscsurg.2015.04.003. Review. PubMed PMID: 26025414

7. Wani ZA, Bhat RA, Bhadoria AS, Maiwall R. Extrahepatic portal vein obstruction and portal vein thrombosis in special situations: need for a new classification. Saudi J Gastroenterol. 2015;21(3):129–38. https://doi.org/10.4103/1319-3767.157550. Review. PubMed PMID: 26021771; PubMed Central PMCID: PMC4455142

8. Varma V, Behera A, Kaman L, Chattopadhyay S, Nundy S. Surgical management of portal cavernoma cholangiopathy. J Clin Exp Hepatol. 2014;4(Suppl 1):S77–84. https://doi.org/10.1016/j.jceh.2013.07.005. Review. PubMed PMID: 25755599; PubMed Central PMCID: PMC4244827

9. Saraswat VA, Rai P, Kumar T, Mohindra S, Dhiman RK. Endoscopic management of portal cavernoma cholangiopathy: practice, principles and strategy. J Clin Exp Hepatol. 2014;4(Suppl 1):S67–76. https://doi.org/10.1016/j.jceh.2013.08.011. Review. PubMed PMID: 25755598; PubMed Central PMCID: PMC4244828

10. Kumar M, Saraswat VA. Natural history of portal cavernoma cholangiopathy. J Clin Exp Hepatol. 2014;4(Suppl 1):S62–6. https://doi.org/10.1016/j.jceh.2013.08.003. Review. PubMed PMID: 25755597; PubMed Central PMCID: PMC42448

11. Kalra N, Shankar S, Khandelwal N. Imaging of portal cavernoma cholangiopathy. J Clin Exp Hepatol. 2014;4(Suppl 1):S44–52. https://doi.org/10.1016/j.jceh.2013.07.004. Review. PubMed PMID: 25755595; PubMed Central PMCID: PMC4244824

12. Duseja A. Portal cavernoma cholangiopathy-clinical characteristics. J Clin Exp Hepatol. 2014;4(Suppl 1):S34–6. https://doi.org/10.1016/j.jceh.2013.05.014. Review. PubMed PMID: 25755593; PubMed Central PMCID: PMC4244822

13. Dhiman RK, Saraswat VA, Valla DC, Chawla Y, Behera A, Varma V, Agarwal S, Duseja A, Puri P, Kalra N, Rameshbabu CS, Bhatia V, Sharma M, Kumar M, Gupta S, Taneja S, Kaman L, Zargar SA, Nundy S, Singh SP, Acharya SK, Dilawari JB. Portal cavernoma cholangiopathy: consensus statement of a working party of the Indian national association for study of the liver. J Clin Exp Hepatol. 2014;4(Suppl1):S2–S14. https://doi.org/10.1016/j.jceh.2014.02.003. Review. PubMed PMID: 25755591; PubMed Central PMCID: PMC4274351

14. Chawla YK, Bodh V. Portal vein thrombosis. J Clin Exp Hepatol. 2015;5(1):22–40. https://doi.org/10.1016/j.jceh.2014.12.008. Epub 2015 Jan 6. Review. PubMed PMID: 25941431; PubMed Central PMCID: PMC4415192

15. Primignani M, Martinelli I, Bucciarelli P, et al. Risk factors for thrombophilia in extrahepatic portal vein obstruction. Hepatology. 2005;41:603–8.

16. Arora A, Sarin SK. Multimodality imaging of primary extrahepatic portal vein obstruction (EHPVO): what every radiologist should know. Br J Radiol. 2015;88(1052):20150008. https://doi.org/10.1259/bjr.20150008. Epub 2015 May 29. PubMed PMID: 26111208; PubMed Central PMCID: PMC4651392

17. Mir TA, Misgar RA, Laway BA, Shah OJ, Shah ZA, Zargar SA. Prevalence and pattern of growth abnormalities in children with extrahepatic portal vein obstruction: Response to shunt surgery. Indian J Endocrinol Metab. 2016;20(6):763–6.

18. Sharma M, Rameshbabu CS. Collateral pathways in portal hypertension. J Clin Exp Hepatol. 2012;2(4):338–52.

19. Poddar U, Borkar V. Management of extra hepatic portal venous obstruction(EHPVO): current strategies. Trop Gastroenterol. 2011;32(2):94–102. Review. PubMed PMID: 21922871

20. Hanif FM, Soomro GB, Akhund SN, Luck NH, Laeeq SM, Abbas Z, Hassan SM, Mubarak M. Clinical presentation of extrahepatic portal vein obstruction: 10-year experience at a tertiary care hospital in Pakistan. J Transl Int Med. 2015;3(2):74–8.

21. Ogren M, Bergqvist D, Bjorck M, Acosta S, Eriksson H, Sternby NH. Portal vein thrombosis: prevalence, patient characteristics and lifetime risk: a population study based on 23,796 consecutive autopsies. World J Gastroenterol. 2006;12:2115–9.

22. Pieri G, Theocharidou E, Burroughs AK. Liver in haematological disorders. Best Pract Res Clin Gastroenterol. 2013;27:513–30.
23. Alvarez F, Bernard O, Brunelle F, Hadchouel P, Odievre M, Alagille D. Portal obstruction in children. I. Clinical investigation and hemorrhage risk. J Pediatr. 1983;103:696–702.
24. Morag I, Epelman M, Daneman A, et al. Portal vein thrombosis in the neonate: risk factors, course, and outcome. J Pediatr. 2006;148:735–9.
25. Kim JH, Lee YS, Kim SH, et al. Does umbilical vein catheterization lead to portal venous thrombosis? Prospective US evaluation in 100 neonates. Radiology. 2001;219:645–50.
26. Janssen HL, Wijnhoud A, Haagsma EB, et al. Extrahepatic portal vein thrombosis: aetiology and determinants of survival. Gut. 2001;49:720–4.
27. Amitrano L, Guardascione MA, Brancaccio V, et al. Risk factors and clinical presentation of portal vein thrombosis in patients with liver cirrhosis. J Hepatol. 2004;40:736–41.
28. Monroe DM, Hoffman M. The coagulation cascade in cirrhosis. Clin Liver Dis. 2009;13:1–9.
29. Kinjo N, Kawanaka H, Akahoshi T, et al. Portal vein thrombosis in liver cirrhosis. World J Hepatol. 2014;6:64–71.
30. Amitrano L, Brancaccio V, Guardascione MA, et al. Inherited coagulation disorders in cirrhotic patients with portal vein thrombosis. Hepatology. 2000;31:345–8.
31. Gatt A, Riddell A, Calvaruso V, Tuddenham EG, Makris M, Burroughs AK. Enhanced thrombin generation in patients with cirrhosis-induced coagulopathy. J Thromb Haemost. 2010;8:1994–2000. 380 Viszeralmedizin 2014;30:375–80
32. Tripodi A, Mannucci PM. Abnormalities of hemostasis in chronic liver disease: reappraisal of their clinical significance and need for clinical and laboratory research. J Hepatol. 2007;46:727–33.
33. Denninger MH, Chaõt Y, Casadevall N, et al. Cause of portal or he- € patic venous thrombosis in adults: the role of multiple concurrent factors. Hepatology. 2000;31:587–91.
34. Janssen HL, Meinardi JR, Vleggaar FP, et al. Factor V Leiden mutation, prothrombin gene mutation, and deficiencies in coagulation inhibitors associated with Budd-Chiari syndrome and portal vein thrombosis: results of a case-control study. Blood. 2000;96:2364–8.
35. Bombeli T, Basic A, Fehr J. Prevalence of hereditary thrombophilia in patients with thrombosis in different venous systems. Am J Hematol. 2002;70:126–32.
36. Bhattacharyya M, Makharia G, Kannan M, Ahmed RPH, Gupta PK, Saxena R. Inherited prothrombotic defects in Budd-Chiari syndrome and portal vein thrombosis – a study from north India. Am J Clin Pathol. 2004;121:844–7.
37. Turnes J, García-Pagan JC, Gonz alez M, et al. Portal hypertension-related complications after acute portal vein thrombosis: impact of early anticoagulation. Clin Gastroenterol Hepatol. 2008;6:1412–7.
38. Rosendaal FR. Venous thrombosis: a multicausal disease. Lancet. 1999;353:1167–73.
39. De Franchis R. Evolving consensus in portal hypertension. Report of the Baveno IV consensus workshop on methodology of diagnosis and therapy in portal hypertension. J Hepatol. 2005;43:167–76.
40. Smalberg JH, Arends LR, Valla DC, Kiladjian JJ, Janssen HLA, Leebeek FWG. Myeloproliferative neoplasms in Budd-Chiari syndrome and portal vein thrombosis: a meta-analysis. Blood. 2012;120:4021–8.
41. Qi X, Yang Z, Bai M, Shi X, Han G, Fan D. Meta-analysis: the significance of screening for JAK2V617F mutation in Budd-Chiari syndrome and portal venous system thrombosis. Aliment Pharmacol Ther. 2011;33:1087–103.
42. Qi X, Zhang C, Han G, et al. Prevalence of the JAK2V617F mutation in Chinese patients with Budd-Chiari syndrome and portal vein thrombosis: a prospective study. J Gastroenterol Hepatol. 2012;27:1036–43.
43. Deepak A, Punamiya S, Patel N, Parekh S, Mehta S, Shah N. Prevalence of JAK2(V617F) mutation in intra-abdominal venous thrombosis. Trop Gastroenterol. 2011;32:279–84.
44. Fisher NC, Wilde JT, Roper J, Elias E. Deficiency of natural anticoagulant proteins C, S, and antithrombin in portal vein thrombosis: a secondary phenomenon? Gut. 2000;46:534–9.

45. D'Amico M, Sammarco P, Pasta L. Thrombophilic genetic factors PAI-1, MTHFRC677T, V Leiden 506Q, and prothrombin 20210A in noncirrhotic portal vein thrombosis and Budd-Chiari syndrome in a population. Int J Vasc Med. 2013;2013:717480. https://doi.org/10.1155/2013/717480. Epub 2013 Dec 18
46. Qi X, De Stefano V, Wang J, et al. Prevalence of inherited antithrombin, protein C, and protein S deficiencies in portal vein system thrombosis and Budd-Chiari syndrome: a systematic review and meta-analysis of observational studies. J Gastroenterol Hepatol. 2013;28:432–42.
47. Condat B, Pessione F, Hillaire S, et al. Current outcome of portal vein thrombosis in adults: risk and benefit of anticoagulant therapy. Gastroenterology. 2001;120:490–7.
48. Poultsides GA, Lewis WC, Feld R, Walters DL, Cherry DA, Ruby ST. Portal vein thrombosis after laparoscopic colectomy: thrombolytic therapy via the superior mesenteric vein. Am Surg. 2005;71:856–60.
49. Bernades P, Baetz A, Levy P, Belghiti J, Menu Y, Fékété F. Splenic and portal venous obstruction in chronic pancreatitis. A prospective longitudinal study of a medical-surgical series of 266 patients. Dig Dis Sci. 1992;37:340–6.
50. Fujita F, Lyass S, Otsuka K, et al. Portal vein thrombosis following splenectomy: identification of risk factors. Am Surg. 2003;69:951–6.
51. Bick RL. Coagulation abnormalities in malignancy: a review. Semin Thromb Hemost. 1992;18:353–72.
52. Plessier A, Darwish-Murad S, Hernandez-Guerra M, et al. Acute portal vein thrombosis unrelated to cirrhosis: a prospective multicenter follow-up study. Hepatology. 2010;51:210–8.
53. Habu D, Nishiguchi S, Shiomi S, et al. Portal vein thrombosis following percutaneous ethanol injection therapy for hepatocellular carcinoma. Indian J Gastroenterol. 2002;21:162–3.
54. Zheng RQ, Kudo M, Inui K, et al. Transient portal vein thrombosis caused by radiofrequency ablation for hepatocellular carcinoma. J Gastroenterol. 2003;38:101–3.
55. Matsumoto K, Yamao K, Ohashi K, et al. Acute portal vein thrombosis after EUS-guided FNA of pancreatic cancer: case report. Gastrointest Endosc. 2003;57:269–71.
56. Langnas AN, Marujo W, Stratta RJ, Wood RP, Shaw BW Jr. Vascular complications after orthotopic liver transplantation. Am J Surg. 1991;161:76–82.
57. Doria C, Marino IR. Acute portal vein thrombosis secondary to donor/recipient portal vein diameter mismatch after orthotopic liver transplantation: a case report. Int Surg 2003;88:184–7.
58. Dorffel T, Wruck T, Ruckert RI, Romaniuk P, Dorffel Q, Wermke W. Vascular complications in acute pancreatitis assessed by color duplex ultrasonography. Pancreas. 2000;21:126–33.
59. Murad SD, Valla DC, de Groen PC, et al. Pathogenesis and treatment of Budd-Chiari syndrome combined with portal vein thrombosis. Am J Gastroenterol. 2006;101:83–90.
60. Anand AC, Sashindran VK, Mohan L. Gastrointestinal problems at high altitude. Trop Gastroenterol. 2006;27:147–53.
61. Sakha SH, Rafeey M, Tarzamani MK. Portal venous thrombosis after umbilical vein catheterization. Indian J Gastroenterol. 2007;26:283–4.
62. Mangia A, Villani MR, Cappucci G, et al. Causes of portal venous thrombosis in cirrhotic patients: the role of genetic and acquired factors. Eur J Gastroenterol Hepatol. 2005;17:745–51.
63. Zocco MA, Di Stasio E, De Cristofaro R, et al. Thrombotic risk factors in patients with liver cirrhosis: correlation with MELD scoring system and portal vein thrombosis development. J Hepatol. 2009;51:682–9.
64. Maruyama H, Okugawa H, Takahashi M, Yokosuka O. De novoportal vein thrombosis in virus-related cirrhosis: predictive factors and long-term outcomes. Am J Gastroenterol. 2013;108:568–74.
65. Francoz C, Belghiti J, Vilgrain V, et al. Splanchnic vein thrombosis in candidates for liver transplantation: usefulness of screening and santi coagulation. Gut. 2005;54:691–7.
66. Luca A, Caruso S, Milazzo M, et al. Natural course of extrahepatic nonmalignant partial portal vein thrombosis in patients with cirrhosis. Radiology. 2012;265:124–32.

67. Englesbe MJ, Kubus J, Muhammad W, et al. Portal vein thrombosis and survival in patients with cirrhosis. Liver Transpl. 2010;16:83–90.
68. Van Gansbeke D, Avni EF, Delcour C, Engelholm L, Struyven J. Sonographic features of portal vein thrombosis. AJR Am J Roentgenol. 1985;144:749–52.
69. Shah SR, Mathur SK. Presentation and natural history of variceal bleeding in patients with portal hypertension due to extrahepatic portal venous obstruction. Indian J Gastroenterol. 2003;22(6):217–20.
70. Garcia-Pag an JC, Hern andez-Guerra M, Bosch J. Extrahepatic portal vein thrombosis. Semin Liver Dis. 2008;28:282–92.
71. Webb LJ, Sherlock S. The aetiology, presentation and natural history of extra-hepatic portal venous obstruction. Q J Med. 1979;48:627–39.
72. Amitrano L, Guardascione MA, Scaglione M, et al. Prognostic factors in noncirrhotic patients with splanchnic vein thromboses. Am J Gastroenterol. 2007;102:2464–70.
73. Haddad MC, Clark DC, Sharif HS, Al Shahed M, Aideyan O, Sammak BM. MR, CT, and ultrasonography of splanchnic venous thrombosis. Gastrointest Radiol. 1992;17:34–40.
74. Merkel C, Bolognesi M, Bellon S, et al. Long-term follow-up study of adult patients with non-cirrhotic obstruction of the portal system: comparison with cirrhotic patients. J Hepatol. 1992;15:299–303.
75. Ganguly S, Sarin SK, Bhatia V, Lahoti D. The prevalence and spectrum of colonic lesions in patients with cirrhotic and noncirrhotic portal hypertension. Hepatology. 1995;21:1226–31.
76. Chawla Y, Dilawari JB. Anorectal varices – their frequency in cirrhotic and non-cirrhotic portalhypertension. Gut. 1991;32:309–11.
77. Chawla Y, Dilawari JB, Katariya S. Gallbladder varices in portal veinthrombosis. AJR Am J Roentgenol. 1994;162:643–5.
78. Sarin SK, Sollano JD, Chawla YK, et al. Consensus on extra-hepatic portal vein obstruction. Liver Int. 2006;26:512–9.
79. Sharma P, Sharma BC, Puri V, Sarin SK. Natural history of minimal hepatic encephalopathy in patients with extrahepatic portal vein obstruction. Am J Gastroenterol. 2009;104:885–90.
80. Mack CL, Superina RA, Whitington PF. Surgical restoration of portal flow corrects proco-agulant and anticoagulant deficiencies associated with extrahepatic portal vein sthrombosis. J Pediatr. 2003;142:197–9.
81. Khuroo MS, Yattoo GN, Zargar SA, et al. Biliary abnormalities associated with extrahepatic portal venous obstruction. Hepatology. 1993;17:807–13.
82. Harmanci O, Bayraktar Y. Portal hypertension due to portal venous thrombosis: etiology, clinical outcomes. World J Gastroenterol. 2007;13:2535–40.
83. Harki J, Plompen EP, van Noord D, Hoekstra J, Kuipers EJ, Janssen HL, Tjwa ET. GI isch-emia in patients with portal vein thrombosis: a prospective cohort study. Gastrointest Endosc. 2016;83(3):627–36.
84. Bajaj JS, Bhattacharjee J, Sarin SK. Coagulation profile and platelet function in patients with extrahepatic portal vein obstruction and non-cirrhotic portal fibrosis. J Gastroenterol Hepatol. 2001;16(6):641–6.
85. Chawla Y, Duseja A, Dhiman RK. Review article: the modern management of portal vein thrombosis. Aliment Pharmacol Ther. 2009;30(9):881–94.
86. Mínguez B, García-Pagán JC, Bosch J, et al. Noncirrhotic portal vein thrombosis exhib-its neuropsychological and MR changes consistent with minimal hepaticencephalopathy. Hepatology. 2006;43:707–14.
87. Tessler FN, Gehring BJ, Gomes AS, et al. Diagnosis of portal vein thrombosis: value of color Doppler imaging. AJR Am J Roentgenol. 1991;157:293–6.
88. Sugiyama M, Hagi H, Atomi Y, Saito M. Diagnosis of portal venous invasion by pancreato-biliary carcinoma: value of endoscopic ultrasonography. Abdom Imaging. 1997;22:434–8.
89. Brugge WR, Lee MJ, Kelsey PB, Schapiro RH, Warshaw AL. The use of EUS to diag-nose malignant portal venous system invasion by pancreatic cancer. Gastrointest Endosc. 1996;43:561–7.

90. Parvey HR, Raval B, Sandler CM. Portal vein thrombosis: imaging findings. AJR Am J Roentgenol. 1994;162:77–81.
91. Mathieu D, Vasile N, Grenier P. Portal thrombosis: dynamic CT features and course. Radiology. 1985;154:737–41.
92. Chou CK, Mak CW, Tzeng WS, Chang JM. CT of small bowel ischemia. Abdom Imaging. 2004;29:18–22.
93. Engel brecht M, Akin O, Dixit D, Schwartz L. Bland and tumor thrombi in abdominal malignancies: magnetic resonance imaging assessment in a large oncologic patient population. Abdom Imaging. 2011;36:62–8.
94. Catalano OA, Choy G, Zhu A, Hahn PF, Sahani DV. Differentiation of malignant thrombus from bland thrombus of the portal vein in patients with hepatocellular carcinoma: application of diffusion-weighted MR imaging. Radiology. 2010;254:154–62.
95. Lee EYP, Khong P-L. The value of 18F-FDG PET/contrast-enhanced CT in detection of tumor thrombus. Clin Nucl Med. 2013;38:e60–5.
96. Qian LJ, Zhu J, Zhuang ZG, et al. Differentiation of neoplastic from bland macroscopic portal vein thrombi using dual-energy spectral CT imaging: a pilot study. Eur Radiol. 2012;22:2178–85.
97. Margini C, Berzigotti A. Portal vein thrombosis: the role of imaging in the clinical setting. Dig Liver Dis. 2017;49(2):113–20.
98. Aytekin C, Boyvat F, Kurt A, Yologlu Z, Coskun M. Catheter-directed thrombolysis with transjugular access in portal vein thrombosis secondary to pancreatitis. Eur J Radiol. 2001;39(2):80.
99. Hollingshead M, Burke CT, Mauro MA, Weeks SM, Dixon RG, Jaques PF. Transcatheter thrombolytic therapy for acute mesenteric and portal vein thrombosis. J Vasc Interv Radiol. 2005;16:651–61.
100. Kercher KW, Sing RF, Watson KW, Matthews BD, LeQuire MH, Heniford BT. Transhepatic thrombolysis in acute portal vein thrombosis after laparoscopic splenectomy. Surg Laparosc Endosc Percutan Tech. 2002;12:131–6.
101. Blum U, Haag K, Rössle M, Ochs A, Gabelmann A, Boos S, Langer M. Noncavernomatous portal vein thrombosis in hepatic cirrhosis: treatment with transjugular intrahepatic portosystemic shunt and local thrombolysis. Radiology. 1995;195:153–7.
102. Villa E, Camma C, Marietta M, Luongo M, Critelli R, Colopi S, Tata C, Zecchini R, Gitto S, Petta S, Lei B, Bernabucci V, Vukotic R, De Maria N, Schepis F, Karampatou A, Caporali C, Simoni L, Del Buono M, Zambotto B, Turola E, Fornaciari G, Schianchi S, Ferrari A, Valla D. Enoxaparin prevents portal vein thrombosis and liver decompensation in patients with advanced cirrhosis. Gastroenterology. 2012;143:1253–60.e1–4.
103. Senzolo M, M Sartori T, Rossetto V, Burra P, Cillo U, Boccagni P, Gasparini D, Miotto D, Simioni P, Tsochatzis E, A Burroughs K. Prospective evaluation of anticoagulation and transjugular intrahepatic portosystemic shunt for the management of portal vein thrombosis in cirrhosis. Liver Int. 2012;32:919–27.
104. Werner KT, Sando S, Carey EJ, Vargas HE, Byrne TJ, Douglas DD, Harrison ME, Rakela J, Aqel BA. Portal vein thrombosis in patients with end stage liver disease awaiting liver transplantation: outcome of anticoagulation. Dig Dis Sci. 2013;58:1776–80.
105. European Association for the Study of the Liver, European Organisation for Research and Treatment of Cancer. EASL/EORTC clinical practice guidelines: management of hepatocellularcarcinoma. J Hepatol. 2012;56:908–43.
106. Intagliata NM, Maitland H, Northup PG, Caldwell SH. Treating thrombosis in cirrhosis patients with new oral agents: ready or not? Hepatology. 2015;61:738–9. https://doi.org/10.1002/hep.27225.
107. Martinez M, Tandra A, Vuppalanchi R. Treatment of acute portal vein thrombosis by nontraditional anticoagulation. Hepatology. 2014;60:425–6. https://doi.org/10.1002/hep.26998.
108. Garcia-Tsao G, Sanyal AJ, Grace ND, Carey W. Prevention and management of gastroesophageal varices and variceal haemorrhage in cirrhosis. Hepatology. 2007;46:922–38. https://doi.org/10.1002/hep.21907.
109. Heidbuchel H, Verhamme P, Alings M, Antz M, Hacke W, Oldgren J, Sinnaeve P, Camm AJ, Kirchhof P. European Heart Rhythm Association Practical Guide on the use of new oral

anticoagulants in patients with non-valvular atrial fibrillation. Europace. 2013;15:625–51. https://doi.org/10.1093/europace/eut083. PMID: 23625942

110. Schulman S, Kearon C, Kakkar AK, Schellong S, Eriksson H, Baanstra D, Kvamme AM, Friedman J, Mismetti P, Goldhaber SZ. Extended use of dabigatran, warfarin, or placebo in venousthromboembolism. N Engl J Med. 2013;368:709–18. https://doi.org/10.1056/NEJMoa1113697. PMID: 23425163

111. Agnelli G, Buller HR, Cohen A, Curto M, Gallus AS, Johnson M, Masiukiewicz U, Pak R, Thompson J, Raskob GE, Weitz JI. Oral apixaban for the treatment of acute venous thrombo-embolism. N Engl J Med. 2013;369:799–808. https://doi.org/10.1056/NEJMoa1302507.

112. Eriksson BI, Borris LC, Friedman RJ, Haas S, Huisman MV, Kakkar AK, Bandel TJ, Beckmann H, Muehlhofer E, Misselwitz F, Geerts W. Rivaroxaban versus enoxaparin for thromboprophylaxis after hip arthroplasty. N Engl J Med. 2008;358:2765–75. https://doi.org/10.1056/NEJMoa0800374. PMID: 18579811

113. Scaglione F. New oral anticoagulants: comparative pharmacology with vitamin K antago-nists. Clin Pharmacokinet. 2013;52:69–82. https://doi.org/10.1007/s40262-012-0030-9. PMID: 23292752

114. Han G, Qi X, He C, Yin Z, Wang J, Xia J, Yang Z, Bai M, Meng X, Niu J, Wu K, Fan D. Transjugular intrahepatic portosystemic shunt for portal vein thrombosis with symptom-atic portal hypertension inliver cirrhosis. J Hepatol. 2011;54:78–88. https://doi.org/10.1016/j.jhep.2010.06.029. PMID: 20932597

115. Perarnau JM, Baju A, D'alteroche L, Viguier J, Ayoub J. Feasibility and long-term evolu-tion of TIPS in cirrhotic patients with portal thrombosis. Eur J Gastroenterol Hepatol. 2010;22:1093–8. https://doi.org/10.1097/MEG.0b013e328338d995. PMID: 20308910

116. Delgado MG, Seijo S, Yepes I, Achécar L, Catalina MV, García-Criado A, Abraldes JG, de la Peña J, Bañares R, Albillos A, Bosch J, García-Pagán JC. Efficacy and safety of antico-agulation on patients with cirrhosis and portal vein thrombosis. Clin Gastroenterol Hepatol. 2012;10:776–83.

117. Webster GJ, Burroughs AK, Riordan SM. Review article: portal vein thrombosis – new insights into aetiology and management. Aliment Pharmacol Ther. 2005;21:1–9.

118. Brearley S, Hawker PC, Dykes PW, Keighley MR. A lethal complication of peripheral vein vasopressin infusion. Hepatogastroenterology. 1985;32:224–5.

119. Celinska-Cedro D, Teisseyre M, Woynarowski M, Socha P, Socha J, Ryzko J. Endoscopic ligation of esophageal varices for prophylaxis of first bleeding in children and adoles-cents with portal hypertension: preliminary results of a prospective study. J Pediatr Surg. 2003;38:1008–11.

120. Spaander MC, Murad SD, van Buuren HR, Hansen BE, Kuipers EJ, Janssen HL. Endoscopic treatment of esophagogastric variceal bleeding in patients with non-cirrhotic extrahepatic portal vein thrombosis: a long-term follow-up study. Gastrointest Endosc. 2008;67:821–7.

121. Orr DW, Harrison PM, Devlin J, et al. Chronic mesenteric venous thrombosis: evalua-tion and determinants of survival during longterm follow-up. Clin Gastroenterol Hepatol. 2007;5:80–6.

122. Wolff M, Hirner A. Current state of portosystemic shunt surgery. Langenbecks Arch Surg. 2003;388:141–9.

123. Dasgupta R, Roberts E, Superina RA, Kim PC. Effectiveness of Rex shunt in the treatment of portal hypertension. J Pediatr Surg. 2006;41:108–12.

124. Krebs-Schmitt D, Briem-Richter A, Grabhorn E, et al. Effectiveness of Rex shunt in children with portal hypertension following liver transplantation or with primary portal hypertension. Pediatr Transpl. 2009;13:540–4.

125. Livingstone AS, Koniaris LG, Perez EA, Alvarez N, Levi JU, Hutson DG. 507 Warren-Zeppa distal splenorenal shunts: a 34-year experience. Ann Surg. 2006;243:884–92.

126. Sharma BC, Singh RP, Chawla YK, et al. Effect of shunt surgery on spleen size, portal pressure and oesophageal varices in patients with non-cirrhotic portal hypertension. J Gastroenterol Hepatol. 1997;12:582–4.

127. Query JA, Sandler AD, Sharp WJ. Use of autogenous saphenous vein as a conduit for mesen-terico-left portal vein bypass. J Pediatr Surg. 2007;42:1137–40.

128. Kim HB, Pomposelli JJ, Lillehei CW, et al. Mesogonadal shunts for extrahepatic portal vein thrombosis and variceal hemorrhage. Liver Transpl. 2005;11:1389–94.
129. Doenecke A, Tsui TY, Zuelke C, et al. Pre-existent portal veinthrombosis in liver transplantation: influence of pre-operative disease severity. Clin Transpl. 2010;24:48–55.
130. Lendoire J, Raffin G, Cejas N, et al. Liver transplantation in adult patients with portal vein thrombosis: risk factors, management and outcome. HPB (Oxford). 2007;9:352–6.
131. Yerdel MA, Gunson B, Mirza D, et al. Portal vein thrombosis inadults undergoing liver transplantation: risk factors, screening, management and outcome. Transplantation. 2000;69:1873–81.
132. Rodriguez-Castro KI, Porte RJ, Nadal E, Germani G, Burra P, Senzolo M. Management of non neoplastic portal vein thrombosis in the setting of liver transplantation: a systematic review. Transplantation. 2012;94:1145–53.
133. Tao YF, Teng F, Wang ZX, et al. Liver transplant recipients with portal vein thrombosis: a single center retrospective study. Hepatobiliary Pancreat Dis Int. 2009;8:34–9.
134. Ni YH, Wang NC, Peng MY, Chou YY, Chang FY. Bacteroides fragilis bacteremia associated with portal vein and superior mesentery vein thrombosis secondary to antithrombin III and protein C deficiency: a case report. J Microbiol Immunol Infect. 2002;35:255–8.
135. Sarin SK, Bansal A, Sasan S, Nigam A. Portal-vein obstruction in children leads to growth retardation. Hepatology. 1992;15:229–33.
136. Mehrotra RN, Bhatia V, Dabadghao P, Yachha SK. Extrahepatic portal vein obstruction in children: anthropometry, growth hormone and insulin-like growth factor I. J Pediatri Gastroenterol Nutr. 1997;25:520–3.
137. Menon P, Rao KL, Bhattacharya A, Thapa BR, Chowdhary SK, Mahajan JK, et al. Extrahepatic portal hypertension: quality of life and somatic growth after surgery. Eur J Pediatr Surg. 2005;15:82–7.
138. Nihal N, Bapat MR, Rathi P, Shah NS, Karvat A, Abraham P, et al. Relation of insulin-like growth factor-1 and insulin-like growth factor binding protein-3 levels to growth retardation in extrahepatic portal vein obstruction. Hepatol Int. 2009;3:305.
139. Lautz TB, Sundaram SS, Whitington PF, Keys L, Superina RA. Growth impairment in children with extrahepatic portal vein obstruction is improved by mesenterico-left portal vein bypass. J Pediatr Surg. 2009;44(11):2067–70.
140. Srčtčhović A, Perlslć V, Vujović D, Opacić D, Vukadinović V, Pavićević P, Radević B. Warren shunt combined with partial splenectomy in children withextra-hepatic portal hypertension, massive splenomegaly and severe hypersplenism. Srp Arh Celok Lek. 2014;142(7-8):419–23.
141. Goel A, Yadav S, Saraswat V, Srivastava A, Thomas MA, Pandey CM, Rathore R, Gupta R. Cerebral oedema in minimal hepatic encephalopathy due to extrahepatic portal venous obstruction. Liver Int. 2010;30(8):1143–51.
142. Srivastava A, Yadav SK, Yachha SK, Thomas MA, Saraswat VA, Gupta RK. Pro-inflammatory cytokines are raised in extrahepatic portal venous obstruction, with minimal hepatic encephalopathy. J Gastroenterol Hepatol. 2011;26(6):979–86.
143. Jha SK, Kumar A, Sharma BC, Sarin SK. Systemic and pulmonary hemodynamics in patients with extrahepatic portal vein obstruction is similar to compensated cirrhotic patients. Hepatol Int. 2009;3(2):384–91.
144. Chandra R, Kapoor D, Tharakan A, Chaudhary A, Sarin SK. Portal biliopathy. J Gastroenterol Hepatol. 2001;16:1086–92.
145. Condat B, Vilgrain V, Asselah T, et al. Portal cavernoma-associated cholangiopathy: a clinical and MR cholangiography coupled with MR portography imaging study. Hepatology. 2003;37:1302–8.
146. Umphress JL, Pecha RE, Urayama S. Biliary stricture caused by portal biliopathy: diagnosis by EUS with Doppler US. Gastrointest Endosc. 2004;60:1021–4.
147. Nery F, Chevret S, Condat B, de Raucourt E, Boudaoud L, Rautou PE, Plessier A, Roulot D, Chaffaut C, Bourcier V, Trinchet JC, Valla DC, Groupe d'Etude et de Traitement du Carcinome Hépatocellulaire. Causes and consequences of portal vein thrombosis in 1,243 patients with cirrhosis: results of a longitudinal study. Hepatology. 2015;61(2):660–7.

148. Cai M, Zhu K, Huang W, et al. Portal vein thrombosis after partial splenic embolization in liver cirrhosis: efficacy of anticoagulation and long-term follow-up. J Vasc Interv Radiol. 2013;24:1808–16.
149. Clavien PA, Selzner M, Tuttle-Newhall JE, Harland RC, Suhocki P. Liver transplantation complicated by misplaced TIPS in the portal vein. Ann Surg. 1998;227:440–5.
150. Rajani R, Björnsson E, Bergquist A, Danielsson A, Gustavsson A, Grip O, Melin T, Sangfelt P, Wallerstedt S, Almer S. The epidemiology and clinical features of portal vein thrombosis: a multicentre study. Aliment Pharmacol Ther. 2010;32:1154–62.
151. Kumar A, Sharma P, Arora A. Review article: portal vein obstruction—epidemiology, pathogenesis, natural history, prognosis and treatment. Aliment Pharmacol Ther. 2015;41(3):276–92.
152. Lopera JE, Correa G, Brazzini A, et al. Percutaneous transhepatic treatment of symptomatic mesenteric venous thrombosis. J Vasc Surg. 2002;36:1058–61.
153. Bauer J, Johnson S, Durham J, Ludkowski M, Trotter J, Bak T, Wachs M. The role of TIPS for portal vein patency in liver transplant patients with portal vein thrombosis. Liver Transpl. 2006;12:1544–51. https://doi.org/10.1002/lt.20869. PMID: 17004250
154. Senzolo M, Tibbals J, Cholongitas E, Triantos CK, Burroughs AK, Patch D. Transjugular intrahepatic portosystemic shunt for portal vein thrombosis with and without cavernous transformation. Aliment Pharmacol Ther. 2006;23:767–75. https://doi.org/10.1111/j.1365-2036.2006.02820.x. PMID: 16556179
155. Wang Z, Zhao H, Wang X, Zhang H, Jiang M, Tsauo J, Luo X, Yang L, Li X. Clinical outcome comparison between TIPS and EBL in patients with cirrhosis and portal vein thrombosis. Abdom Imaging. 2014. https://doi.org/10.1007/s00261-014-0320-9. PMID: 25504374 [Epub ahead of print]
156. D'Avola D, Bilbao JI, Zozaya G, Pardo F, Rotellar F, Iñarrairaegui M, Quiroga J, Sangro B, Herrero JI. Efficacy of transjugular intrahepatic portosystemic shunt to prevent total portal vein thrombosis in cirrhotic patients awaiting for liver transplantation. Transplant Proc. 2012;44:2603–5. https://doi.org/10.1016/j.transproceed.2012.09.050. PMID: 23146469
157. Luca A, Miraglia R, Caruso S, Milazzo M, Sapere C, Maruzzelli L, Vizzini G, Tuzzolino F, Gridelli B, Bosch J. Short- and longterm effects of the transjugular intrahepatic portosystemic shunt on portal vein thrombosis in patients with cirrhosis. Gut. 2011;60:846–52. https://doi.org/10.1136/gut.2010.228023. PMID: 21357252
158. Thomas V, Jose T, Kumar S. Natural history of bleeding after esophageal variceal eradication in patients with extrahepatic portal venous obstruction; a 20-year follow-up. Indian J Gastroenterol. 2009;28(6):206–11.
159. Sarin SK, Kumar A. Noncirrhotic portal hypertension. Clin Liver Dis. 2006;10:627–51. x
160. Tantemsapya N, Superina R, Wang D, Kronauer G, Whitington PF, Melin-Aldana H. Hepatic histology and morphometric measurements in idiopathic extrahepatic portal vein thrombosis in children, correlated to clinical outcome of Meso-Rex Bypass.Ann Surg. Epub 2016 Dec 30.
161. Sharma P, Sharma BC. Lactulose for minimal hepatic encephalopathy in patients with extrahepatic portal vein obstruction. Saudi J Gastroenterol. 2012;18(3):168–72.
162. El-Karaksy HM, Afifi O, Bakry A, Kader AA, Saber N. A pilot study using lactulose in management of minimal hepatic encephalopathy in children with extrahepatic portal vein obstruction. World J Pediatr. 2017;13(1):70–5.
163. Sogaard KK, Astrup LB, Vilstrup H, Gronbaek H. Portal vein thrombosis; risk factors, clinical presentation and treatment. BMC Gastroenterol. 2007;7:34.
164. Romano F, Caprotti R, Conti M, et al. Thrombosis of the splenoportal axis after splenectomy. Langenbecks Arch Surg. 2006;391:483–8.
165. Condat B, Pessine T, Helene DM, Hillaire S, Valla D. Recent portal or mesenteric venous thrombosis, increased recognition and frequent recanalisation on anticoagulant therapy. Hepatology. 2000;32:466–70.
166. Garcovich MZM, Ainora ME, Annicchiarico BE, Ponziani FR, Cesario V, et al. Clinical outcome of portal vein thrombosis (PVT) in cirrhotic patients: observe or treat? Hepatology. 2011;54:1261A–2A.

167. Chung JW, Kim GH, Lee JH, et al. Safety, efficacy, and response predictors of anticoagulation for the treatment of nonmalignant portal-vein thrombosis in patients with cirrhosis: a propensity score matching analysis. Clin Mol Hepatol. 2014;20:384–91.
168. Risso ASD, Martini S, Rizzetto M, Salizzoni M. Liver transplantation in cirrhotic patients with portal vein thrombosis: a single centre experience. Dig Liver Dis. 2014;46:e40.
169. Chen H, Liu L, Qi X, et al. Efficacy and safety of anticoagulation in more advanced portal vein thrombosis in patients with liver cirrhosis. Eur J Gastroenterol Hepatol. 2016;28:82–9.
170. Wang Z, Jiang MS, Zhang HL, et al. Is post-TIPS anticoagulation therapy necessary in patients with cirrhosis and portal vein thrombosis? a randomized controlled trial. Radiology. 2016;279:943–51.
171. Englesbe MJ, Schaubel DE, Cai S, Guidinger MK, Merion RM. Portal vein thrombosis and liver transplant survival benefit. Liver Transpl. 2010;16:999–1005. https://doi.org/10.1002/lt.22105. PMID: 20677291
172. Sringeri R. Incidental portal vein thrombosis: does it impact the surgical outcomes following liver transplantation? Liver Transpl. 2013;19:S289.
173. Ravaioli M, Zanello M, Grazi GL, Ercolani G, Cescon M, DelGaudio M, Cucchetti A, Pinna AD. Portal vein thrombosis andliver transplantation: evolution during 10 years of experience at the University of Bologna. Ann Surg. 2011;253:378–84. https://doi.org/10.1097/SLA.0b013e318206818b. PMID: 21183851

Idiopathic Portal Hypertension (Portosinusoidal Disease)

19

Virginia Hernández-Gea, Ernest Belmonte,
Angeles García-Criado, and Juan Carlos García-Pagán

Idiopathic portal hypertension is a rare cause of intrahepatic portal hypertension (PH) of uncertain etiology and frequently misdiagnosed. Commonly the diagnosis is made when PH related complications such as ascites and variceal bleeding appear in the absence of cirrhosis, portal vein thrombosis or other specific liver diseases.

The nomenclature of this entity has been very ambiguous and has made difficult the advance in the knowledge of its pathophysiology. For years it has received different names such as hepato-portal sclerosis, non-cirrhotic portal fibrosis, idiopathic portal hypertension, incomplete septal cirrhosis and regenerative nodular hyperplasia. In addition, some of the liver histology features observed in PSD are relatively frequent in patients in whom liver biopsy has been done for mild liver tests abnormalities in the absence of portal hypertension, and only some of these patients will develop a full-blown PSD during the follow-up. To address this problem and unify the diagnostic criteria the international committee of the monothematic conference organized by VALDIG (Vascular Liver Disease Group) in Ascona in 2017 proposed a new name for the disease: **PortoSinusoidal Disease (PSD)**. This term has the advantage of not mentioning the presence of portal hypertension and mentioning the anatomical site where the injury is thought to occur.

As previously mentioned, PSD can be diagnosed at liver biopsy in an asymptomatic patient submitted for the study of a mild alteration in liver enzymes, usually ASAT and/or ALAT. However, even when portal hypertension is already present, the clinical presentation of the disease varies form an asymptomatic state to severe

V. Hernández-Gea • J.C. García-Pagán (✉)
Hepatic Hemodynamic Laboratory, Liver Unit, Hospital Clinic, IDIBAPS, Universitat de Barcelona, Barcelona, Spain

Centro de Investigación Biomédica en Red de Enfermedades Hepáticas y Digestivas, CIBERehd, Instituto de Salud Carlos III, Madrid, Spain
e-mail: JCGARCIA@clinic.cat

E. Belmonte • A. García-Criado
Department of Radiology, Hospital Clinic, Universitat de Barcelona, Barcelona, Spain

© Springer International Publishing AG, part of Springer Nature 2018
A. Berzigotti, J. Bosch (eds.), *Diagnostic Methods for Cirrhosis and Portal Hypertension*, https://doi.org/10.1007/978-3-319-72628-1_19

Table 19.1 Diagnostic criteria for PSD

Presence of clinical signs of portal hypertension
Cirrhosis excluded by hepatic biopsy
Exclusion of chronic liver diseases leading to cirrhosis or non-cirrhotic portal hypertension
Exclusion of diseases causing non-cirrhotic portal hypertension
Patent portal and hepatic veins (checked by Doppler ultrasound or CT scanning)

complications of portal hypertension (PH). Portal hypertension-related bleeding mainly due to esophageal varices is the most frequent clinical presentation [1], whereas asymptomatic patients are commonly diagnosed due to thrombocytopenia and/or splenomegaly [2]. Ascites development is associated with bad prognosis and hepatic encephalopathy although rarely can develop, usually due to the massive presence of porto-systemic collaterals [3]; other PH-related complications rarely occur.

Currently, in patients with PSD and no portal hypertension, the diagnosis is based on liver histology, and the ability to recognize subtle changes is highly related to the experience of the pathologist and to the availability of a high-quality and large liver sample. Liver biopsy should demonstrate the presence of the typical lesions such as phlebosclerosis, nodular regeneration, sinusoidal dilatation, para-portal venous anastomosis and perisinusoidal fibrosis [4]. In patients with PSD-associated portal hypertension, it is mandatory to exclude other pathologies causing portal hypertension and to demonstrate a patent portal venous axis in addition to the findings of the liver biopsy.

Non-invasive diagnosis of PSD still remains a challenge due to the absence of a specific diagnostic test; nevertheless here we describe how some minimally invasive and non-invasive methods may help in the diagnostic work-up and decision-making (Table 19.1).

19.1   Non-invasive Methods

19.1.1 Doppler Ultrasonography

Ultrasonography is usually the first-line approach for the study of symptomatic patients or after liver test abnormalities detection. Frequent findings although not specific for PSD, more frequently detected when portal hypertension is present, are the presence of soft or slightly irregular liver surface, caudal lobe hypertrophy, right hepatic lobe atrophy and thickening of the portal vein walls and intrahepatic portal vein radicle irregularities [5]. Large splenomegaly [4] is more frequently found than in cirrhosis.

Contrast harmonic US with perflubutane micro bubble agent (Sonazoid™) has been suggested as a useful tool for PSD diagnosis. Sonazoid, contrary to other purely intravascular agents (SonoVue® or Definity®), has the property of accumulating in the liver parenchyma. In patients with PSD a delayed peri-portal parenchymal enhancement (differences in the onset time of portal contrast enhancement and different signal intensity) has been described [6, 7]. A plausible explanation for this abnormal distribution of microbubbles may be due to narrowing and/or obstruction in the peripheral portal vein branches that impairs liver hemodynamics and perfusion. This technique has been proposed as a microflow imaging that may help to evaluate the spatial continuity between portal vein branches and depict vascular morphology. Although initially promising, these signs described in Asian population have not been yet validated.

19.1.2 Liver and Spleen Stiffness

Elastography is very useful discriminating between liver cirrhosis and PSD. Liver stiffness values measured by Transient elastography (Fibroscan) [8] and Acoustic radiation force impulse Elastography (ARFI) [9] are significantly lower in PSD than in patients with cirrhosis with similar clinical signs of portal hypertension. Values of liver stiffness <14 kPa in the presence of clear signs of portal hypertension should give rise to PSD suspicion [8]. By contrast, spleen stiffness is increased and even higher in PSD than in cirrhosis. As a consequence, the ratio spleen/liver stiffness is markedly elevated in PSD patients and can be used to differentiate PSD from cirrhosis [9].

19.1.3 Computed Tomography (CT)

Most of the patients with PSD have extra and/or intrahepatic portal venous abnormalities, heterogeneous hepatic enhancement and morphologic changes in the liver at CT that may help to differentiate from cirrhosis. An accurate evaluation of the peripheral intrahepatic portal branch is indispensable and requires thin sections acquisition and postprocessing reconstruction.

Another radiological finding characteristic of PSD, observed in both CT and Magnetic Resonance Imaging, is the approximation of medium caliber portal vessels and/or hepatic veins to the hepatic surface as a consequence of a subcapsular parenchymal atrophy secondary to an insufficient portal circulation [10].

Sudden narrowing of second-degree intrahepatic portal vein branches is the most common finding in CT angiography and can progress to vessel disappearance [5, 11]. Abnormalities range from caliber reduction to vessel disappearance due to venous sclerosis. Portography show intrahepatic paucity of medium-sized portal branches, obtuse angle division of the most peripheral portal branches, abrupt vascular interruptions and lack of opacification of some of the main intrahepatic branches.

Around 45% of patients present increased arterial hepatic inflow responsible in part of the high prevalence of perfusion disorders and parenchymal heterogeneity [11, 12]. This increased arterial inflow is frequently accompanied of diminished portal perfusion especially at the periphery. These hemodynamic abnormalities explain the elevated incidence of benign hypervascular nodules in patients with PSD. Nodular regenerative hyperplasia is the most common histological finding that can be found in around 15% of the patients [11].

Although only in form of a case report, a reduction in Tc-99m galactosyl human serum albumin evaluated by single photon emission CT with has been associated with PSD [13]. All these findings have been reported in patients with PSD and portal hypertension and their presence in patients without PSD has not been explored yet.

19.1.4 Magnetic Resonance Imaging (MRI)

An increase in intrahepatic periportal signal intensity in T2-weighted images has been associated with abnormalities in the portal tracts, presence of fibrosis and increased vascular channels. It can also identify small vessels parallel to the second-order branches of the intrahepatic portal vein (portal collateral pathways) [14].

A periportal enhancement has also been described in the hepatobiliary phase of hepato-specific contrast gadolinium ethoxybenzyl diethylenetriamine pentaacetic acid (Gd-EOB-DTPA). The incidence of periportal high intensity observed on hepatobiliary phase images of EOB-enhanced MRI was significantly higher in cases with primary biliary cirrhosis (PBC) and idiopathic portal hypertension than in those with chronic liver disease and hepatic cirrhosis. It is assumed that in liver diseases such as PBC and Idiopathic portal hypertension, periportal hepatocytes show regenerative changes and present a relatively increased uptake of EOB compared to the damaged background liver, which shows a decrease uptake of EOB [15].

19.2   (Minimally) Invasive Methods

19.2.1 Hepatic Vein Catheterization

Hepatic venous pressure gradient (HVPG) is the gold standard method to diagnose portal hypertension in cirrhosis. A finding of an HVPG usually normal or slightly elevated but below the threshold required for developing portal hypertension related complications (10 mmHg) in a patient with clear signs of portal hypertension and an imaging study discarding portal vein thrombosis should rise the suspicion of PSD. In addition, around 50% of the patients with PSD develop hepatic vein-to-vein communications (HVVC), a finding more frequently found in PSD patients than in patients with cirrhosis (50% vs less than 10%) ([8, 16, 17]). The presence of HVVC may prevent a proper occlusion of the hepatic vein, and in this case the HVPG can be underestimated. However, a proper occlusion of the hepatic vein in a point where HVVC are not present is usually possible and allows to measure the wedged hepatic vein pressure properly, and to confirm that the HVPG is normal or at most slightly elevated.

19.2.2 Liver Biopsy

Liver biopsy remains a mandatory examination to get the diagnosis of PSD. It must exclude liver cirrhosis and it can found some histological findings that are associated to PSD.

The most common histological finding is the narrowing or obliteration of small portal vein branches (obliterative portal venopathy), but other usual morphological changes are: increased number of portal vascular channels, dilated portal veins with herniation into the parenchyma (paraportal shunts), sinusoidal dilatation, and thin fibrous septa and fibrotic portal tracts in the absence of cirrhosis [4, 18–20]. Development of benign nodules due to hyperplasia in the best-perfused areas and atrophic borders in the areas with reduced portal venous blood supply represent the typical morphological change in PSD [20, 21]. Two kind of benign nodular lesions can be identified in patients with PSD: nodular regenerative hyperplasia (central hyperplasia and atrophic border without fibrosis) and partial nodular transformation (parenchymal nodules in the perihiliar region around large portal tracts in the absence of cirrhosis) [22, 23].

19.3   Future Diagnostic Tools

19.3.1 Metabolomics

Innovative research using high-throughput technology has allowed the identification of metabolic biomarkers able to differentiate PSD patients with portal hypertension from patients with cirrhosis with similar signs of portal hypertension or healthy individuals. A proof of concept, phase 2 diagnostic study evaluated 33 patients with PSD and matched controls (both healthy volunteers and patients with cirrhosis) and metabolomic analysis of plasma samples was performed using mass spectrometry. Authors could demonstrate a discriminative plasmatic metabolic profile on patients with PSD [24]. Moreover, using an untargeted approach analysis the same authors could identify a specific metabolomic signature that allows the diagnosis of PSD from patients with cirrhosis or healthy individuals, with high specificity and sensibility [25]. Based on this pioneering data, metabolomics may represent an excellent non-invasive diagnostic tool. However, the potential value of this tool needs to be validated in other cohorts of PSD patients with and without portal hypertension.

Conclusions

Diagnosis of PSD remains a clinical unmet need and so far there are no specific diagnostic tests and therefore excluding other causes of PHT is mandatory. However research in the last decade has shed light into the field and findings in non-invasive methods or minimally invasive technics such as hepatic vein catheterization definitely have a complementary role to liver biopsy in the diagnosis of PSD (Fig. 19.1 and Table 19.2). Innovation and evidence-based research may lead to the discovery of new diagnostic tools able to unravel the actual challenge of PSD diagnosis.

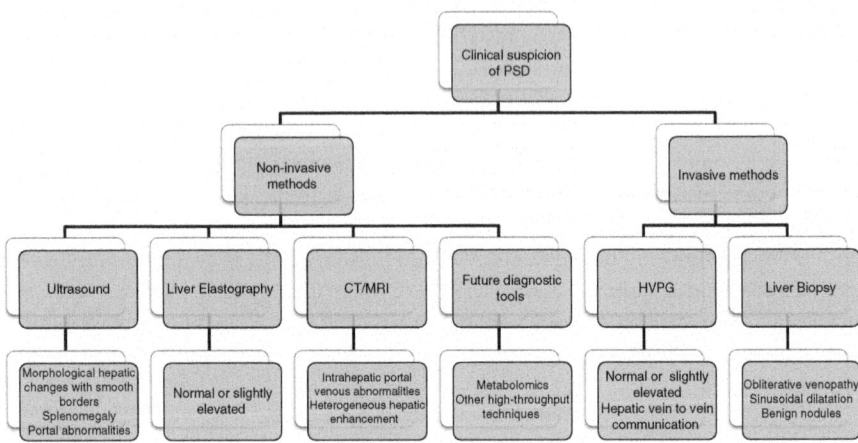

Fig. 19.1 Flowchart summarizing how the different imaging methods can help in the diagnosis of PSD

Table 19.2 Common finding in patients with PSD

Technique	Finding
Invasive methods	
Hepatic catheterization	Hepatic vein-to-vein communications – HVPG normal or slightly elevated
Liver biopsy	– Obliteraitve portal venopathy – Paraportal shunts – Sinusoidal dilatation – Periportal/perisinusoidal fibrosis
Non-invasive methods	
US	– Soft or slightly irregular liver surface – Caudal lobe hypertrophy and right hepatic lobe atrophy – Thickening of the portal vein walls and intrahepatic portal vein radicle irregularities – Large splenomegaly
CT	– Extra and/or intrahepatic portal venous abnormalities. – Heterogeneous hepatic enhancement – Elevated incidence of benign hypervascular nodules
MRI	– Increase in intrahepatic periportal signal intensity in T2-weighted images – Periportal enhancement in the hepatobiliary phase of hepato-specific contrast
Elastography	– Values of liver stiffness <14 kPa in the presence of clear signs of portal hypertension – Spleen stiffness has been described to be higher in PSD than in cirrhosis and the ratio spleen/liver stiffness significantly lower

References

1. Schouten JN, Francque S, Van Vlierberghe H, Colle I, Nevens F, Delwaide J, Adler M, et al. The influence of laboratory-induced MELD score differences on liver allocation: more reality than myth. Clin Transpl. 2012;26:E62–70.
2. Siramolpiwat S, Seijo S, Miquel R, Berzigotti A, Garcia-Criado A, Darnell A, Turon F, et al. Idiopathic portal hypertension: natural history and long-term outcome. Hepatology. 2014;59:2276–85.
3. Krasinskas AM, Eghtesad B, Kamath PS, Demetris AJ, Abraham SC. Liver transplantation for severe intrahepatic noncirrhotic portal hypertension. Liver Transpl. 2005;11:627–34. discussion 610–21
4. Hillaire S, Bonte E, Denninger MH, Casadevall N, Cadranel JF, Lebrec D, Valla D, et al. Idiopathic non-cirrhotic intrahepatic portal hypertension in the west: a re-evaluation in 28 patients. Gut. 2002;51:275–80.
5. Dhiman RK, Chawla Y, Vasishta RK, Kakkar N, Dilawari JB, Trehan MS, Puri P, et al. Non-cirrhotic portal fibrosis (idiopathic portal hypertension): experience with 151 patients and a review of the literature. J Gastroenterol Hepatol. 2002;17:6–16.
6. Maruyama H, Shimada T, Ishibashi H, Takahashi M, Kamesaki H, Yokosuka O. Delayed periportal enhancement: a characteristic finding on contrast ultrasound in idiopathic portal hypertension. Hepatol Int. 2012;6:511–9.
7. Maruyama H, Ishibashi H, Takahashi M, Imazeki F, Yokosuka O. Effect of signal intensity from the accumulated microbubbles in the liver for differentiation of idiopathic portal hypertension from liver cirrhosis. Radiology. 2009;252:587–94.
8. Seijo S, Reverter E, Miquel R, Berzigotti A, Abraldes JG, Bosch J, Garcia-Pagan JC. Role of hepatic vein catheterisation and transient elastography in the diagnosis of idiopathic portal hypertension. Dig Liver Dis. 2012;44:855–60.
9. Furuichi Y, Moriyasu F, Taira J, Sugimoto K, Sano T, Ichimura S, Miyata Y, et al. Noninvasive diagnostic method for idiopathic portal hypertension based on measurements of liver and spleen stiffness by ARFI elastography. J Gastroenterol. 2013;48:1061–8.
10. Jha P, Poder L, Wang ZJ, Westphalen AC, Yeh BM, Coakley FV. Radiologic mimics of cirrhosis. AJR Am J Roentgenol. 2010;194:993–9.
11. Glatard AS, Hillaire S, d'Assignies G, Cazals-Hatem D, Plessier A, Valla DC, Vilgrain V. Obliterative portal venopathy: findings at CT imaging. Radiology. 2012;263:741–50.
12. Waguri S, Kohmura M, Kanamori S, Watanabe T, Ohsawa Y, Koike M, Tomiyama Y, et al. Different distribution patterns of the two mannose 6-phosphate receptors in rat liver. J Histochem Cytochem. 2001;49:1397–405.
13. Nishida T, Hayakawa K, Ogasawara H, Katsuma Y. Interesting RI accumulation in hepatic images with Tc-99m GSA SPECT scintigraphy in idiopathic portal hypertension. Ann Nucl Med. 2001;15:53–5. discussion 52
14. Krishnan P, Fiel MI, Rosenkrantz AB, Hajdu CH, Schiano TD, Oyfe I, Taouli B. Hepatoportal sclerosis: CT and MRI appearance with histopathologic correlation. AJR Am J Roentgenol. 2012;198:370–6.
15. Kobayashi S, Matsui O, Gabata T, Koda W, Minami T, Kozaka K, Kitao A, et al. Intrahepatic periportal high intensity on hepatobiliary phase images of Gd-EOB-DTPA-enhanced MRI: imaging findings and prevalence in various hepatobiliary diseases. Jpn J Radiol. 2013;31:9–15.
16. Okuda K, Kono K, Ohnishi K, Kimura K, Omata M, Koen H, Nakajima Y, et al. Clinical study of eighty-six cases of idiopathic portal hypertension and comparison with cirrhosis with splenomegaly. Gastroenterology. 1984;86:600–10.
17. Futagawa S, Fukazawa M, Musha H, Isomatsu T, Koyama K, Ito T, Horisawa M, et al. Hepatic venography in noncirrhotic idiopathic portal hypertension. Comparison with cirrhosis of the liver. Radiology. 1981;141:303–9.
18. Sciot R, Staessen D, Van Damme B, Van Steenbergen W, Fevery J, De Groote J, Desmet VJ. Incomplete septal cirrhosis: histopathological aspects. Histopathology. 1988;13:593–603.

19. Schouten JN, Garcia-Pagan JC, Valla DC, Janssen HL. Idiopathic noncirrhotic portal hypertension. Hepatology. 2011;54:1071–81.
20. Ludwig J, Hashimoto E, Obata H, Baldus WP. Idiopathic portal hypertension. Hepatology. 1993;17:1157–62.
21. Wanless IR. Micronodular transformation (nodular regenerative hyperplasia) of the liver: a report of 64 cases among 2,500 autopsies and a new classification of benign hepatocellular nodules. Hepatology. 1990;11:787–97.
22. International Working P. Terminology of nodular hepatocellular lesions. Hepatology. 1995;22:983–93.
23. Sherlock S, Feldman CA, Moran B, Scheuer PJ. Partial nodular transformation of the liver with portal hypertension. Am J Med. 1966;40:195–203.
24. Seijo S, Lozano JJ, Alonso C, Reverter E, Miquel R, Abraldes JG, Martinez-Chantar ML, et al. Metabolomics discloses potential biomarkers for the noninvasive diagnosis of idiopathic portal hypertension. Am J Gastroenterol. 2013;108:926–32.
25. Seijo S, Lozano JJ, Alonso C, Miquel R, Berzigotti A, Reverter E, Turon F, et al. Metabolomics as a diagnostic tool for idiopathic non-cirrhotic portal hypertension. Liver Int. 2016;36:1051–8.

Hereditary Hemorrhagic Telangiectasia (Osler-Weber-Rendu Syndrome) and Liver Vascular Malformations

20

Elisabetta Buscarini and Guido Manfredi

Hereditary hemorrhagic telangiectasia (HHT) is an autosomal dominant disorder with an estimated incidence of 1/5000, characterized by recurrent epistaxis, cutaneous telangiectasia and visceral arteriovenous malformations (VMs) that affect many organs, including the lungs, gastrointestinal tract, liver and brain.

Telangiectasia is the elementary lesion of HHT, arising from the dilation of a postcapillary venule that fuses directly with an arteriole, bypassing the capillary system. Vascular malformations (VMs) in HHT are direct arterio-venous or veno-venous connections with complex architecture; in the case of an arterio-venous VM upstream and downstream hemodynamic consequences are expected. Clinical presentation of HHT varies greatly, depending on the number, type and location of telangiectases or vascular malformations (VMs) with potential morbidity and mortality.

Diagnosis is based on the Curaçao criteria [1] and is considered definite if at least three criteria are present. The criteria are: (1) spontaneous and recurrent epistaxis, (2) telangiectasia, (3) family history and (4) visceral lesions. Two genes from different families are associated with HHT: HHT type 1 results from mutations in *ENG* on chromosome 9 (coding for endoglin), and HHT type 2 results from mutations in *ACRLV1* on chromosome 12 (coding for the activin receptor-like kinase 1, ALK-1). Mutations to either of these genes account for most, but not all, clinical cases. In addition, mutations to *MADH4* (encoding SMAD4) [2] that cause juvenile polyposis/HHT overlap syndrome have been described. All three identified HHT genes encode endothelial cell transmembrane proteins, which appear to be components of the receptor complexes for growth factors from the Transforming Growth Factor-beta superfamily (TGF-beta). The penetrance of HHT is age related with the disease signs expressed generally by the age of 40.

E. Buscarini (✉) • G. Manfredi
Gastroenterology and Endoscopy Department, HHT Reference Center, Crema, Italy
e-mail: elisabetta.buscarini@hcrema.it; ebuscarini@rim.it

© Springer International Publishing AG, part of Springer Nature 2018
A. Berzigotti, J. Bosch (eds.), *Diagnostic Methods for Cirrhosis and Portal Hypertension*, https://doi.org/10.1007/978-3-319-72628-1_20

Liver involvement occurs more frequently in HHT type 2 [3]. The mean age of patients with symptoms of hepatic VMs is around 50 [3, 4]. Literature data show a strong predominance of hepatic VMs in females with HHT, with a male/female ratio of 1/4.5.

Liver VMs unique to HHT are spread throughout the liver, can evolve in a continuum from small telangiectases to large VMs, occur in 41–74% of patients with HHT [5, 6].

Three different types of intrahepatic shunting are recognized: hepatic artery to hepatic veins, hepatic artery to portal vein and portal vein to hepatic veins. These shunts may lead to either high output cardiac failure (HOCF), or portal hypertension, or encephalopathy, or biliary ischemia, or mesenteric ischemia [4–8]; the two latter are due to a blood flow steal through arteriovenous shunting. Perfusion abnormality can also entail hepatocellular regenerative activity, either diffuse or partial, leading to focal nodular hyperplasia (FNH), which has a 100-fold greater prevalence in HHT patients than in the general population, or to nodular regenerative hyperplasia [6–9]. Arterio-hepatic shunting is associated with increased cardiac preload and decreased peripheral vascular resistances, leading to an increase of cardiac output, which over time entails adaptive modifications of cardiac structure and hemodynamics, possibly up to the final stage of heart failure. A correlation is observed between cardiac output and hepatic artery diameter [10].

Anicteric cholestasis is observed in one-third of patients with liver VMs [4]; its degree is generally correlated with the severity of vascular malformations. Of note, liver synthetic function is normal even in liver VMs with portal hypertension [8].

Only 8% of patients with liver VMs are symptomatic at baseline as shown by cross-sectional surveys [5, 6]. On the other hand the data about natural history of liver VMs in HHT have demonstrated that 21% of patients had an increasing size and complexity of liver VMs over a median follow-up of 44 months; hepatic VM-related morbidity and mortality occurred in 25% and 5% of patients respectively, with incidence rates of complications and death of 3.6 and 1.1 per 100 person-years, respectively. HOCF represented the predominant complication associated with HHT, but complicated PH occurred at a rate comparable to that of HOCF (1.4 and 1.2 respectively per 100 person-years); HOCF and complicated PH accounted each for about a half of hepatic VM–associated fatalities [4, 8].

According to available data, treatment is recommended exclusively for symptomatic liver VMs in HHT [8]. The specific approach has to be intensive and depends on the type of complication. HOCF is first treated by administration of diuretics and beta blockers. If indicated, measures are taken to correct anemia and manage any arrhythmia, such as atrial fibrillation. Management of portal hypertension is analogous to that recommended in patients with cirrhosis. Biliary necrosis, which is associated with a poor prognosis, is treated with antibiotics and all necessary supportive measures.

Looking for a potential alternative to invasive therapies for cure of symptomatic liver VMs in HHT, recently bevacizumab (an antivascular endothelial growth factor monoclonal antibody) was evaluated in HHT patients with severe liver involvement [11]. These preliminary data suggested that bevacizumab may be a therapeutic option in the treatment of complicated liver VMs in HHT; however, potential adverse events related to bevacizumab, its rates of no or partial response, and the symptoms/signs recurrence after drug withdrawal are to be weighed carefully, depending on whether patients are candidate to OLT or not [12].

Amongst invasive therapies considered in patients refractory to first-line treatment, embolization of arteriovenous hepatic fistulas [13] is not currently recommended because it is palliative and can entail ominous complications, such as hepatic or biliary necrosis [14]; it can be considered for patients who are not candidates for OLT [8].

Nowadays OLT remains the only definitive curative option for patients with HHT who have refractory cardiac failure, biliary ischemia and/or complicated portal hypertension due to liver VMs. Outcomes of OLT for liver VMs in HHT are excellent [8]. In HHT, liver VMs do not progress to cirrhosis, and even in more severe cases they are not associated to liver insufficiency. In fact HHT is included in MELD (Model for End Stage Liver Disease) exceptions [8, 15] with a score of 22 for intractable HOCF/PH, and 40 for ischemic biliary necrosis. On the basis of available literature and expert consensus OLT can be discussed in the HHT patients with otherwise intractable liver VMs, with a priority based on the predictors of bad outcome [8].

20.1   Diagnosis of Liver VMs in HHT

Investigations for liver VMs are to be completed in HHT patients with symptoms/ signs suggestive of complicated liver VMs and in all subjects at risk for HHT, as liver VMs diagnosis and staging offer the advantages of a proper patient management and follow-up [8].

20.2   Doppler US

At Doppler US exam hepatic artery dilation is a prominent feature of liver VMs in HHT since very early stages; dilation of the hepatic artery has been described in patients with cirrhosis or hypervascular liver tumors; however, in patients with HHT hepatic artery flow may increase to values greatly exceeding the upper normal limit, and hepatic artery larger than 10 mm has been repeatedly reported (Fig. 20.1).

The diameter of the hepatic artery (inner diameter of the common hepatic artery measured 10–20 mm distal to the celiac trunk) is above normal limit of 5 mm ± 1 (Fig. 20.1) without overlap between HHT patients with liver involvement or patients with HHT without liver VMs, patients with cirrhosis, healthy subjects; it represents a very sensitive diagnostic parameter for hepatic VMs in HHT. The intra-hepatic dilated artery branches appear as tubular structures either parallel to portal branches (double-channel aspect) or tortuous and tangled in more severe liver involvement. The unique ability of pulsed and color Doppler US over other imaging modalities is to allow a rapid analysis of flow pattern of hepatic VMs, including qualitative

Fig. 20.1 (**a**) In grade 1 liver VMs transverse sonogram of upper abdomen shows celiac trunk (ct): hepatic artery (ha) is slightly dilated (diameter 6.4 mm), without normal tapering. *Pv* portal vein, *sa* splenic artery, *vc* vena cava, *a* aorta. (**b**) Marked dilation (18.7 mm) of hepatic artery in grade 4 liver VMs. *Pv* portal vein, *sa* splenic artery, *vc* vena cava, *a* aorta, * VMs

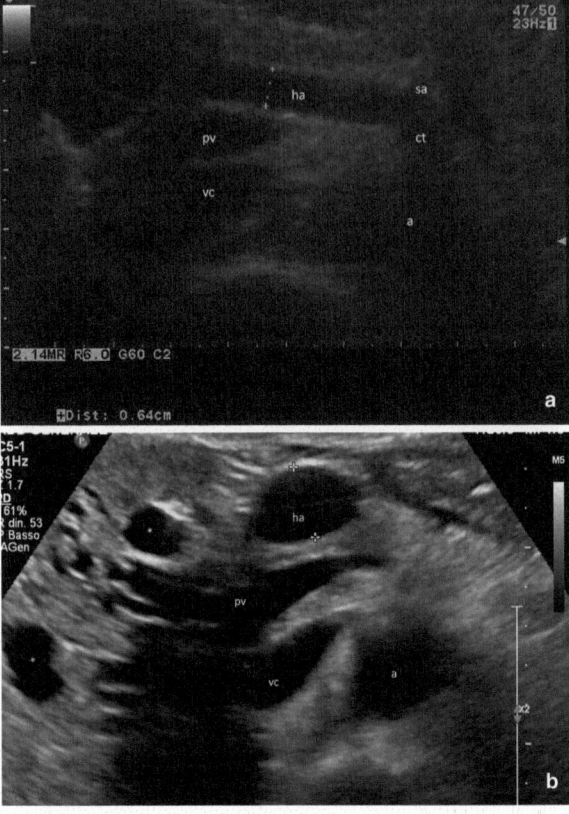

parameters, as flow direction and turbulence, quantitative parameters as the angle-corrected (60°) flow velocities (peak flow velocity in hepatic artery, mean velocity in portal vein, diastolic peak flow velocity in hepatic veins) and semi-quantitative measures as Resistivity Index (RI) and Pulsatility Index (PI). The spectral analysis show high-velocity flow (even aliased or turbulent) in the hepatic artery and its branches with high diastolic phase due to low parenchymal resistances, with RI and PI values lower than in controls; RI shows an inverse correlation with the entity of intrahepatic shunt, and is particularly low where shunt is predominantly arterioportal [5, 16, 17] (Fig. 20.2).

Intrahepatic and particularly peripheral hypervascularization (Fig. 20.3) can be detected with different color Doppler analysis modalities [5, 16]. At color Doppler analysis of liver parenchyma color-spots or spider-like vessels, with a high-velocity arterial blood flow and low resistivity index, identify small VMs [5, 17].

Hepatic artery to portal vein shunts cause pulsatility of portal flow possibly with phasic or continuous reversal. Hepatic artery to hepatic vein shunts cause changes in the Doppler waveform of the hepatic veins, with prominence of diastolic peak and with shift from triphasic to biphasic in more severe cases. The diameter of

Fig. 20.2 Doppler US analysis of hepatic artery flow in HHT liver VMs. (**a**) Longitudinal sonogram of liver demonstrates a prominent hepatic artery below liver margin, with spectrally broadened, high-velocity flow (peak flow velocity: 321 cm/s). (**b**) Color Doppler with spectral analysis of prominent intrahepatic branches of hepatic artery shows high-velocity flow, both systolic and diastolic, with low RI (0.52)

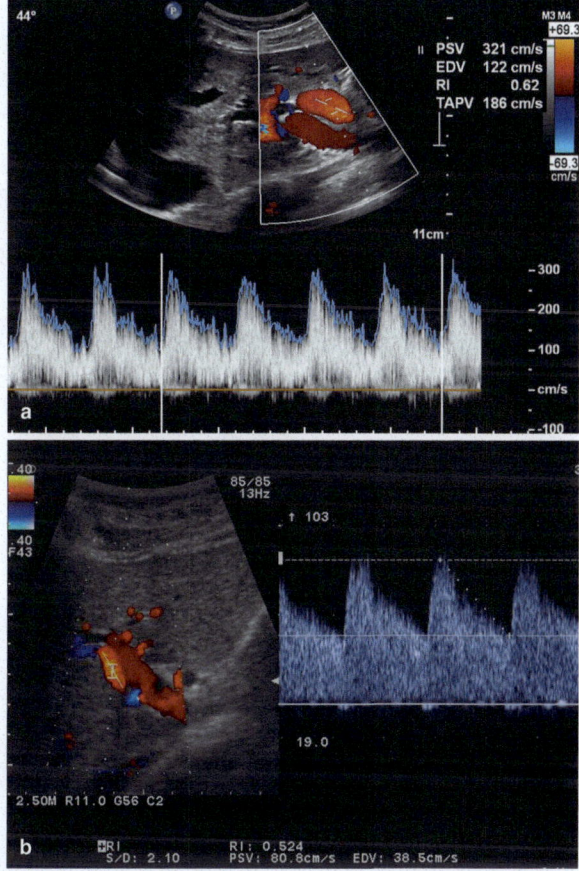

portal vein and/or of hepatic veins is dilated in severe and decompensated liver arteriovenous shunt (Figs. 20.4, 20.5, and 20.6). Portosystemic shunts can also be found (Fig. 20.7).

Liver size can be enlarged (length at midclavicular line >15 cm) in liver VMs in HHT, whereas spleen size is usually normal (bipolar diameter <13 cm). US evaluation of liver parenchyma can show either focal isoechoic lesions compatible with FNH (Fig. 20.8) or, in more severe VMs, a nodular liver surface and coarse, heterogeneous echo pattern (Figs. 20.3 and 20.6). Ascites can be associated with severe decompensated liver VMs (Fig. 20.6).

Combination of different features of liver VMs have been proposed as US criteria for the hepatic involvement in HHT. Anomalies of liver vessels have been classified with Doppler ultrasound which is the only imaging technique able to give a severity grading (from 0.5 to 4) (Table 20.1) of liver VMs [5]. Caselitz et al. [16] have defined two major criteria as dilated common hepatic artery >7 mm and intrahepatic arterial hypervascularization whereas minor criteria are either Vmax in hepatic artery >110 cm/s, or RI of the proper hepatic artery <0.60, or Vmax of the

Fig. 20.3 (a) Intrahepatic hypervascularization is demonstrated by color Doppler as color spots and tangles of vessels (arrowhead) and, (b), as "spider-like" vessels; liver margins are nodular (arrows) and parenchymal echotexture is coarse

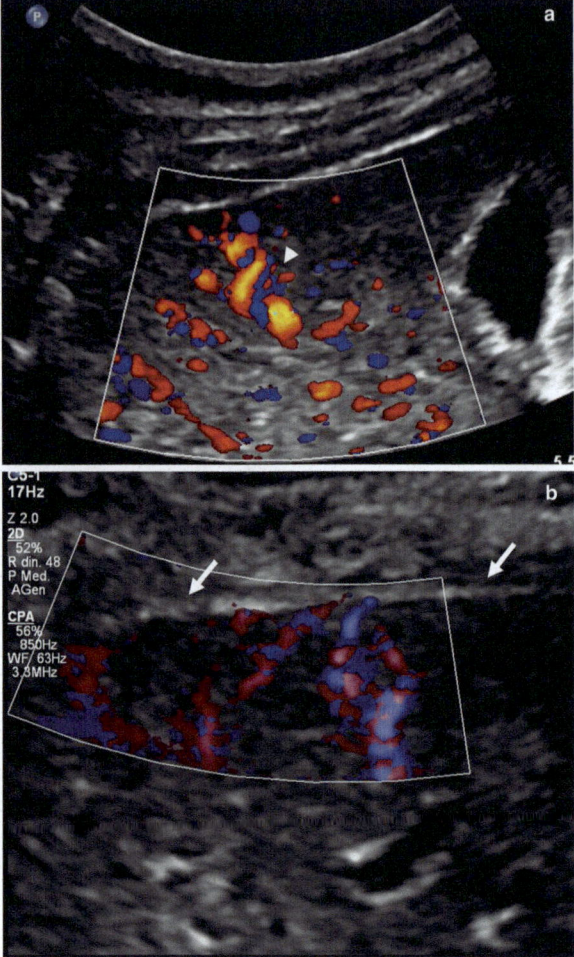

portal vein >25 cm/s or tortuous course of the extrahepatic hepatic artery; two major criteria, or one major and two minor would to be required for the diagnosis of liver VMs in HHT.

Sensitivity of different Doppler US criteria [5, 16, 17] has been recently compared, using CT or MR as standard of reference, in a series of 18 patients; the Caselitz and Buonamico criteria missed 16% and 27% respectively of liver VMs, the Buscarini criteria did not miss any [18].

As Doppler US plays a pivotal role in the diagnosis of hepatic VMs, observer agreement on the parameters for identifying VMs is crucial, all the more so as Doppler US is an operator-dependent imaging technique. Interobserver agreement on Doppler US diagnosis of liver VMs in HHT was evaluated in a controlled interobserver study: a very good interobserver agreement was found on diagnosing the presence/absence of liver VMs, with K value 0.85–0.93 [19].

Fig. 20.4 Grade 4 liver VMs with predominant artero-hepatic shunt. (**a**) Color US analysis with substraction of liver parenchyma shows markedly dilated hepatic veins (hv), surrounded by prominent and tortuous hepatic artery branches (arrows). (**b**) In dilated hepatic vein a biphasic flow with high diastolic peak is shown

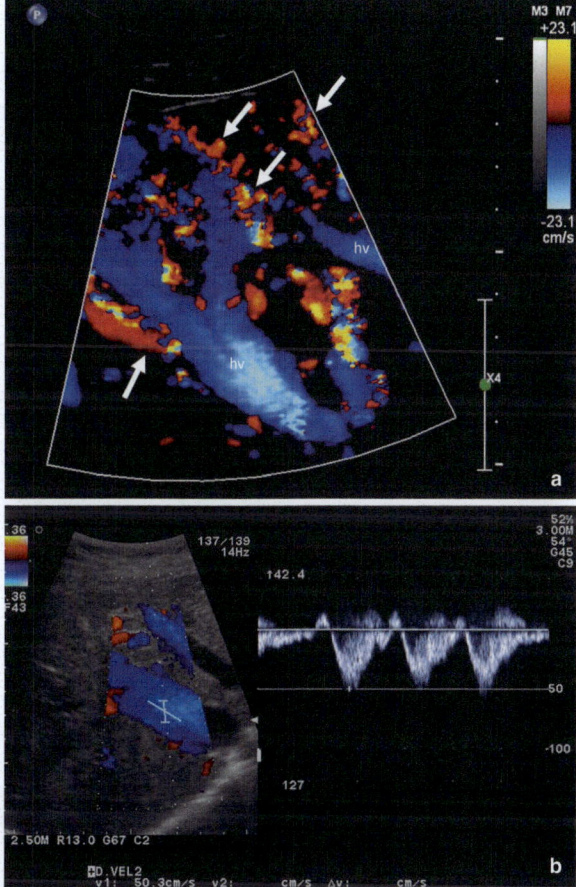

The Doppler US severity grading of liver VMs [5] has been shown to be a predictor of clinical outcome [4], and insofar it is very important to allow a tailored patient management and follow-up.

Contrast enhanced US (CEUS) findings with the use of a sulfur hexafluoride-filled microbubble contrast agent have been reported in 18 HHT patients with liver VMs. The study demonstrated significant lowest time to peak (69.8%) and a 100% AUC values in the hepatic artery [18]. However, the use of sulfur hexafluoridefilled microbubble contrast is contraindicated by the manufacturer in patients with right-to-left shunt, and could thus represent a hazard in HHT subjects who can have pulmonary VMs in a high percentage of cases [14]; furthermore CEUS appears a pointless add to Doppler US evaluation of liver VMs, as the same study has shown that also Doppler US criteria [5] had a 100% accuracy.

Doppler US sensitivity for liver VMs compares favourably with multislice CT (86% vs 84%) in a series of 153 patients [17]. Important advantages of Doppler US on contrast enhanced CT/MR are the ability to stage liver VMs

Fig. 20.5 Grade 4 liver
VMs with predominant
artero-portal shunt. (**a, b**)
Marked dilatation of portal
vein (pv) with prominent
arterial branches (arrows):
(**c**) Spectral analysis of
portal flow shows a
pulsatile hepatopetal flow

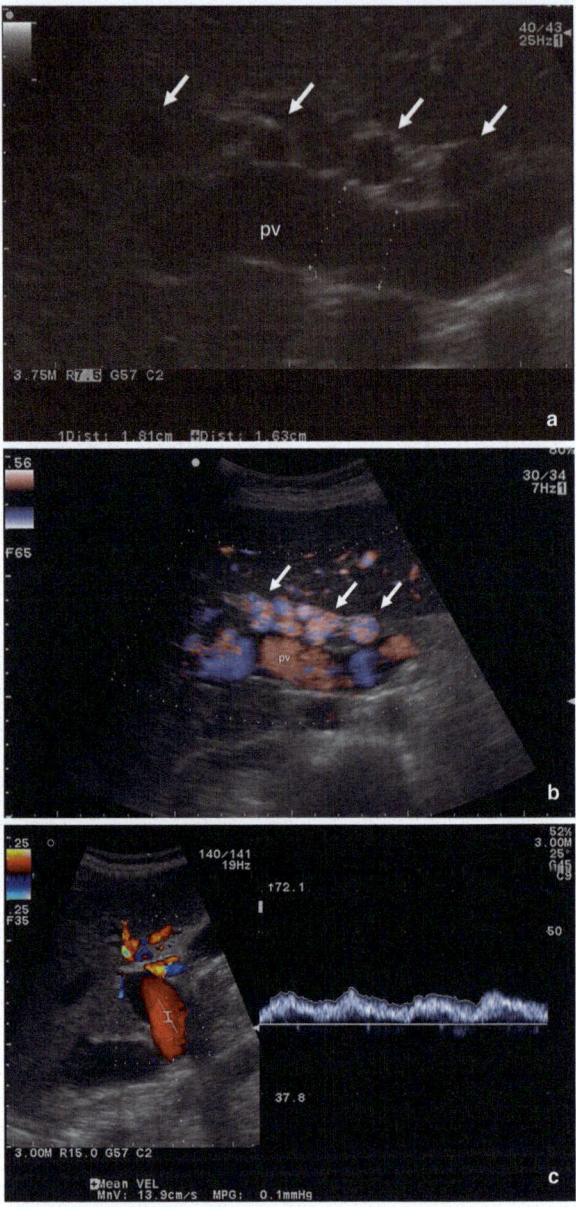

severity and a better identification of parenchymal nodularity and FNH in presence of diffuse VMs [9, 20].

Due to its non-invasiveness, safety, tolerability at any age and condition, lack of ionizing radiation, real-time evaluation without contrast material, accuracy for the detection of liver VMs, and low costs, Doppler US has been proposed as the ideal first line investigation for the assessment of liver VMs [8].

Fig. 20.6 Grade 4 liver VMs with predominant artero-portal shunt. (**a**) Inversion of flow in portal vein (pv) surrounded by tangles of tortuous arterial branches (arrows); liver surface is nodular (arrowheads), conspicuous ascites (A) is found; (**b**) Spectral analysis shows a pulsatile and continuous flow reversal in portal vein; (**c**) Spectral analysis of hepatic artery branches shows high velocity flow with notably low RI (0.45)

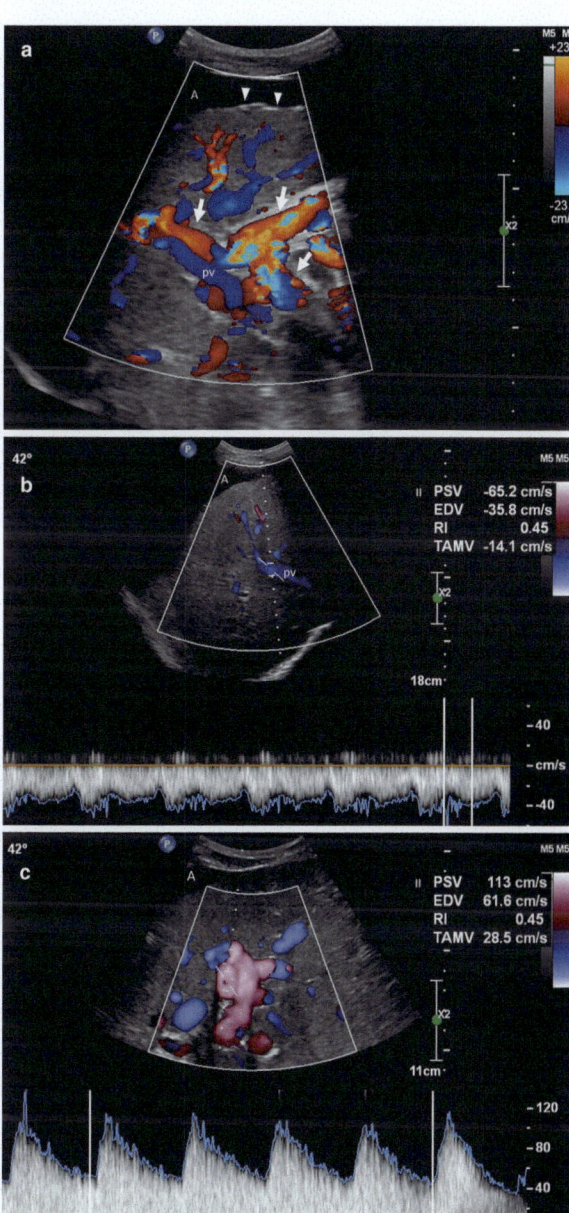

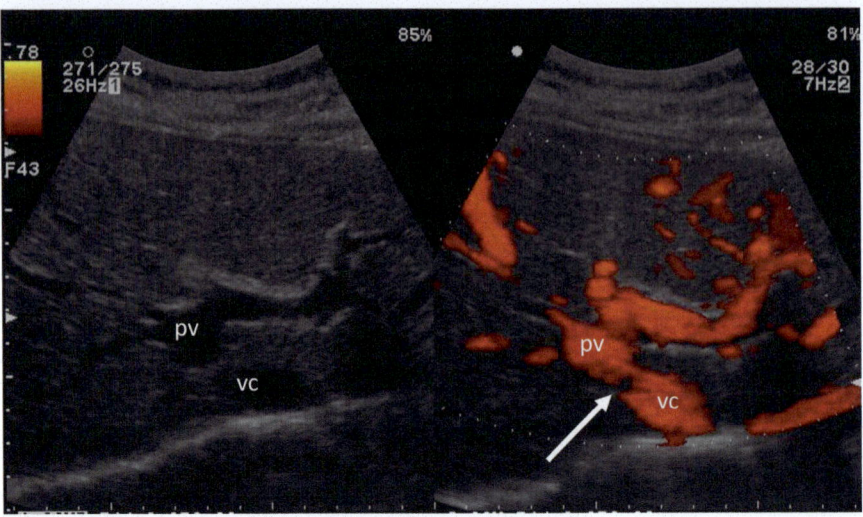

Fig. 20.7 Transverse sonogram of liver shows the aneurismatic dilation of right inferior branch of portal vein (pv) with shunt (arrow) to the vena cava (vc)

Fig. 20.8 In a HHT patient with grade 2 liver VMs US shows dilation of hepatic artery (ha) (8.8 mm) and a isoechoic oval lesion (arrow) of left liver lobe (2.2 cm), confirmed as FNH with MR. *sa* splenic artery, *ct* celiac trunk, *a* aorta

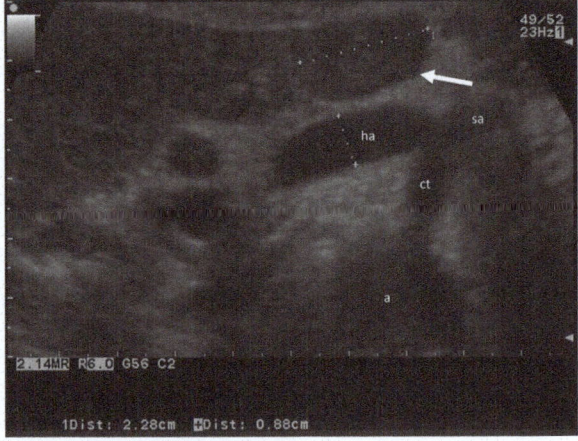

20.3 Non Invasive and Invasive Assessment of Cardiac Hemodynamics

Echocardiographic evaluation of cardiac function and morphology, particularly cardiac index and pulmonary arterial pressures, is crucial to estimate non-invasively the haemodynamic impact of liver VMs; even though quantitative assessments are an estimate, this method is the only acceptable in asymptomatic HHT patients, allowing repeated evaluations either to the diagnosis or during follow-up, in contrast with invasive measurement of cardiac hemodynamics by cardiac catherization [10, 21]. Moreover, a close correlation has been demonstrated between

Table 20.1 Doppler US grading of severity of hepatic VMs in HHT (modified from Buscarini et al., Ultrashall 2004)

VMs grade	Schema	Doppler US findings
0+		• HA diameter >5 <6 mm, and/or • PFV > 80 cm/s, and/or • RI < 0.55, and/or • Peripheral hepatic hypervascularization
1		• HA dilatation, only extrahepatic >6 mm, and • PFV > 80 cm/s, and/or • RI < 0.55
2		• HA dilatation, extra- and intrahepatic ("double channel" aspect) and • PFV > 80 cm/s • Possibly associated with moderate flow abnormality of hepatic and/or portal veins
3		• Complex changes in hepatic artery and its branches (tortuous and tangled) with marked flow abnormalities • Abnormality of hepatic and/or portal vein flow
4		Decompensation of arteriovenous shunt with: • Dilatation of hepatic and/or portal vein • Marked flow abnormalities in both arteries and vein/s

Veno-venous shunts may be found as well and do not necessarily imply a VM up-grading. Nodular transformation of hepatic parenchyma progresses along with liver VMs severity, and it is typically found in grade 4

HA hepatic artery, *PV* portal vein, *HV* hepatic vein

echocardiography and cardiac catheterization in assessing cardiac output in a series of HHT patients with liver VMs [16].

Echocardiography in HHT patients may suggest pulmonary hypertension (i.e., right ventricular enlargement and increased tricuspid regurgitant peak velocity) [22, 23] Increased pulmonary artery pressures invariably accompany and likely predispose to high output cardiac failure, entail a severe condition that significantly reduces survival on HHT patients, and should be screened in all HHT patients with liver VMs [8].

Right heart catheterization is always to be done in HHT patients with complicated liver VMs who are evaluated for OLT: specific pulmonary hemodynamic patterns with normal or reduced pulmonary vascular resistances are consistent with secondary pulmonary hypertension which accompanies liver VMs in HHT, that is a post-capillary pulmonary hypertension with pulmonary artery systolic pressure >40 mmHg; OLT is allowed with pulmonary vascular resistance <240 dynes.s.cm^{-5} [8].

Right heart catheterization is also essential in differentiating a form of primary pre-capillary pulmonary artery hypertension characterized by very high pulmonary vascular resistances which can be associated to HHT [22, 24].

20.4 CT/MR

Contrast-enhanced multiphase multirow CT shows a prominent hepatic artery possibly associated with dilated hepatic and/or portal veins. CT scans of the hepatic hilus and hepatic veins show the filling kinetics of the hepatic artery, portal vein, and hepatic veins. Multirow CT and reconstructions depict the complex hepatic vascular alterations typical of HHT, different types of shunt, parenchymal perfusion disorders, together with evaluation of spleen, gastroesophageal varices and other venous collaterals [6, 25] (Fig. 20.9). X-ray exposure and potential adverse reaction to contrast make multiphase CT recommendable wherever expertise of Doppler US is lacking to investigate symptomatic liver VMs in HHT; CT may be also required depending either on the presence of focal liver lesions or on the severity of liver VMs and their haemodynamic impact; it is always used in complicated liver VMs considered for OLT [8].

MR imaging can also show hepatic VMs. The abnormalities are depicted better on MR angiograms and dynamic MR images. Dynamic contrast-enhanced MR angiography provide a map of anomalous vessels: MR images obtained after the injection of paramagnetic contrast material allow analysis of filling kinetics, and the technique has been proven to be as accurate as multirow CT, on which it has the advantage of the absence of ionising radiation. MR can thus be considered for diagnosis and follow-up of liver VMs, wherever expertise of Doppler US is lacking [25, 26].

20.5 Celiac Angiography

Angiography, once considered the gold standard for the diagnosis of liver VMs, has been replaced by less invasive CT or MR angiograms.

Fig. 20.9 (**a**) Contrast enhanced CT scan: prominent and tangled hepatic artery (ha) with enhancement of hepatic veins (hv) in arterial phase in a patient with grade 4 liver VMs, predominantly artero-hepatic: note enlarged heart (H), marked liver enlargement, with nodular margins, and diffuse VMs throughout the liver. (**b**) Contrast enhanced CT, MIP reconstruction of arterial phase shows dilated hepatic artery (ha) with substantial intrahepatic tangles, with enhancement of hepatic veins (hv) in arterial phase

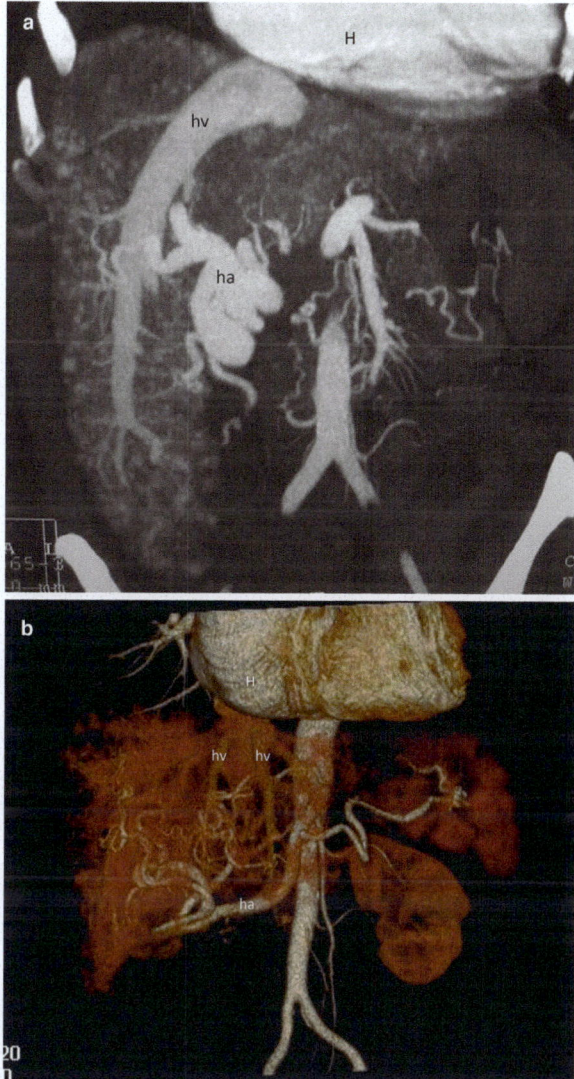

20.6 Endoscopy and Invasive Evaluation of Portal Hypertension

GI bleeding in HHT patients with portal hypertension due liver VMs is generally caused by GI telangiectases rather than to gastroesophageal varices [4], which are seldom found in these patients probably because of spontaneous liver portosystemic shunts; upper endoscopy in this setting fundamentally aims to treat bleeding telangiectases.

Portal pressure measurement with hepatic venous pressure gradient is reserved to selected patients with complicated liver VMs when evaluated for OLT [8].

20.7   Liver Biopsy

Liver biopsy is not necessary in the diagnosis of hepatic VMs related to HHT; if it is necessary for other reasons, in a patient with known or suspected HHT, the risk of increased bleeding with percutaneous transcapsular route has to be considered in view of the high prevalence of liver VMs in HHT [8].

Characterization of a liver mass in the context of HHT can be made non-invasively by weighing epidemiological (high prevalence of FNH in HHT), clinical and laboratory data (including serum tumor markers, hepatitis B and C markers) as well as imaging (at least two examinations—whether Doppler ultrasound, MR or CT—showing suggestive findings) [8].

References

1. Shovlin CL, Guttmacher AE, Buscarini E, Faughnan ME, Hyland RH, Westermann CJ, Kjeldsen AD, Plauchu H. Diagnostic criteria for hereditary hemorrhagic telangiectasia (Rendu-Osler-Weber syndrome). Am J Med Genet. 2000;91:66–7. PubMed PMID: 10751092
2. Gallione CJ, Repetto GM, Legius E, Rustgi AK, Schelley SL, Tejpar S, Mitchell G, Drouin E, Westermann CJ, Marchuk DA. A combined syndrome of juvenile polyposis and hereditary haemorrhagic telangiectasia associated with mutations in MADH4 (SMAD4). Lancet. 2004;363:852–9. PubMed PMID: 15031030
3. Lesca G, Olivieri C, Burnichon N, Pagella F, Carette MF, Gilbert-Dussardier B, Goizet C, Roume J, Rabilloud M, Saurin JC, Cottin V, Honnorat J, Coulet F, Giraud S, Calender A, Danesino C, Buscarini E, Plauchu H. French-Italian-Rendu-Osler Network. Genotype-phenotype correlations in hereditary hemorrhagic telangiectasia: data from the French-Italian HHT network. Genet Med. 2007;9:14–22. PubMed PMID: 17224686
4. Buscarini E, Leandro G, Conte D, Danesino C, Daina E, Manfredi G, Lupinacci G, Brambilla G, Menozzi F, De Grazia F, Gazzaniga P, Inama G, Bonardi R, Blotta P, Forner P, Olivieri C, Perna A, Grosso M, Pongiglione G, Boccardi E, Pagella F, Rossi G, Zambelli A. Natural history and outcome of hepatic vascular malformations in a large cohort of patients with hereditary hemorrhagic teleangiectasia. Dig Dis Sci. 2011;56:2166–78. https://doi.org/10.1007/s10620-011-1585-2. PubMed Central PMCID: PMC3112486
5. Buscarini E, Danesino C, Olivieri C, Lupinacci G, De Grazia F, Reduzzi L, Blotta P, Gazzaniga P, Pagella F, Grosso M, Pongiglione G, Buscarini L, Plauchu H, Zambelli A. Doppler ultrasonographic grading of hepatic vascular malformations in hereditary hemorrhagic telangiectasia – results of extensive screening. Ultraschall Med. 2004;25:348–55. PubMed PMID: 15368138
6. Memeo M, Stabile Ianora AA, Scardapane A, Buonamico P, Sabbà C, Angelelli G. Hepatic involvement in hereditary hemorrhagic telangiectasia: CT findings. Abdom Imaging. 2004;29:211–20. PubMed PMID: 15290948
7. Garcia-Tsao G, Korzenik JR, Young L, Henderson KJ, Jain D, Byrd B, Pollak JS, White RI Jr. Liver disease in patients with hereditary hemorrhagic telangiectasia. N Engl J Med. 2000;343:931–6. PubMed PMID: 11006369

8. Garcia-Pagàn JC, Buscarini E, Janssen HL, Leebeck FW, Plessier A, Rubbia-Brandt L, Senzolo M, Schouten JN, Tripodi A, Valla DC. European Association for the Study of the Liver. Vascular diseases of the liver. J Hepatol. 2016;64:179–202. https://doi.org/10.1016/j.jhep.2015.07.040. PubMed PMID: 26516032

9. Buscarini E, Danesino C, Plauchu H, de Fazio C, Olivieri C, Brambilla G, Menozzi F, Reduzzi L, Blotta P, Gazzaniga P, Pagella F, Grosso M, Pongiglione G, Cappiello J, Zambelli A. High prevalence of hepatic focal nodular hyperplasia in subjects with hereditary hemorrhagic telangiectasia. Ultrasound Med Biol. 2004;30:1089–97. PubMed PMID: 15550313

10. Gincul R, Lesca G, Gelas-Dore B, Rollin N, Barthelet M, Dupuis-Girod S, Pilleul F, Giraud S, Plauchu H, Saurin JC. Evaluation of previously nonscreened hereditary hemorrhagic telangiectasia patients shows frequent liver involvement and early cardiac consequences. Hepatology. 2008;48:1570–6. PubMed PMID: 18972447

11. Dupuis-Girod S, Ginon I, Saurin JC, Marion D, Guillot E, Decullier E, Roux A, Carette MF, Gilbert-Dussardier B, Hatron PY, Lacombe P, Lorcerie B, Rivière S, Corre R, Giraud S, Bailly S, Paintaud G, Ternant D, Valette PJ, Plauchu H, Faure F. Bevacizumab in patients with hereditary hemorrhagic telangiectasia and severe hepatic vascular malformations and high cardiac output. JAMA. 2012;307:948–55. PubMed PMID: 22396517

12. Dupuis-Girod S, Buscarini E. Response to Bevacizumab for the treatment of Rendu-Osler disease—a note of caution. Liver Int. 2017;37(6):928. PubMed PMID: 28544692

13. Caselitz M, Wagner S, Chavan A, Gebel M, Bleck JS, Wu A, Schlitt HJ, Galanski M, Manns MP. Clinical outcome of transfemoral embolisation in patients with arteriovenous malformations of the liver in hereditary haemorrhagic telangiectasia (Weber-Rendu-Osler disease). Gut. 1998;42:123–6. PubMed PMID: 9505897

14. Faughnan ME, Palda VA, Garcia-Tsao G, Geisthoff UW, McDonald J, Proctor DD, Spears J, Brown DH, Buscarini E, Chesnutt MS, Cottin V, Ganguly A, Gossage JR, Guttmacher AE, Hyland RH, Kennedy SJ, Korzenik J, Mager JJ, Ozanne AP, Piccirillo JF, Picus D, Plauchu H, Porteous ME, Pyeritz RE, Ross DA, Sabba C, Swanson K, Terry P, Wallace MC, Westermann CJ, White RI, Young LH, Zarrabeitia R, HHT Foundation International – Guidelines Working Group. International guidelines for the diagnosis and management of hereditary haemorrhagic telangiectasia. J Med Genet. 2011;48:73–87. https://doi.org/10.1136/jmg.2009.069013. PubMed PMID: 19553198

15. Garcia-Tsao G, Gish RG, Punch J. Model for end-stage liver disease (MELD) exception for hereditary hemorrhagic telangiectasia. Liver Transpl. 2006;12(Suppl 3):S108–9.

16. Caselitz M, Bahr MJ, Bleck JS, Chavan A, Manns MP, Wagner S, Gebel M. Sonographic criteria for the diagnosis of hepatic involvement in hereditary hemorrhagic telangiectasia (HHT). Hepatology. 2003;37:1139–46. PubMed PMID: 12717395

17. Buonamico P, Suppressa P, Lenato GM, Pasculli G, D'Ovidio F, Memeo M, Scardapane A, Sabbà C. Liver involvement in a large cohort of patients with hereditary hemorrhagic telangiectasia: echo-color-Doppler vs multislice computed tomography study. J Hepatol. 2008;48:811–20. https://doi.org/10.1016/j.jhep.2007.12.022.

18. Schelker RC, Barreiros AP, Hart C, Herr W, Jung EM. Macro- and microcirculation patterns of intrahepatic blood flow changes in patients with hereditary hemorrhagic telangiectasia. World J Gastroenterol. 2017;23:486–95. PubMed PMID: 28210085

19. Buscarini E, Gebel M, Ocran K, Manfredi G, Del Vecchio Blanco G, Stefanov R, Olivieri C, Danesino C, Zambelli A. Interobserver agreement in diagnosing liver involvement in hereditary hemorrhagic telangiectasia by Doppler ultrasound. Ultrasound Med Biol. 2008;34:718–25. https://doi.org/10.1016/j.ultrasmedbio.2007.11.007. PubMed PMID: 18207308

20. Siddiki H, Doherty MG, Fletcher JG, Stanson AW, Vrtiska TJ, Hough DM, Fidler JL, McCollough CH, Swanson KL. Abdominal findings in hereditary hemorrhagic telangiectasia: pictorial essay on 2D and 3D findings with isotropic multiphase CT. Radiographics. 2008;28:171–84.

21. Buscarini E, Buscarini L, Danesino C, Piantanida M, Civardi G, Quaretti P, Rossi S, Di Stasi M, Silva M. Hepatic vascular malformations in hereditary hemorrhagic telangiectasia: Doppler sonographic screening in a large family. J Hepatol. 1997;26:111–8. PubMed PMID: 9148001
22. Olivieri C, Lanzarini L, Pagella F, Semino L, Corno S, Valacca C, Plauchu H, Lesca G, Barthelet M, Buscarini E, Danesino C. Echocardiographic screening discloses increased values of pulmonary artery systolic pressure in 9 of 68 unselected patients affected with hereditary hemorrhagic telangiectasia. Genet Med. 2006;8:183–90.
23. Sopeña B, Pérez-Rodríguez MT, Portela D, Rivera A, Freire M, Martínez-Vázquez C. High prevalence of pulmonary hypertension in patients with hereditary hemorrhagic telangiectasia. Eur J Intern Med. 2013;24:30–4.
24. Trembath RC, Thomson JR, Machado RD, Morgan NV, Atkinson C, Winship I, Simonneau G, Galie N, Loyd JE, Humbert M, Nichols WC, Morrell NW, Berg J, Manes A, McGaughran J, Pauciulo M, Wheeler L. Clinical and molecular genetic features of pulmonary hypertension in patients with hereditary hemorrhagic telangiectasia. N Engl J Med. 2001;345:325–34.
25. Buscarini E, Buscarini L, Civardi G, Arruzzoli S, Bossalini G, Piantanida M. Hepatic vascular malformations in hereditary hemorrhagic telangiectasia: imaging findings. AJR Am J Roentgenol. 1994;163:1105–10. PubMed PMID: 7976883
26. Scardapane A, Stabile Ianora A, Sabbà C, Moschetta M, Suppressa P, Castorani L, Angelelli G. Dynamic 4D MR angiography versus multislice CT angiography in the evaluation of vascular hepatic involvement in hereditary haemorrhagic telangiectasia. Radiol Med. 2012;117:29–45.

Diagnostic Methods of Cirrhosis and Portal Hypertension: Specifics of the Pediatric Population

21

Daniel H. Leung, Milton J. Finegold, and Benjamin L. Shneider

21.1 Introduction

Fibrosis and portal hypertension (PHT) in children are quite distinct from adults often with unusually rapid progression (Fig. 21.1) and as such our approaches to these important problems should be modified in pediatrics. Critical differences exist at several levels: diagnosis, etiopathogenesis, prognosis, available therapies and evidence supporting surveillance or prophylaxis. In light of these fundamental issues, the rationale for and advantage of pre-clinical identification of cirrhosis and portal hypertension in children is less well understood and/or established.

The etiopathogenesis of progressive liver disease in childhood is remarkably different than in adults. Table 21.1 lists several common pediatric liver diseases along with multi-center reports of the prevalence of cirrhosis or portal hypertension among these disorders. The most clinically relevant disorders in the context of cirrhosis and portal hypertension are primarily biliary in origin, including but not limited to biliary atresia, sclerosing cholangitis, cystic fibrosis and congenital hepatic fibrosis (Figs. 21.1 and 21.2). In direct contrast to liver disease in adults, hepatocellular diseases (e.g. nonalcoholic fatty liver disease, hepatitis B and C) are much less common causes of advanced liver disease in childhood. However, even the histologic presentation of NASH related fibrosis in children

D.H. Leung, M.D. (✉) • B.L. Shneider, M.D.
Section of Pediatric Gastroenterology, Hepatology and Nutrition, Department of Pediatrics, Baylor College of Medicine, Texas Children's Hospital, Houston, TX, USA
e-mail: dhleung@bcm.edu; Benjamin.Shneider@bcm.edu

M.J. Finegold, M.D.
Department of Pathology and Immunology, Baylor College of Medicine, Houston, TX, USA
e-mail: MJFINEGO@texaschildrens.org

Fig. 21.1 Liver explant of
an 8 month old with biliary
atresia that displays diffuse
micronodular cirrhosis
with extensive bile duct
proliferation and
cholangitis among broad
bands of scar tissue (×25
magnification; Trichrome
stain)

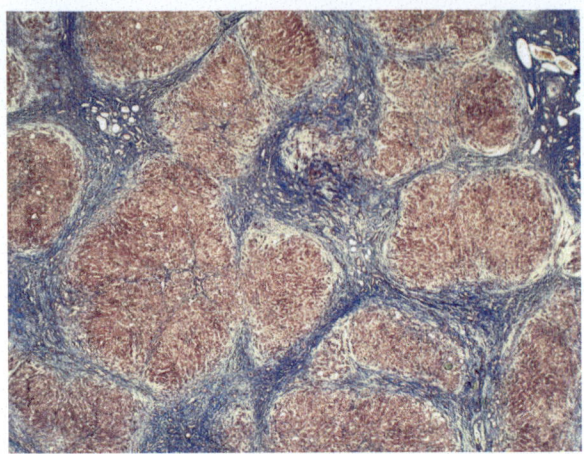

Table 21.1 Prevalence of cirrhosis and/or portal hypertension in multicenter investigations of pediatric liver diseases

Diagnosis	# studied	% positive	Features of disease	Reference	Research infrastructure; comments
Alpha-1 antitrypsin deficiency	208	29	Splenomegaly[a] or Thrombocytopenia[b]	[1]	ChiLDReN Network
Biliary atresia	163	66	Splenomegaly[a] or Thrombocytopenia[b]	[2]	ChiLDReN Network
Congenital hepatic fibrosis/ ARPKD	56 31	62 48	Splenomegaly on imaging Varices on endoscopy	[3]	NIH
Cystic fibrosis	35,516	3.6	Clinician report	[4]	CF Foundation Patient Registry
Hepatitis B	343	4.5	Thrombocytopenia <160,000	[5]	Hepatitis B Network
Hepatitis C	121	1.6	Histologic cirrhosis	[6]	PEDS-C Network Excluded severe disease
Nonalcoholic fatty liver disease	776	1.6	Histologic cirrhosis	[7]	NASH-CRN
Sclerosing cholangitis	781	5.0	Clinical complications of portal hypertension	[8]	International Registry

[a]Spleen palpable >2 cm below left costal margin
[b]Platelets <150,000

is distinct from the adult form of NASH (Fig. 21.2). These underlying differences in etiology and pathogenesis have profound implications for the predicted prognosis of these disorders. In general, advanced fibrosis in pediatric biliary

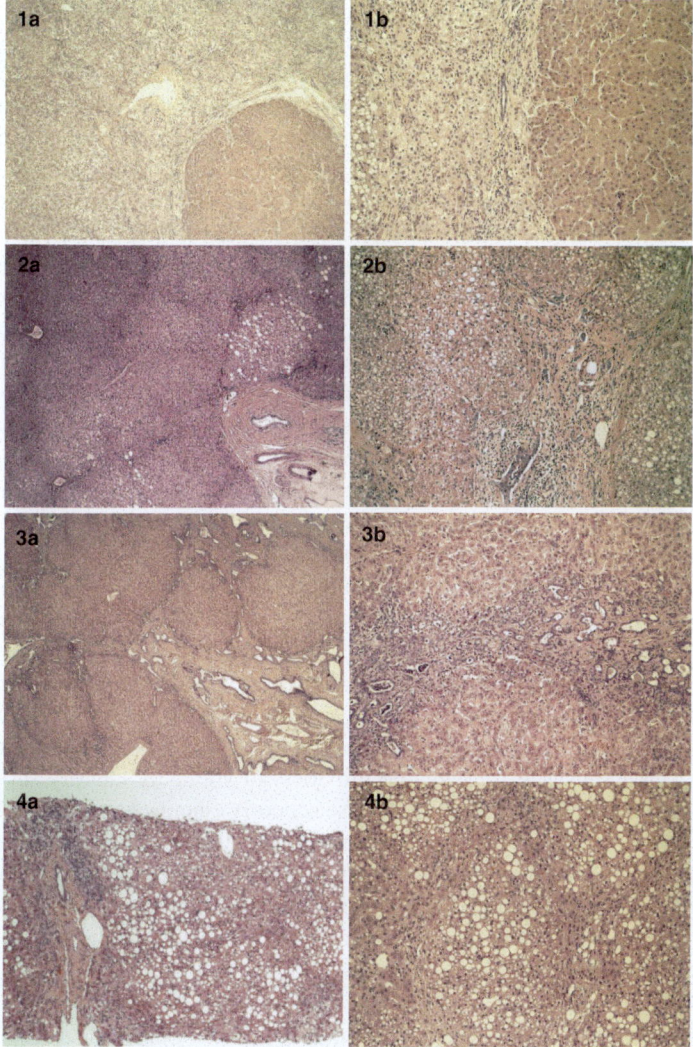

Fig. 21.2 (**1a**) **Tyrosinemia** at 6 months. Multinodularity in a cirrhotic liver with modest steato-sis in most hepatocytes but missing from distinct nodule on the right ×25. (**1b**) Moderate dysplasia in the right -sided nodule on the path to carcinoma ×125. (**2a**) **Cystic fibrosis** in a 9 year old. A medium sized bile duct has a collar of collagen resembling sclerosing cholangitis. Small tracts are unremarkable. Lobular architecture is focally altered, with macrosteatosis in some nodules, ×50. (**2b**) Scarred portal tract and bridging fibrosis separating steatotic nodules. Acute cholangitis is evident, ×100. (**3a**) **Congenital hepatic fibrosis** at age 4 associated with polycystic kidneys (ARPKD). Multiple large, deformed and displaced bile ducts with focal ductal-plate malforma-tion, ×25. (**3b**) Secondary acute cholangitis and bile retention, ×100. (**4a**) **Non-alcoholic steato-hepatitis** (NASH) in a 5 year old with bridging portal fibrosis and extensive portal inflammation. The macrosteatosis is more abundant in lobular zone 1 than 3 in children, ×62. (**4b**) Nodularity is exceptionally advanced for the age, ×125

disorders occurs much earlier compared to common hepatocellular diseases in adults. In biliary atresia, compensated cirrhosis can exist at the time of diagnosis in the first months of life and can notably persist for years if not decades in some cases. In congenital hepatic fibrosis, decompensated liver disease is distinctly uncommon and it is a misnomer to label the fibrotic process as cirrhosis. Cystic fibrosis is also a distinct form of liver disease with multilobular involvement, abnormal vasculature and quite pronounced portal hypertension with and without cirrhosis in the setting of well-compensated liver disease [9, 10]. The multi-organ involvement of cystic fibrosis, namely pulmonary disease, has a profound effect on survival, potentially limiting the impact of liver fibrosis on overall outcome.

Distinct etiopathogenesis and prognosis of pediatric liver diseases potentially translates into fundamental differences in the therapeutic relevance of pre-clinical identification of cirrhosis and portal hypertension. In adults, three major rationales for noninvasive screening include: (1) disease specific treatment and surveillance for and primary prophylaxis of (2) esophageal varices and (3) hepatocellular carcinoma. Unfortunately for many of these pediatric biliary disorders, disease-specific therapies are limited or non-existent (Table 21.2). Surveillance for and/or primary prophylaxis of varices in children remains a very contentious debate [11–14]. Proponents point to the ability to endoscopically identify and treat esophageal varices, while opponents question the evidence for prevention of mortality and suggest that the risks associated with these procedures may be higher in early childhood. Data regarding time to transplant or first variceal bleed in children with cirrhosis and portal hypertension is also disease-specific and very limited. Clinically, this may dampen enthusiasm for pediatric providers to vigilantly identify sub-clinical cirrhosis when the natural history of disease is poorly elucidated. Foreknowledge of an untreatable condition often raises a socio-ethical dilemma.

Hepatocellular carcinoma is an important issue that is largely unexplored and poorly understood in these pediatric disorders. Small case series of hepatocellular

Table 21.2 Available disease-specific interventions for advanced fibrosis or cirrhosis in pediatric liver disease

Diagnosis	Advanced fibrosis	Cirrhosis
Alpha-1 antitrypsin deficiency	None	None
Biliary atresia	None	None
Congenital hepatic fibrosis/ ARPKD	None	None
Cystic fibrosis	None	None
Hepatitis B	Nucleos(t)ide analogues (NA)	Nucleos(t)ide analogues (NA)
Hepatitis C	Direct acting-antivirals (DAA)[a]	Direct acting-antivirals (DAA)[a]
Nonalcoholic fatty liver disease	Weight loss[a]; bariatric surgery	Bariatric surgery
Sclerosing cholangitis	None; UDCA[a]	None

[a]Therapy independent of fibrosis stage may be indicated

carcinoma in biliary atresia exist [15, 16], while much less information is available for diseases like cystic fibrosis (n = 3 between ages 18–34) [17–19] and congenital hepatic fibrosis (n = 1 at age 27 and n = 1 unconfirmed age) [20, 21]. It is highly likely that the prevalence of hepatobiliary cancer in childhood liver disease is much less than hepatocellular diseases in adults. The efficacy and cost-effectiveness of extrapolating hepatocellular cancer screening programs used in adults to children is unproven and probably significantly reduced.

21.2 Cirrhosis Is Different in Children

The definition of cirrhosis in pediatrics is surprisingly poorly elaborated upon in the literature, despite being widely used in clinical practice. Cirrhosis has typically referred to a histologic stage of disease that was once considered irreversible and was manifest by transformation of the liver into diffuse regenerative nodularity and fibrosis. Advances in therapeutics, especially in adults, now call into question the irreversibility of the histologic lesion. In pediatrics, depending upon the underlying etiology and duration of the disease, there is considerable diversity and extent of the nodularity and fibrosis (Fig. 21.2). Differentiation of advanced fibrosis and "cirrhosis" may be more theoretical rather than practical. There have been very few attempts to assess the inter-rater agreement on histologic findings of grading of fibrosis/cirrhosis in pediatrics. In a multi-center study of neonatal cholestasis, the interobserver agreement for stage of fibrosis in needle biopsies was 58% [22]. Despite guidance from widely accepted scoring systems for assessment of fibrosis or predetermined standards for bile duct paucity/proliferation or ductal plate malformation (findings unique to pediatrics), chance-corrected concordance measures are less than ideal, ranging from 0.56–0.81 [23].

Many of the pediatric disorders that lead to progressive fibrosis or cirrhosis are characterized by patchy distribution of the lesions. This is particularly true for diseases such as biliary atresia and cystic fibrosis. In addition, many of the relevant disorders may not be manifest by "classical" cirrhosis but instead by lesions that have significant overlap with conditions defined as developmental rather than acquired, such as congenital hepatic fibrosis. Because of the natural tendency to limit invasive procedures, such as liver biopsy in children, the collective experience in pediatrics is significantly reduced compared to the experience in adults. At Texas Children's Hospital over the past 48 years, 682 cases of cirrhosis (<1%) were diagnosed amongst 82,234 liver biopsies, of which half had a biliary etiology. As might be expected, many of these cirrhotic cases were confirmed by explants taken at the time of liver transplantation. Thus in pediatrics, the gold standard of liver biopsy alone for defining cirrhosis is unproven. The existing literature is limited, the lesions are diverse and the reliability of the histologic findings is suspect because many of the diseases are patchy in their distribution. In many ways there is a greater need in pediatrics for noninvasive methods to ascertain fibrosis stage, although the "catch-22" may be the lack of a true gold standard.

Pediatric clinical practice often equates cirrhosis with clinical portal hypertension. While practical, this is not entirely scientific. Portal hypertension itself is ill defined in pediatrics and problematic to reliably assess. Direct operative measurements of portal pressure in biliary atresia have demonstrated its presence in infancy [24], although this is neither practical nor a standard of care. Hepatic venous pressure gradient (HVPG) is not often utilized in pediatrics as a means of assessing portal pressure and is limited in its prognosis for variceal development and clinical outcomes [25]. A great deal of the safety and feasibility with HVPG measurement in pediatrics stems from interventional radiology and transjugular intrahepatic portosystemic shunt placement [26]. An important proviso in this experience and the other literature related to HVPG is the necessity for general anesthesia for the procedure. There is no information on the impact of general anesthesia on portal pressure in pediatric liver disease. In addition venovenous collaterals in biliary atresia make HVPG measurements potentially unreliable [27]. As such, HVPG remains investigational or of limited utility in documenting portal hypertension in pediatrics.

The concept of clinically significant portal hypertension (CSPH) is an attractive construct in pediatrics but is not yet developed [14]. Essentially, this is what most clinicians use as an indication of "cirrhosis" in pediatrics, although there is marked variability in what clinical features constitute CSPH in pediatrics. The variability stems in part from differences in clinical practice [28]. Some have proposed that the finding of esophageal varices or other endoscopic features of portal hypertension be the definition of CSPH in pediatrics [29, 30]. This is an approach espoused by those that routinely perform surveillance endoscopy in children with features of "advanced" liver disease, but is not applicable for those who do not. Features of hypersplenism have been advanced by others as a defining feature of CSPH [31]. For research purposes, a spleen palpable greater than 2 cm below the costal margin and platelet count <150,000 has been used in biliary atresia [31] and alpha-1 antitrypsin deficiency [1]. While seemingly straight-forward, this approach too has its own limitations. Are both features required or just one? What about presence or absence of clinically detectable ascites? Infants with complications of portal hypertension may have platelet counts >150,000 and assessment of spleen size by physical examination is not always straight-forward in pediatrics, especially in uncooperative infants and children.

Another critical difference between pediatric and adult cirrhosis is the stage of disease at onset and the related implications, namely on prognosis. The biliary nature of most of the predisposing pediatric disorders leads to very early portal hypertension, presumably due to direct distortion of the portal triad by biliary injury and inflammation. As such, compensated cirrhosis is the rule and not an exception in pediatric cirrhosis. The cirrhotic histology in Fig. 21.1 is from an 8 month old infant with biliary atresia who had no ascites and preserved hepatic synthetic function. Survival for 5–20 years after the documentation of cirrhosis in these pediatric disorders is not uncommon [32]. The hepatic reserve and lack of co-morbidities limits the mortality associated with first variceal hemorrhage in many children and thus potentially alters the relative benefit of primary prophylaxis.

Pre-emptive knowledge of the presence or absence of advanced fibrosis or cirrhosis in pediatrics may not confer the same benefits as in adults (Table 21.2). As noted above, a general consensus for the use of primary prophylaxis of variceal hemorrhage does not exist in pediatrics. Screening programs for hepatocellular or hepatobiliary cancer have also not been proven to be beneficial for children. While deadly, HCC is exceedingly rare in children. North American and European Population—and tumor based registry studies (i.e. Surveillance, Epidemiology, and End Results (SEER) program and West Midlands Regional Children's Tumour Registry Profile) have reported age-adjusted rates (95% confidence intervals) of HCC to range from only 0.09–0.5 per 1,000,000 between the ages of 0 up to 19 years with a 5-year survival of only 18% [33, 34]. Based on a US population-based registry study by Darbari et al. [33], it was estimated that HCC caused only 16 deaths per year between 1979 and 1996. Interestingly, of the 918 deaths reported in the multiple cause-of-death database, less than 6% had an associated liver disease such as biliary atresia, congenital hepatic fibrosis, Byler disease, or Wilson disease documented. This suggests that clinically apparent cirrhotic liver disorders are an infrequent cause of pediatric HCC. While cirrhosis associated HCC is one of the most common indications for adult liver transplantation, in children it is one of the least [35]. Only a few published series have focused on the outcome of HCC in children [36–38]. Hepatocellular malignancy arising from cirrhosis in children is not only infrequent but, sometimes discovered only incidentally in an explant (<1%) [39]. In a multi-national natural history study of primary sclerosing cholangitis in 781 children for example, 8 (1%) developed cholangiocarcinoma between the ages of 15–18 years of age within a median of 6 years following diagnosis [8]. There are certain cirrhosis causing diseases where the risk of hepatobiliary cancer is significant—tyrosinemia [40, 41] (Fig. 21.2) and bile salt export pump disease [42, 43] (Progressive Familial Intrahepatic Cholestasis, type 2) [37] both of which have an underlying metabolic and genetic background that likely predisposes to the risk of cancer. Intensive screening for HCC is warranted in children with these disorders independent of stage of fibrosis. As disease-specific therapies evolve, early and pre-emptive identification of advanced fibrosis or cirrhosis becomes an opportunity for certain therapeutic options. This unfortunately is not commonly the case in pediatrics with the potential exceptions of hepatitis B and hepatitis C.

In contrast to adults, Child-Pugh stage specific prognosis in pediatrics have not been clearly delineated for many of the common pediatric disorders that lead to advanced fibrosis/cirrhosis in childhood. While the MELD score is used to functionally categorize severity of cirrhosis and determine prognosis and the necessity of liver transplantation in adults, it is not a tool that is used or validated in children less than 12 year of age. With childhood acquired hepatobiliary diseases, our experience is that even among those with established cirrhosis, there are varying histological stages of severity. Might this correlate with functional severity (compensated vs decompensated cirrhosis) or clinical outcomes such as risk or frequency of variceal bleeding, time to transplantation, or death? In children, fibrosis stage subclassifications beyond METAVIR stage 4 (i.e. 4a–c) or Ishak stage 6 (i.e. 6a–c) may be relevant.

The more important question is "Will diagnosing histologic cirrhosis change management?" Earlier counseling of families regarding signs of portal hypertension and sooner listing for liver transplantation may offer clinical benefit to the child with sub-clinical cirrhosis. Recently, a CF Foundation Patient Registry (CFFPR) study of over 900 subjects with reported cirrhosis determined that variceal bleeding is an uncommon complication of CF cirrhosis, (a 10-year cumulative rate of 6.6%) and can herald the diagnosis, but does not affect all-cause mortality compared to those without bleeding. Variceal prophylaxis or surveillance for HCC without sufficient data to justify the practice may introduce unnecessary medical and emotional risk without a clear benefit in morbidity or mortality.

21.3   Non-invasive Diagnostic Approaches in Children

In light of all of these challenges, one wonders why we should try to advance noninvasive determination of advanced fibrosis/cirrhosis in pediatrics. There are several compelling reasons. First, liver biopsy, while a historical cornerstone in staging fibrosis may not be as reliable or safe in pediatrics, with a post biopsy hematoma incidence of 5% [44, 45] and neurocognitive concerns about early and repeated exposure to general anesthesia [46, 47]. Second, CSPH has not been well delineated in pediatrics. Third, the field needs additional information to delineate stages of cirrhotic liver disease and their prognosis in children. As such, development of noninvasive markers is critical. They should be linked to objective measures of disease severity and correlated with future prognosis. Biomarkers may also yield interesting insights into distinct and disease-specific pathogenic mechanisms of cirrhosis in children. Finally, these markers may ultimately be extremely important in assessing evolving novel therapies for pediatric liver disease, particularly anti-fibrotics.

21.3.1 Biomarker Indices

The validation of noninvasive tests to diagnose esophageal varices is a priority in children due to the invasive nature of endoscopic evaluations and neurodevelopmental consequences of repeated exposure to general anesthesia [48, 49]. Both single [50] and multi-center studies [51] have found that biomarker indices such as the clinical prediction rule (CPR = ((0.75× platelets (×109/L))/ (SSAZ + 5)) + 2.5 × albumin(g/dL)) have an AUROC of 0.80–0.93 in predicting esophageal varices of any size with sensitivity 81–94%, specificity 73–81%, and positive predictive value 0.83–0.87 in children with chronic liver disease or portal vein thrombosis. Notably, CPR appears to correlate with changes in varix size in a subset of children who underwent repeat endoscopy. In a multi-center validation study, standard of care tests, namely platelet count (cut-off value 115) also performed quite well to detect esophageal varices in children, with an AUROC of 0.79 and sensitivity and specificity of 81% and 70%, respectively [51]. In a large UK single-center study of 124 treatment-naïve children with suspected portal hypertension or gastrointestinal bleeding undergoing their first EGD, a newly developed prediction score (King's = (3 × albumin ([g/dL]) − (2 − equivalent adult spleen size [cm])) to detect clinically significant varices (defined as grade II or higher) demonstrated an AUROC of 0.77 with sensitivity and specificity of 72% and 73%, respectively using an optimal cut-off value of 76 [52].

A recent study in which 51 children with cystic fibrosis liver disease (CFLD) underwent liver biopsy was compared to 104 age and sex matched children without CFLD (CFnoLD) suggests that the indices APRI and FIB-4 may be non-invasive clinical tools that can provide information which may increase vigilance in screening [53]. Among those with CFLD, APRI had an AUROC of 0.81 (p < 0.0001) for predicting severe fibrosis, defined as ≥F3 (Metavir) and a score >0.462 indicated a sevenfold increased odds of severe liver fibrosis (F3–F4). In the small sample size of patients who developed portal hypertension (n = 14), only FIB-4 predicted portal hypertension at diagnosis (AUROC 0.76; p < 0.001).

In a study of over 250 children with BA, Grieve et al. found that an APRI >1.22 identified cirrhosis with an AUROC of 0.83 [54]. Further, using APRI as a marker for survival, patients with an APRI of <0.43 had the highest transplant-free survival and as a clinical predictor, no patients with an APRI >3 at the time of Kasai hepatoportoenterotomy (KP) cleared their bilirubin. In fact, all progressed to liver transplantation. APRI at time of KP may be a clinically informative adjunct in evaluating cirrhosis in BA at presentation. In a small, liver biopsy-validated study of 29 BA subjects, those requiring transplant (n = 10) had higher APRI at presentation (1.34 vs. 0.77, P = 0.017) vs those who survived with native liver (n = 19) with an AUROC of 0.77 (p = 0.017) [55]. However, APRI at the time of KP did not correlate with Metavir fibrosis stage or collagen immunohistochemistry.

21.3.2 Serum Panels and Biomarkers

Fibrotest™ has been studied in a case controlled analysis of 24 children with CFLD vs 82 CFnoLD. Notably, haptoglobin, a component of Fibrotest™, significantly correlated with C-reactive-protein (r = 0.38, p = 0.000083). Given the prevalence of chronic inflammation due to lung injury in CF, this reduced the diagnostic accuracy of Fibrotest to 64% (95% CI: 49%; 78%) and Fibrotest™ underestimated liver fibrosis (6.6%) in CF-patients compared with transient elastography (TE) and acoustic radiation force impulse (ARFI) (16%), highlighting that certain diseases may confound the utility of a biomarker.

Collagen and matrix-based serum markers such as TIMP-1 (tissue inhibitor of matrix metalloproteinase (MMP), PH (prolyl hydroxylase), and periostin have been studied in canonical hepatobiliary diseases such as CF [56] and biliary atresia [57]. In CFLD, a combination of PH and TIMP-1 resulted in an AUROC of 0.85 (p = 0.02) to identify CFLD patients with no fibrosis (stage 0) vs. any fibrosis (stages 1–4) and an AUROC of 0.83 (p = 0.01) to distinguish Early (stages 0–1) vs. Extensive (stages 2–4) fibrosis. Periostin, a matricellular protein that actively contributes to tissue injury and fibrosis [58]; and autotaxin, a phosphodiesterase found to be elevated in patients with cholestasis associated pruritus [59] are both significantly increased in BA patients with jaundice and correlated with liver stiffness as measured by TE, reflecting severity of disease and potentially fibrosis [57, 60]. It is highly likely that a combination of biomarkers, rather than a single one, will increase discriminative ability when correlating with fibrosis stage in children.

Given the critical roles in disease function that micro RNA's (miRNAs) play through RNA silencing and post-transcriptional regulation of gene expression, they are an attractive biomarker to study. However, finding a miRNA signature that is expressed in the liver, can differentiate between stages of liver fibrosis and has biologically relevant downstream targets of stellate cell activation has been challenging [61, 62], not withstanding the many variables which may result in over or underexpression of miRNA.

While the search for an ideal, growth independent serum biomarker of fibrosis continues in children, two routine biochemical tests, namely bilirubin and GGT may provide important prognostic implications that will direct our clinical monitoring. In a prospective, multicenter study within the Childhood Liver Disease Research Network, infants with BA undergoing KP between 2004–2011 with an elevated bilirubin 3 months after KP did not fare well. A total bilirubin >2 mg/dL dichotomized nearly all who would die, require LT, or who would develop early complications such as ascites and thrombocytopenia [63]. In a retrospective analysis of patients with CF with macronodularity and splenomegaly (n = 19) vs those without (n = 236), patients with a persistently "high-normal" GGT (>35 U/L) in the 2 years prior had an odds ratio of 39 for developing CF cirrhosis [64].

21.4   Imaging

There are limited large-scale cross-sectional data on the correlation of gray scale ultrasound, transient elastography (TE), and magnetic resonance elastography (MRE) in children with clinical status and outcome. There is even less data on changes in TE-based liver stiffness over time in pediatric liver diseases.

However, a recent study of 36 German children with CF followed for up to 5 years with repeated TE measurements found that a mean increase in TE of 0.38 kPa/year predicted those who would develop both clinical CFLD [65] and a final LSM value >6.2 which has been published to discriminate for CFLD portal hypertension [66]. One of the major limitations is the lack of liver biopsy validation. In a French study of 116 children with TE LSM's, only 28% had correlative liver biopsies for comparison [67]. Despite this, TE and fibrosis stage demonstrated a strong correlation (AUROC 0.88 [0.68–0.95]) and in another small study, TE could be used as a tool to detect those at risk for development of esophageal varices (EV) (22.4 kPa vs. 7.9 kPa, p = 0.01) [68]. A recent cross sectional study of 31 Chinese children with BA comparing LSM with Metavir fibrosis stage demonstrated a similar AUROC of 0.87 for ≥F4, proposing a cut-off value of 15 kPa for ≥F4, with a sensitivity, specificity, positive predictive value and negative predictive value of 0.86, 0.92, 0.75, and 0.96, respectively [69]. In addition, LSM in children with BA following KP appears to correlate with clinical features of PHT, including spleno-megaly and/or the presence of esophageal varices (EV) or gastric varices (GV). In a study from Thailand, patients with BA were compared to normal controls; the LSM of 73 patients with BA was significantly higher than 50 controls (27.37 ± 22.48 vs 4.69 ± 1.03 kPa; $p < 0.001$) [70]. Further, patients with EV or GV also had signifi-cantly higher LSM than those without (37.7 ± 21.6 [n = 39] vs 11.0 ± 8.7 [n = 34], $p < 0.001$). For the diagnosis of EV or GV, the AUC's were 0.89 (95% CI, 0.80–0.98) for TE and 0.87 (95% CI, 0.78–0.96) for APRI, respectively. The sensitivity (and specificity) of TE using a cut-off value of 12.7 kPa and APRI, using a cut-off value of 1.92, in predicting EV/GV were 84%/77% and 84%/83%, respectively. Interestingly, the sensitivity (and specificity) of splenomegaly in predicting EV/GV were 92% (85%). TE among obese children has also predicted clinically significant fibrosis ($\geq$F2) well in a cohort of children with nonalcoholic fatty liver disease, although none of the children had cirrhosis [65].

Much of the data on magnetic resonance elastography (MRE) in children has come from feasibility studies. In a pilot study, Siegel et al. reported that in six chil-dren with cystic fibrosis, a cutoff of >3.38 kPa was both 100% sensitive and specific for the detection of cirrhosis compared to four healthy controls [71]. In a case series of 35 children with a spectrum of different chronic liver diseases, a cutoff of 2.71 kPa had a sensitivity of 88% and specificity of 85% in discriminating fibrosis stages 0–1 from 2–4 [72].

However in a prospective, multi-center study of 2D-MRE in children with NAFLD using two reading centers, thresholds for classifying the presence of fibro-sis and of advanced fibrosis were computed and cross-validated [73]. The study fail rate was 16% due to breathing/imaging artifacts or too small of a region of interest. In 90 children of whom MRE was obtained, a cut-point of 2.7 kPa demonstrated low sensitivity (44.4–47.2%) but high specificity (88.9–90.7%) depending on the center. MRE in children underperforms compared to adult studies. For example, in a series of 117 adults with NAFLD, a cutoff of 3.02 kPa had a sensitivity of 0.55 and speci-ficity of 0.91 for identifying ANY fibrosis; for advanced fibrosis (F3–F4), a cutoff of 3.64 had a sensitivity of 0.86 and specificity of 0.91 [74]. Importantly, stiffness measurements from the two pediatric centers correlated with each other (r = 0.83) and significantly correlated with stages of fibrosis ($\rho = 0.53$ for Center 1, $\rho = 0.55$ for Center 2, both $p < 0.001$) [73]. It should also be acknowledged that MRE cutoffs derived from adult studies may not be applicable to children with NAFLD. For example, in a study of 142 adults with NAFLD, a cut-off of 4.15 kPa had a sensitiv-ity of 0.85 and specificity of 0.93 for identifying advanced fibrosis (F3–F4) [75]. Further, liver stiffness values in children are lower and more stable than in adults, increasing with age during normal development and do not reach adult values until adolescence [76]. We must be very cautious about using adult baseline values to detect pediatric liver mechanical abnormalities. For the reasons mentioned above, it may lead to underestimation of severity.

There are ongoing multi-center studies incorporating TE and MRE into its study protocols to establish pediatric specific cut-points. The FibroScan™ in Pediatric Cholestatic Liver Disease (FORCE, NCT02922751) study within the Childhood

Liver Disease Research Network includes the collection of serum and plasma at the time of liver stiffness measurement (LSM) in an effort to promote future investigations to correlate LSM with known and to be identified serum biomarkers of fibrosis. The ability of these biomarkers to predict change in LSM over time will be assessed and correlated with clinical features and outcomes within the study. ELASTIC (Longitudinal Assessment of Transient Elastography in Cystic Fibrosis, NCT03001388) is an ancillary study within the Cystic Fibrosis Liver Disease Network, which is capturing liver stiffness in patients to determine if the combination of TE with ultrasound pattern can improve the prediction of progression to a nodular pattern or cirrhosis.

Conclusion

The etiopathogenesis, biology and clinical course of liver disease in children are distinct from adults, which significantly affects the "value" of preclinical knowledge of an advanced fibrotic or cirrhotic state. Clinical practice approaches of surveillance for varices and HCC impact on the relevance of this knowledge. The importance of a meticulous physical exam, history and laboratory/imaging review in infants and young children with liver disease cannot be overstated as portal hypertension (which is often equated with cirrhosis) in children is a clinical diagnosis.

Fibrosis scores may provide improved discrimination to differentiate liver disease and predict significant clinical outcomes, but may be less discriminatory as surrogates of liver fibrosis. Commercially available and biologically relevant markers of fibrosis are likely to be "disease-specific", "growth dependent", and may be confounded by states of inflammation. The advent of non-invasive imaging such as TE and MRE, while currently considered research techniques, likely will soon be integrated into our standard of care for children once validated thresholds that predict clinically relevant outcomes are established.

It is clear there are differences in the way pediatricians process the word cirrhosis. No doubt there are challenges in the diagnosis of cirrhosis and even more so from a therapeutic perspective. Histology has been a cornerstone of defining cirrhosis, but as we are learning, it is and can no longer be the only method. Complemented by multiple disciplines such as radiology, pathology, biochemistry, and clinical medicine, the ultimate goal is to identify fibrosis far before it progresses to cirrhosis with the hopes that disease-specific interventions to reverse inflammation and scarring are developed and approved.

References

1. Teckman JH, Rosenthal P, Abel R, Bass LM, Michail S, Murray KF, et al. Baseline analysis of a young alpha-1-antitrypsin deficiency liver disease cohort reveals frequent portal hypertension. J Pediatr Gastroenterol Nutr. 2015;61(1):94–101. PubMed PMID: 25651489. Pubmed Central PMCID: 4692167
2. Shneider BL, Abel B, Haber B, Karpen SJ, Magee JC, Romero R, Schwarz K, et al. Portal hypertension in children and young adults with biliary atresia. J Pediatr Gastroenterol Nutr. 2012;55:567–73.

3. Gunay-Aygun M, Font-Montgomery E, Lukose L, Tuchman Gerstein M, Piwnica-Worms K, Choyke P, Daryanani KT, et al. Characteristics of congenital hepatic fibrosis in a large cohort of patients with autosomal recessive polycystic kidney disease. Gastroenterology. 2013;144:112–121.e112.

4. Ye W, Narkewicz M, Leung DH, Karnsakul W, Murray KF, Alonso E, Magee J, et al. Variceal hemorrhage and adverse liver outcomes in patients with cystic fibrosis cirrhosis. J Pediatr Gastrotenterol Nutr. 2017 [Epub ahead of print].

5. Schwarz KB, Cloonan YK, Ling SC, Murray KF, Rodriguez-Baez N, Schwarzenberg SJ, Teckman J, et al. Children with chronic hepatitis B in the United States and Canada. J Pediatr. 2015;167:1287–1294.e1282.

6. Goodman ZD, Makhlouf HR, Liu L, Balistreri W, Gonzalez-Peralta RP, Haber B, Jonas MM, et al. Pathology of chronic hepatitis C in children: liver biopsy findings in the Peds-C Trial. Hepatology. 2008;47:836–43.

7. Africa JA, Behling CA, Brunt EM, Zhang N, Luo Y, Wells A, Hou J, et al. In children with nonalcoholic fatty liver disease, zone 1 steatosis is associated with advanced fibrosis. Clin Gastroenterol Hepatol. 2017 Mar 7 [Epub ahead of primt].

8. Deneau MR, El-Matary W, Valentino PL, Abdou R, Alqoaer K, Amin M, et al. The natural history of primary sclerosing cholangitis in 781 children: a multicenter, international collaboration. Hepatology. 2017;66(2):518–27. PubMed PMID: 28390159

9. Witters P, Libbrecht L, Roskams T, Boeck KD, Dupont L, Proesmans M, et al. Noncirrhotic presinusoidal portal hypertension is common in cystic fibrosis-associated liver disease. Hepatology. 2011;53(3):1064–5. PubMed PMID: 21374682

10. Witters P, Libbrecht L, Roskams T, De Boeck K, Dupont L, Proesmans M, et al. Liver disease in cystic fibrosis presents as non-cirrhotic portal hypertension. J Cyst Fibros. 2017;16(5):e11–e3. PubMed PMID: 28347603

11. Duche M, Ducot B, Ackermann O, Guerin F, Jacquemin E, Bernard O. Portal hypertension in children: high-risk varices, primary prophylaxis and consequences of bleeding. J Hepatol. 2017;66(2):320–7. PubMed PMID: 27663417

12. Duche M, Ducot B, Tournay E, Fabre M, Cohen J, Jacquemin E, et al. Prognostic value of endoscopy in children with biliary atresia at risk for early development of varices and bleeding. Gastroenterology. 2010;139(6):1952–60. PubMed PMID: 20637201

13. Shneider BL. Tacit consensus. J Pediatr Gastroenterol Nutr. 2017;64(4):497. PubMed PMID: 28118292

14. Shneider BL, de Ville de Goyet J, Leung DH, Srivastava A, Ling SC, Duche M, et al. Primary prophylaxis of variceal bleeding in children and the role of MesoRex Bypass: summary of the Baveno VI Pediatric Satellite Symposium. Hepatology. 2016;63(4):1368–80. PubMed PMID: 26358549

15. Hadzic N, Quaglia A, Portmann B, Paramalingam S, Heaton ND, Rela M, et al. Hepatocellular carcinoma in biliary atresia: King's College Hospital experience. J Pediatr. 2011;159(4):617–22.e1. PubMed PMID: 21489554

16. Hirzel AC, Madrazo B, Rojas CP. Two rare cases of hepatocellular carcinoma after Kasai procedure for biliary atresia: a recommendation for close follow-up. Case Rep Pathol. 2015;2015:982679. PubMed PMID: 26339518. Pubmed Central PMCID: 4539070

17. Kelleher T, Staunton M, O'Mahony S, McCormick PA. Advanced hepatocellular carcinoma associated with cystic fibrosis. Eur J Gastroenterol Hepatol. 2005;17(10):1123–4. PubMed PMID: 16148560

18. McKeon D, Day A, Parmar J, Alexander G, Bilton D. Hepatocellular carcinoma in association with cirrhosis in a patient with cystic fibrosis. J Cyst Fibros. 2004;3(3):193–5. PubMed PMID: 15463908

19. O'Donnell DH, Ryan R, Hayes B, Fennelly D, Gibney RG. Hepatocellular carcinoma complicating cystic fibrosis related liver disease. J Cyst Fibros. 2009;8(4):288–90. PubMed PMID: 19473889

20. Bauman ME, Pound DC, Ulbright TM. Hepatocellular carcinoma arising in congenital hepatic fibrosis. Am J Gastroenterol. 1994;89(3):450–1. PubMed PMID: 8122667

21. Ghadir MR, Bagheri M, Ghanooni AH. Congenital hepatic fibrosis leading to cirrhosis and hepatocellular carcinoma: a case report. J Med Case Rep. 2011;5:160. PubMed PMID: 21513523. Pubmed Central PMCID: 3105948

22. Russo P, Magee JC, Boitnott J, Bove KE, Raghunathan T, Finegold M, et al. Design and validation of the biliary atresia research consortium histologic assessment system for cholestasis in infancy. Clin Gastroenterol Hepatol. 2011;9(4):357–62.e2. PubMed PMID: 21238606. Pubmed Central PMCID: 3400532

23. Russo P, Magee JC, Anders RA, Bove KE, Chung C, Cummings OW, et al. Key histopathologic features of liver biopsies that distinguish biliary atresia from other causes of infantile cholestasis and their correlation with outcome: a multicenter study. Am J Surg Pathol. 2016;40(12):1601–15. PubMed PMID: 27776008. Pubmed Central PMCID: 5123664

24. Duche M, Fabre M, Kretzschmar B, Serinet MO, Gauthier F, Chardot C. Prognostic value of portal pressure at the time of Kasai operation in patients with biliary atresia. J Pediatr Gastroenterol Nutr. 2006;43(5):640–5. PubMed PMID: 17130742

25. Shalaby A, Makin E, Davenport M. Portal venous pressure in biliary atresia. J Pediatr Surg. 2012;47(2):363–6. PubMed PMID: 22325391

26. Woolfson J, John P, Kamath B, Ng VL, Ling SC. Measurement of hepatic venous pressure gradient is feasible and safe in children. J Pediatr Gastroenterol Nutr. 2013;57(5):634–7. PubMed PMID: 23799453

27. Miraglia R, Luca A, Maruzzelli L, Spada M, Riva S, Caruso S, et al. Measurement of hepatic vein pressure gradient in children with chronic liver diseases. J Hepatol. 2010;53(4):624–9. PubMed PMID: 20615572

28. Gana JC, Valentino PL, Morinville V, O'Connor C, Ling SC. Variation in care for children with esophageal varices: a study of physicians', patients', and families' approaches and attitudes. J Pediatr Gastroenterol Nutr. 2011;52(6):751–5. PubMed PMID: 21593647

29. Celinska-Cedro D, Teisseyre M, Woynarowski M, Socha P, Socha J, Ryzko J. Endoscopic ligation of esophageal varices for prophylaxis of first bleeding in children and adolescents with portal hypertension: preliminary results of a prospective study. J Pediatr Surg. 2003;38(7):1008–11. PubMed PMID: 12861528

30. Goncalves ME, Cardoso SR, Maksoud JG. Prophylactic sclerotherapy in children with esophageal varices: long-term results of a controlled prospective randomized trial. J Pediatr Surg. 2000;35(3):401–5. PubMed PMID: 10726678

31. Ling SC, Walters T, McKiernan PJ, Schwarz KB, Garcia-Tsao G, Shneider BL. Primary prophylaxis of variceal hemorrhage in children with portal hypertension: a framework for future research. J Pediatr Gastroenterol Nutr. 2011;52(3):254–61. PubMed PMID: 21336158. Pubmed Central PMCID: 3728696

32. Lykavieris P, Chardot C, Sokhn M, Gauthier F, Valayer J, Bernard O. Outcome in adulthood of biliary atresia: a study of 63 patients who survived for over 20 years with their native liver. Hepatology. 2005;41(2):366–71. PubMed PMID: 15660386

33. Darbari A, Sabin KM, Shapiro CN, Schwarz KB. Epidemiology of primary hepatic malignancies in U.S. children. Hepatology. 2003;38(3):560–6. PubMed PMID: 12939582

34. Mann JR, Kasthuri N, Raafat F, Pincott JR, Parkes SE, Muir KR, et al. Malignant hepatic tumours in children: incidence, clinical features and aetiology. Paediatr Perinat Epidemiol. 1990;4(3):276–89. PubMed PMID: 2374747

35. Rawal N, Yazigi N. Pediatric liver transplantation. Pediatr Clin N Am. 2017;64(3):677–84. PubMed PMID: 28502445

36. Arikan C, Kilic M, Nart D, Ozgenc F, Ozkan T, Tokat Y, et al. Hepatocellular carcinoma in children and effect of living-donor liver transplantation on outcome. Pediatr Transplant. 2006;10(1):42–7. PubMed PMID: 16499586

37. Romano F, Stroppa P, Bravi M, Casotti V, Lucianetti A, Guizzetti M, et al. Favorable outcome of primary liver transplantation in children with cirrhosis and hepatocellular carcinoma. Pediatr Transplant. 2011;15(6):573–9. PubMed PMID: 21797955

38. Zhang XF, Liu XM, Wei T, Liu C, Li MX, Long ZD, et al. Clinical characteristics and outcome of hepatocellular carcinoma in children and adolescents. Pediatr Surg Int. 2013;29(8):763–70. PubMed PMID: 23794023

39. Abdelfattah MR, Abaalkhail F, Al-Manea H. Misdiagnosed or incidentally detected hepatocellular carcinoma in explanted livers: lessons learned. Ann Transplant. 2015;20:366–72. PubMed PMID: 26124187

40. Koelink CJ, van Hasselt P, van der Ploeg A, van den Heuvel-Eibrink MM, Wijburg FA, Bijleveld CM, et al. Tyrosinemia type I treated by NTBC: how does AFP predict liver cancer? Mol Genet Metab. 2006;89(4):310–5. PubMed PMID: 17008115

41. van Ginkel WG, Pennings JP, van Spronsen FJ. Liver cancer in tyrosinemia type 1. Adv Exp Med Biol. 2017;959:101–9. PubMed PMID: 28755188

42. Knisely AS, Strautnieks SS, Meier Y, Stieger B, Byrne JA, Portmann BC, et al. Hepatocellular carcinoma in ten children under five years of age with bile salt export pump deficiency. Hepatology. 2006;44(2):478–86. PubMed PMID: 16871584

43. Lagana SM, Salomao M, Remotti HE, Knisely AS, Moreira RK. Bile salt export pump: a sensitive and specific immunohistochemical marker of hepatocellular carcinoma. Histopathology. 2015;66(4):598–602. PubMed PMID: 25378077

44. Almeida P, Schreiber RA, Liang J, Mujawar Q, Guttman OR. Clinical characteristics and complications of pediatric liver biopsy: a single centre experience. Ann Hepatol. 2017;16(5):797–801. PubMed PMID: 28809725

45. Bolia R, Matta J, Malik R, Hardikar W. Outpatient liver biopsy in children: safety, feasibility, and economic impact. J Pediatr Gastroenterol Nutr. 2017;65(1):86–8. PubMed PMID: 28644355

46. Glatz P, Sandin RH, Pedersen NL, Bonamy AK, Eriksson LI, Granath F. Association of anesthesia and surgery during childhood with long-term academic performance. JAMA Pediatr. 2017;171(1):e163470. PubMed PMID: 27820621

47. McCann ME, Soriano SG. General anesthetics in pediatric anesthesia: influences on the developing brain. Curr Drug Targets. 2012;13(7):944–51. PubMed PMID: 22512394. Pubmed Central PMCID: 4172352

48. Bong CL, Allen JC, Kim JT. The effects of exposure to general anesthesia in infancy on academic performance at age 12. Anesth Analg. 2013;117(6):1419–28. PubMed PMID: 24132012

49. Wang X, Xu Z, Miao CH. Current clinical evidence on the effect of general anesthesia on neurodevelopment in children: an updated systematic review with meta-regression. PLoS One. 2014;9(1):e85760. PubMed PMID: 24465688. Pubmed Central PMCID: 3896404

50. Gana JC, Turner D, Roberts EA, Ling SC. Derivation of a clinical prediction rule for the noninvasive diagnosis of varices in children. J Pediatr Gastroenterol Nutr. 2010;50(2):188–93. PubMed PMID: 19966576

51. Gana JC, Turner D, Mieli-Vergani G, Davenport M, Miloh T, Avitzur Y, et al. A clinical prediction rule and platelet count predict esophageal varices in children. Gastroenterology. 2011;141(6):2009–16. PubMed PMID: 21925123

52. Witters P, Hughes D, Karthikeyan P, Ramakrishna S, Davenport M, Dhawan A, et al. King's variceal prediction score: a novel noninvasive marker of portal hypertension in pediatric chronic liver disease. J Pediatr Gastroenterol Nutr. 2017;64(4):518–23. PubMed PMID: 27749613

53. Leung DH, Khan M, Minard CG, Guffey D, Ramm LE, Clouston AD, et al. Aspartate aminotransferase to platelet ratio and fibrosis-4 as biomarkers in biopsy-validated pediatric cystic fibrosis liver disease. Hepatology. 2015;62(5):1576–83. PubMed PMID: 26223427

54. Grieve A, Makin E, Davenport M. Aspartate aminotransferase-to-platelet ratio index (APRi) in infants with biliary atresia: prognostic value at presentation. J Pediatr Surg. 2013;48(4):789–95. PubMed PMID: 23583135

55. Suominen JS, Lampela H, Heikkila P, Lohi J, Jalanko H, Pakarinen MP. APRi predicts native liver survival by reflecting portal fibrogenesis and hepatic neovascularization at the time of portoenterostomy in biliary atresia. J Pediatr Surg. 2015;50(9):1528–31. PubMed PMID: 25783319

56. Pereira TN, Lewindon PJ, Smith JL, Murphy TL, Lincoln DJ, Shepherd RW, et al. Serum markers of hepatic fibrogenesis in cystic fibrosis liver disease. J Hepatol. 2004;41(4):576–83. PubMed PMID: 15464237

57. Honsawek S, Udomsinprasert W, Vejchapipat P, Chongsrisawat V, Phavichitr N, Poovorawan Y. Elevated serum periostin is associated with liver stiffness and clinical outcome in biliary atresia. Biomarkers. 2015;20(2):157–61. PubMed PMID: 25980529

58. Sen K, Lindenmeyer MT, Gaspert A, Eichinger F, Neusser MA, Kretzler M, et al. Periostin is induced in glomerular injury and expressed de novo in interstitial renal fibrosis. Am J Pathol. 2011;179(4):1756–67. PubMed PMID: 21854746. Pubmed Central PMCID: 3181392

59. Wunsch E, Krawczyk M, Milkiewicz M, Trottier J, Barbier O, Neurath MF, et al. Serum autotaxin is a marker of the severity of liver injury and overall survival in patients with cholestatic liver diseases. Sci Rep. 2016;6:30847. PubMed PMID: 27506882. Pubmed Central PMCID: 4978954

60. Udomsinprasert W, Honsawek S, Anomasiri W, Chongsrisawat V, Vejchapipat P, Poovorawan Y. Serum autotaxin levels correlate with hepatic dysfunction and severity in postoperative biliary atresia. Biomarkers. 2015;20(1):89–94. PubMed PMID: 25536867

61. Cook NL, Pereira TN, Lewindon PJ, Shepherd RW, Ramm GA. Circulating microRNAs as noninvasive diagnostic biomarkers of liver disease in children with cystic fibrosis. J Pediatr Gastroenterol Nutr. 2015;60(2):247–54. PubMed PMID: 25625579

62. Zahm AM, Hand NJ, Boateng LA, Friedman JR. Circulating microRNA is a biomarker of biliary atresia. J Pediatr Gastroenterol Nutr. 2012;55(4):366–9. PubMed PMID: 22732895. Pubmed Central PMCID: 3459263

63. Shneider BL, Magee JC, Karpen SJ, Rand EB, Narkewicz MR, Bass LM, et al. Total serum bilirubin within 3 months of hepatoportoenterostomy predicts short-term outcomes in biliary atresia. J Pediatr. 2016;170:211–7.e1–2. PubMed PMID: 26725209. Pubmed Central PMCID: 4826612

64. Bodewes FA, van der Doef HP, Houwen RH, Verkade HJ. Increase of serum gamma-glutamyltransferase associated with development of cirrhotic cystic fibrosis liver disease. J Pediatr Gastroenterol Nutr. 2015;61(1):113–8. PubMed PMID: 25658056

65. Klotter V, Gunchick C, Siemers E, Rath T, Hudel H, Naehrlich L, et al. Assessment of pathologic increase in liver stiffness enables earlier diagnosis of CFLD: results from a prospective longitudinal cohort study. PLoS One. 2017;12(6):e0178784. PubMed PMID: 28575039. Pubmed Central PMCID: 5456384

66. Aqul A, Jonas MM, Harney S, Raza R, Sawicki GS, Mitchell PD, et al. Correlation of transient elastography with severity of cystic fibrosis-related liver disease. J Pediatr Gastroenterol Nutr. 2017;64(4):505–11. PubMed PMID: 27782957

67. de Ledinghen V, Le Bail B, Rebouissoux L, Fournier C, Foucher J, Miette V, et al. Liver stiffness measurement in children using FibroScan: feasibility study and comparison with Fibrotest, aspartate transaminase to platelets ratio index, and liver biopsy. J Pediatr Gastroenterol Nutr. 2007;45(4):443–50. PubMed PMID: 18030211

68. Malbrunot-Wagner AC, Bridoux L, Nousbaum JB, Riou C, Dirou A, Ginies JL, et al. Transient elastography and portal hypertension in pediatric patients with cystic fibrosis transient elastography and cystic fibrosis. J Cyst Fibros. 2011;10(5):338–42. PubMed PMID: 21550861

69. Shen QL, Chen YJ, Wang ZM, Zhang TC, Pang WB, Shu J, et al. Assessment of liver fibrosis by Fibroscan as compared to liver biopsy in biliary atresia. World J Gastroenterol. 2015;21(22):6931–6. PubMed PMID: 26078570. Pubmed Central PMCID: 4462734

70. Chongsrisawat V, Vejapipat P, Siripon N, Poovorawan Y. Transient elastography for predicting esophageal/gastric varices in children with biliary atresia. BMC Gastroenterol. 2011;11:41. PubMed PMID: 21501480. Pubmed Central PMCID: 3089784

71. Siegel MJPA, Bolster B, Kotyk JJ. Pediatric MR elastography of the liver. Clin Pediatr Imaging. 2012:108–11.

72. Xanthakos SA, Podberesky DJ, Serai SD, Miles L, King EC, Balistreri WF, et al. Use of magnetic resonance elastography to assess hepatic fibrosis in children with chronic liver disease. J Pediatr. 2014;164(1):186–8. PubMed PMID: 24064151. Pubmed Central PMCID: 3872246

73. Schwimmer JB, Behling C, Angeles JE, Paiz M, Durelle J, Africa J, et al. Magnetic resonance elastography measured shear stiffness as a biomarker of fibrosis in pediatric nonalcoholic fatty liver disease. Hepatology. Epub 2017 May 11. PubMed PMID: 28493388.
74. Loomba R, Wolfson T, Ang B, Hooker J, Behling C, Peterson M, et al. Magnetic resonance elastography predicts advanced fibrosis in patients with nonalcoholic fatty liver disease: a prospective study. Hepatology. 2014;60(6):1920–8. PubMed PMID: 25103310. Pubmed Central PMCID: 4245360
75. Kim D, Kim WR, Talwalkar JA, Kim HJ, Ehman RL. Advanced fibrosis in nonalcoholic fatty liver disease: noninvasive assessment with MR elastography. Radiology. 2013;268(2):411–9. PubMed PMID: 23564711. Pubmed Central PMCID: 3721049
76. Etchell E, Juge L, Hatt A, Sinkus R, Bilston LE. Liver stiffness values are lower in pediatric subjects than in adults and increase with age: a multifrequency MR elastography study. Radiology. 2017;283(1):222–30. PubMed PMID: 27755913

The manufacturer's authorised representative in the EU is Springer
Nature Customer Service Centre GmbH, Europaplatz 3, 69115 Heidelberg,
Germany. If you have any concerns regarding our products, please
contact ProductSafety@springernature.com

Printed and bound by CPI Group (UK) Ltd, Croydon, CR0 4YY
29/04/2026
02099519-0002